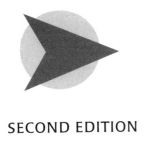

SECOND EDITION

Core Curriculum *for* INTRAVENOUS NURSING

INTRAVENOUS NURSES SOCIETY
CAMBRIDGE, MASSACHUSETTS

EDITORS

Ann Corrigan, CRNI, BSN, MS
Manager, IV Therapy
Wellstar Health System
Austell, Georgia

Gloria Pelletier, CRNI
Coordinator, Pharmacy/IV Programs
Southern New Hampshire Medical Center
Nashua, New Hampshire

Mary Alexander, CRNI
Chief Executive Officer
Intravenous Nurses Society
Cambridge, Massachusetts

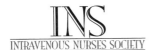

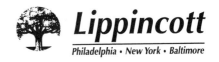
Lippincott
Philadelphia • New York • Baltimore

Editor: Margaret Zuccarini
Production Editor: Karen M. Ruppert

Copyright © 2000 Lippincott Williams & Wilkins

351 West Camden Street
Baltimore, Maryland 21201-2436 USA

227 East Washington Square
Philadelphia, PA 19106

Printed in the United States of America

First Edition, 1984

Library of Congress Cataloging-in-Publication Data

Core curriculum for intravenous nursing / Intravenous Nurses Society ;
  [edited by] Ann Corrigan, Gloria Pelletier, Mary Alexander. — 2nd ed.
      p.   cm.
    Includes bibliographical references and index.
    ISBN 0-7817-2116-4
    1. Intravenous therapy Outlines, syllabi, etc. 2. Nursing Outlines, syllabi,
  etc. I. Corrigan, Ann, 1948– . II. Pelletier, Gloria. III. Alexander, Mary,
  1955– .
    [DNLM: 1. Infusions, Parenteral—nursing Outlines. 2. Curriculum
  Outlines. 3. Fluid Therapy—nursing Outlines. 4. Parenteral Nutrition—
  nursing Outlines.   WY 18.2 C7963 1999]
  RM170.C67 1999
  615.8′55—dc21
  DNLM/DLC   99–21557
  for Library of Congress   CIP

To purchase additional copies of this book, call our customer service department at **(800) 638-3030** or fax orders to **(301) 824-7390**. International customers should call **(301) 714-2324**.

00 01 02 03 04
1 2 3 4 5 6 7 8 9 10

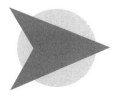

Contributors

TECHNOLOGY AND CLINICAL APPLICATION

Maxine B. Perdue, CRNI, BSN, MHA, MBA
Director of Clinical Support Services
High Point Regional Health System
High Point, North Carolina

FLUID AND ELECTROLYTE BALANCE

Judy Hankins, BSN, CRNI
IV Admixture Coordinator
Moses H. Cone Memorial Hospital
Greensboro, North Carolina

PHARMACOLOGY

Sharon M. Weinstein, MS, CRNI
Director, Office of Internal Affairs
PREMIER, Inc.
Westchester, Illinois

INFECTION CONTROL

Roxanne R. Perucca, MSN, CRNI
IV Therapy Clinical Nurse Specialist
University of Kansas Hospital
Kansas City, Kansas

PEDIATRICS

Viki Patch Shutak, ADN, BSN, MS(c), CRNI
Director, IV Program
Visiting Nurse Association/Vermont and
    New Hampshire
White River Junction, VT

President
IV Therapy Care Consultants
Enfield, New Hampshire

TRANSFUSION THERAPY

Ann Corrigan, CRNI, BSN, MS
Manager, IV Therapy
Wellstar Health System
Austell, Georgia

AND

Gloria Pelletier, CRNI
Coordinator, Pharmacy/IV Programs
Southern New Hampshire Medical Center
Nashua, New Hampshire

ANTINEOPLASTIC THERAPY

Michaelle M. Wetteland, CRNI, BA
Director, Clinical Infusion Management
Olsten Health Services
Eagan, Minnesota

PARENTERAL NUTRITION

Leslie Baranowski, BSN, CRNI
(1958–1998)

QUALITY ASSURANCE

Deborah B. Benvenuto, CRNI
Nurse Educator, Intravenous Therapy
Intravenous Nurses Society
Cambridge, Massachusetts

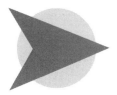

Preface

The Intravenous Nurses Society (INS) is committed to the specialty practice of intravenous nursing and to advancing the quality of intravenous care delivery. Two methods of meeting these commitments are through education and certification. The *Core Curriculum for Intravenous Nursing* provides an opportunity to educate the practitioner by providing the basic knowledge required to obtain certification in the intravenous specialty.

The goal of this revised edition of the *Core Curriculum* is to provide information related to new technological advances and the expansion of the specialty practice. This information is presented in an expanded outline format.

The *Core Curriculum* is divided into the nine content areas of the specialty: Technology and Clinical Application, Fluid and Electrolyte Balance, Pharmacology, Infection Control, Pediatrics, Transfusion Therapy, Antineoplastic Therapy, Parenteral Nutrition, and Quality Assurance.

The information contained in each chapter provides a basis for the development of test questions for the certification examination. References are supplied to provide the nurse with additional resources for continuing education and professional development.

The *Core Curriculum for Intravenous Nursing* is designed for use as a comprehensive, preparatory resource for the Intravenous Nurses Certification Corporation (INCC) Certification Examination and a framework from which courses in intravenous therapy may be designed.

Competency in intravenous nursing requires mastering the information contained in this book, as well as extensive clinical experience in the specialty. This combination of knowledge and skill allows intravenous nurse specialists to provide optimal infusion care and develop a broader understanding of the specialty practice.

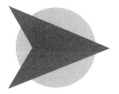

Acknowledgments

The second edition of the *Core Curriculum for Intravenous Nursing* represents the accumulation of effort by many infusion therapy colleagues. We would like to take this opportunity to thank these individuals for their contributions.

We especially would like to thank the chapter authors for their expertise and commitment to both this revision and the specialty practice of intravenous nursing. We are indebted to these professionals for their time and dedication to this project. We would also like to thank Nancy Delisio, CRNI, and Jane Weir, BSN, CRNI, for their contribution to the Transfusion Therapy chapter.

In addition, we appreciate the continued support of the Intravenous Nurses Society Board of Directors and the Intravenous Nurses Certification Corporation Board of Directors.

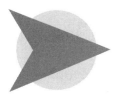

Scope of Practice

Specialization marks the advancement of nursing practice. It signifies that nursing has moved from a global approach to a focus on defined areas within the practice that require specialized knowledge and skills. The foundation of specialty practice is based on the knowledge gained from general nursing education and a concentrated study in a selected clinical area of nursing. Consequently, a specialist is also a generalist, but a generalist has not acquired the knowledge and skill in a defined area to be designated a specialist.

The intravenous nurse specialist is a registered nurse who, through study and supervised practice and validation of competency, has acquired knowledge and developed skills necessary for the practice of intravenous nursing. Intravenous nursing practice is a dynamic process. The scope of intravenous nursing is defined by anatomy and physiology as well as treatment modalities and technology; it encompasses the intravenous therapy patient, nurse, and setting in which intravenous nursing is practiced.

Patients receiving intravenous therapy represent a diversity of diagnoses and varying severity of illness. These patients represent all age groups, from the premature infant to the geriatric person. The care of the patient receiving intravenous therapy extends to the patient's family and significant others.

The intravenous nurse may be a registered nurse (RN) or a licensed practical/vocational nurse (LPN/LVN) who has acquired knowledge and skill in intravenous nursing. The intravenous nurse is committed to providing safe, quality intravenous nursing care and is accountable for practicing within the defined scope of practice for the RN or LPN/LVN. The intravenous nurse's practice is based on the following:

- Autonomy and accountability within the specific scope of practice;
- Knowledge of anatomy and physiology;
- Specific knowledge and understanding of the vascular system and its relationship to other body systems and intravenous treatment modalities;
- Attainment of skills necessary for the administration of intravenous therapies;
- Knowledge of advanced technologies associated with intravenous therapies;

- Knowledge of psychosocial aspects, including but not limited to sensitivity to the patient's wholeness, uniqueness, significant social relationships, and awareness of community and economic resources;
- Interaction and collaboration with members of the healthcare team and participation in the clinical decision-making process.

To advance the specialty practice of intravenous nursing, the intravenous nurse should actively participate in education, research, and development of new technologies. The sharing of information is critical to the advancement of the profession. Thus, the intravenous nurse is encouraged to share information by communicating with colleagues through official nursing publications and other forums.

The intravenous therapy setting is defined as any environment in which intravenous therapy is delivered. Intravenous therapies are administered in a variety of settings, which include but are not limited to the hospital, home, clinic, physician's office, and ambulatory infusion centers.

The intravenous nurse should develop, implement, and adhere to intravenous policies and procedures, which are presented in the INS-established professional *Intravenous Nursing Standards of Practice*. The intravenous nurse should collaborate with and/or participate in committees that regulate the practice of intravenous nursing and should interact with other members of the healthcare team to provide safe, quality intravenous therapy.

The scope of practice statements provide a definition and framework for the practice of intravenous nursing. The *Intravenous Nursing Standards of Practice* represent an extension of the scope of practice and offer specific criteria essential to the delivery of safe, quality intravenous therapy.

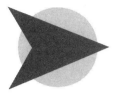

The Nine Core Areas of Intravenous Therapy

CURRICULUM DESCRIPTION

Theoretical

The theoretical aspect of intravenous nursing includes the intravenous nurse's knowledge and understanding of general institutional and intravenous department policies. The nurse will be cognizant of his or her responsibilities to the patient, employer, nursing profession, and to other healthcare professionals, the community, and the intravenous department.

The *Core Curriculum for Intravenous Nursing* consists of nine content areas:

1. **Technology and Clinical Application.** Provides information about the vascular and neurological systems and their relationships to other body systems and to intravenous nursing; proper function, usage, care, and maintenance of supplies and equipment used in the delivery of parenteral therapies; and potential hazards and possible complications related to intravenous therapies and the equipment used. Hands-on practice sessions should be used. The instruction of skills and techniques should be interactive.

2. **Fluid and Electrolyte Balance.** Promotes understanding of the nature, pathophysiology, clinical manifestations, and principles of maintenance, replacement, and/or corrective therapy as they relate to the fluid and electrolyte balance.

3. **Pharmacology.** Presents information about intravenous medications, including indications for use, pharmacological properties, dosing, clinical mathematics, anticipated side effects, potential complications/antidotal therapy, compatibilities, stabilities, and methods of administration.

4. **Infection Control.** Provides a general overview of microbiology with emphasis on microorganisms pertaining to intravenous therapy, transmission of disease-causing organisms, surveillance, preventive measures, precautions, and aseptic technique.

5. **Pediatrics.** Addresses administration of parenteral therapy to the pediatric patient. Includes information on growth and development, psychosocial implications, fluid and electrolyte balance, special considerations in equipment and delivery systems, dosing, site selection, and solutions used.

6. **Transfusion Therapy.** Provides information related to immunohematology, blood grouping, blood/blood components, administration equipment and techniques, and potential adverse reactions.

7. **Antineoplastic Therapy.** Provides an overview of cancer therapies as they relate to the cell cycle, purpose of therapy, and effects on body systems. Includes information on the intravenous antineoplastic agents, as well as indications for use, dosing, anticipated side effects, potential complications, administration, and safe handling techniques.

8. **Parenteral Nutrition.** Addresses the types of parenteral nutrition, including indications for use, compositions of solutions, patient assessment, administration and termination techniques, and potential complications.

9. **Quality Assurance.** Provides an overview of the structural components and legal aspects of quality management/performance improvement as they relate to the process of delivering optimal intravenous therapy.

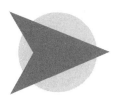

Contents

CHAPTER 1

Technology and Clinical Application

Maxine B. Perdue, CRNI, BSN, MHA, MBA

PART ONE **ANATOMY AND PHYSIOLOGY**

I. VASCULAR SYSTEM ANATOMY AND PHYSIOLOGY

A. Cardiac Circulation (circulation through the heart)

1. Heart
   a. Is a hollow muscular organ made of four chambers that functions as a two-sided pump
      1) Right side is a low-pressure system pumping venous or deoxygenated blood to the lung
      2) Left side is a high-pressure system pumping arterial or oxygenated blood to systemic circulation
   b. Right atrium (RA) is a thin-walled muscle that acts as a receiving chamber
      1) Receives systemic venous blood from superior vena cava, which drains blood from upper part of body, and from inferior vena cava, which drains blood from lower extremities
      2) Receives blood from myocardial circulation by the coronary sinus
      3) Blood flow to RA occurs during inspiration
         • RA pressure drops below the pressure in veins outside the chest cavity
         • Blood flows from area of high pressure to area of low pressure
   c. Right ventricle (RV) is the most anterior chamber of the heart, lying directly beneath the sternum
      1) Functions as both an inflow and an outflow tract
      2) During diastole, blood enters RV through the tricuspid valve and is ejected into pulmonary circulation through the pulmonic valve
      3) Because of pulmonary resistance, systolic or ejection pressures of the RV are low

     d. Left atrium (LA) is the most posterior chamber of the heart
- 1) Receives oxygenated blood from lungs via the right and left pulmonary veins
- 2) Wall is slightly thicker than that of the RA and exerts a pressure of 5 to 10 mm Hg with little breathing variation

     e. Left ventricle (LV) is the chamber that lies posterior to and to the left of the RV
- 1) Wall is made of thick muscular tissue, two to three times thicker than that of the RV
- 2) Increased muscular mass is necessary to generate pressure to move blood into circulation

2. Cardiac valves
- a. The heart's efficiency as a pump depends on the integrity of the cardiac valves, whose sole purpose is to ensure one-way forward blood flow
- b. Atrioventricular (AV) valves: positioned along the AV groove separating the atria from the ventricles
  - 1) Tricuspid valve: located between the RA and the RV
    - Larger and thinner than the mitral valve with three separate leaflets: anterior, posterior, and septal
    - Anterior and posterior leaflets associated with RV lateral wall function
    - Septal leaflet attached to portions of the interventricular septum sitting in close proximity to the AV node
  - 2) Mitral valve: located between the LA and the LV; composed of two cusps
    - Anterior leaflet descends deep into the LV during diastole and rises quickly in systole to meet the posterior leaflet
    - Posterior leaflet is smaller and more restricted in its motion
- c. Semilunar valves: smaller than AV valves
  - 1) Aortic semilunar valves: located above the outflow tract of the LV; composed of a fibrous supporting ring called the annulus and three valve leaflet cusps that are thicker than those of the AV valves
  - 2) Pulmonic semilunar valve: located above the outflow tract of the LA at the junction of the pulmonary artery and the LA; composed of a fibrous supporting ring called the annulus and three valve leaflet cusps

3. Nerve conduction
- a. Involves a special system consisting of atypical muscle fibers that transmit and coordinate electrical impulses throughout the heart
- b. Sinoatrial (SA) or sinus node: located at the border of the superior vena cava and the RA
  - 1) Gives rise to a self-generating impulse known as the heartbeat
  - 2) Primary pacemaker of the heart, generating impulses at a rate of 60 to 100 beats/minute
  - 3) Innervated by sympathetic and parasympathetic nerve fibers
- c. AV node: located in the RA

1) Forms conduction system of the heart
2) Filters atrial impulses as they pass through to the ventricles
3) Innervated by the autonomic nervous system

d. Bundle of His: located along the two sides of the intraventricular system, dividing into the right and left bundle branches and providing infranodal conduction

e. The right and left bundle branches: located in the outer walls of the ventricles
1) Conduction system of heart working with the bundle of His and the Purkinje fibers to produce contraction of the ventricles
2) Terminate in a fine network of conductive tissue called Purkinje fibers

f. Purkinje fibers: fibers extending to the papillary muscles and lateral walls of the ventricles; located in the upper outer walls of the ventricles

B. Pulmonary Circulation

1. Blood flows from the RV to the lungs via pulmonary arteries and from the lungs to the LA via pulmonary veins
2. Major purpose is to deliver blood to the alveoli
   a. Oxygen is taken in
   b. Carbon dioxide is removed

C. Systemic Circulation

1. Blood flows from the LV through the aorta and all its branches (arteries) to the capillaries of the tissues
2. Blood returns to the heart through veins and the vena cavae, which empties into the RA
3. Arteries
   a. Layers (Fig. 1.1)
      1) Tunica intima: inner elastic endothelial lining consisting of smooth layers of flat cells
      2) Tunica media: middle layer consisting of muscular and elastic tissue
         • Strong layer that withstands pressure, preventing collapse of vessels
         • Location of nerve fibers for vasoconstriction and vasodilation
         • Responsive to stimulation of chemical irritation by producing spasms that may cause a contraction, cutting off blood flow to surrounding tissues and resulting in necrosis and gangrene
      3) Tunica adventitia: thick outer layer that provides protection consisting of areolar connective tissue
   b. Characteristics
      1) Contain bright red blood
      2) Pulsate
      3) Do not contain valves
      4) Branches terminate in arterioles, which form arterial capillaries

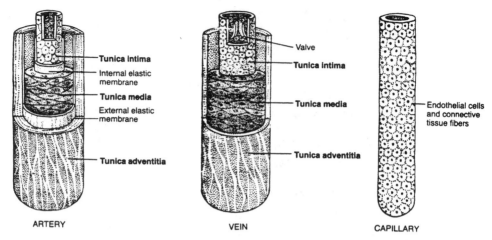

FIGURE 1-1 Microscopic anatomy of an artery, vein, and capillary. (*Reprinted with permission from Ignatavicius DD, Bayne MV. Medical-Surgical Nursing: A Nursing Process Approach. Philadelphia, PA: Saunders, 1991:2083.*)

   c. Location
      1) Usually deep in tissue protected by muscle
      2) Aberrant
         • Located superficially in an unusual place
         • Administration of chemicals causing spasms results in permanent damage
   d. Nerve conduction
      1) Sympathetic innervation: direct effect on arteries
         • Control of contraction and relaxation of muscle fibers within the vessels; vasoconstrictor fibers constrict vascular smooth muscle; vasodilator fibers relax vascular smooth muscle
         • Vascular reflexes aided by chemical actions in regulating diameter of vessels to distribute blood properly to tissues
         • Transmitter substance, norepinephrine (noradrenalin), secreted by postganglionic nerve terminals
      2) Parasympathetic innervation: indirect effect on arteries
         • Baroceptors located in the carotid sinus and the aortic arch
         • Activated by impulses to heart stimulating parasympathetic fibers
         • Causes decrease in heart rate and dilation of arterioles
         • Transmitter substance, acetylcholine, secreted by both preganglionic and postganglionic fibers
   e. Arteries appropriate for vascular access
      1) Radial artery
         • Direct continuation of the brachial artery beginning 1 cm distal to the bend of the elbow, descending along the lateral side of the forearm to the wrist

- Usually considered site of choice
- Superficial and easy to enter; location at wrist making artery easy to stabilize for quick entry
- Allen's test: used to assure adequacy of collateral circulation before use; radial and ulnar arteries located and compressed; blanching of the hand indicates successful compression with good color return to the entire hand when releasing only the ulnar artery pressure; ulnar artery capable of supplying blood to the entire hand by collateral circulation, if thrombosis occurs
- Easy to apply a post-puncture pressure dressing

2) Ulnar artery
- Large terminal branch of the brachial artery beginning just distal to the elbow and reaching the medial side of the forearm midway between the elbow and the wrist, and passes vertically, crossing the flexor retinaculum lateral to the ulnar bone
- Larger, much deeper, and more difficult to stabilize than the radial artery
- Should not be used if radial artery of same arm has been used

3) Femoral artery
- Artery located midway between the anterior superior spine of the ilium and the symphysis pubis
- Largest accessible artery; easily palpated, stabilized, and entered
- Difficult to maintain an intact dry dressing
- Digital pressure required for post-puncture pressure
- Limb- or life-threatening condition possible if post-puncture thrombosis occurs

4) Pulmonary arteries
- Arteries leading away from the heart to the lungs
- Shorter and smaller than the right, the left pulmonary artery runs horizontally in front of the descending aorta and the left principal bronchus to the left hilum, dividing into upper and lower lobar branches
- Longer and larger, the right pulmonary artery runs horizontally to the right behind the ascending aorta, superior vena cava, and upper right pulmonary vein, then in front of the plexus
- Access obtained by insertion of Swan-Ganz catheter via subclavian vein with passage through RA and RV and into the pulmonary artery, providing assessment of both right and left heart pressures

f. Advantages of use
1) Diagnosis
- Measurement of carbon dioxide and oxygen levels
- Measurement of bicarbonate blood levels
2) Continuous arterial monitoring
- Systolic, diastolic, and mean arterial pressure readings
- Assessment of cardiovascular effects of vasopressor and/or vasodilator drugs during treatment of shock

  • Simultaneous drawing of arterial blood for arterial blood gases
    (ABGs)
g. Disadvantages of use
  1) Thrombosis with resultant loss of limb or life
  2) Arterial spasms with resultant loss of circulation to an extremity
  3) Threat of infection and septicemia
  4) Cardiac arrhythmias if catheter is placed in the RA
4. Veins
  a. Layers (Fig. 1.1)
    1) Tunica intima: inner elastic endothelial lining consisting of smooth lay-
      ers of flat cells
      • Semilunar folds of endothelium form valves
      • Trauma during venipuncture encourages thrombosis whereby cells
        and platelets adhere to vessel wall
    2) Tunica media: middle layer consisting of muscular and elastic tissue
      • Not as strong as in arteries; tends to collapse or distend as pressure
        within vein falls or rises
      • Location of nerve fibers for vasoconstriction and vasodilation: cold
        solutions result in spasms, impeding blood flow and causing pain;
        heat promotes vasodilation, relieving spasm, improving blood flow,
        and relieving pain; heat promotes dilation of vessels, reducing inflam-
        mation of vessel wall by increasing blood flow and diluting irritating
        medications and/or solutions
    3) Tunica adventitia: outer layer consisting of areolar connective tissue
      providing vessel protection; not as thick as in the artery
  b. Characteristics
    1) Contain dark blood
    2) Do not pulsate
    3) Located superficially
    4) Venous capillaries unite to form venules, which unite to form veins
  c. Nerve conduction
    1) Sympathetic innervation: direct effect on veins
      • Innervation by postganglionic efferent and primary afferent
        nerves
      • Controls contraction and relaxation of muscle fibers within vessel
        walls; vasoconstrictor fibers constrict vascular smooth muscle;
        vasodilator fibers relax vascular smooth muscle
      • Transmitter substance, norepinephrine, secreted by postganglionic
        nerve terminals
    2) Parasympathetic innervation: indirect effect on veins
      • Baroreceptors located in carotid sinus and aortic arch
      • Activated by impulses to heart stimulating parasympathetic fibers
        and causing heart rate to decrease and venules to dilate
  d. Veins appropriate for peripheral intravenous therapy (Fig. 1.2)
    1) Digital veins
      • Flow along lateral portions of fingers

- From adjacent sides of digits unite to form three metacarpal veins
- Last resort for therapy

2) Metacarpal veins
- Formed by union of digital veins found on dorsal aspect of hand
- Usually well adapted for intravenous therapy
- Occasionally contraindicated in the elderly because of inadequate tissue and thin skin in the area
- Use in initial therapy enables successive venipunctures above previous sites, promoting availability of veins without inflammation and pain

3) Cephalic vein
- Large vein formed by metacarpal veins and located in radial part of dorsal venous network, flowing upward along radial border of forearm
- Excellent for transfusion therapy
- Provides a natural splint

4) Basilic vein
- Originates in ulnar part of dorsal venous network, ascending along ulnar portion of forearm
- Visualization promoted by flexing elbow and bending arm upward

5) Median antebrachial vein
- Arises from venous plexus on palm of hand and extends upward along ulnar side of front of forearm
- Varies as to size and visibility

6) Intermediate (median) cephalic vein
- Large vein located in the antecubital fossa
- Used for blood withdrawal
- Cautious use necessary because vessel crosses in front of brachial artery

7) Intermediate (median) basilic vein
- Located outside antecubital fossa on ulnar curve of arm
- Least desirable vessel for venipuncture

e. Peripheral veins appropriate for central intravenous therapy
1) Cephalic vein
- Ascends along outer border of biceps muscle to upper third of arm, passing in the space between pectoralis major and deltoid muscles, terminating in the axillary vein with a descending curve just below the clavicle
- Occasional connection with external jugular or subclavian vein by a branch that passes from it upward in front of the clavicle

2) Basilic vein
- Passes upward in a smooth path along inner side of biceps muscle and terminates in the axillary vein
- Larger than the cephalic vein

f. Central veins appropriate for central intravenous therapy

(*text continues on page 9*)

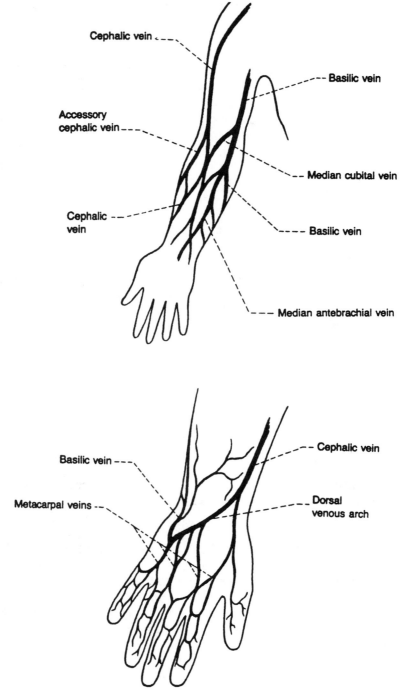

FIGURE 1-2 Superficial veins of the dorsal aspect of the hand and of the forearm. (*Reprinted with permission from Weinstein S. Plumer's Principles and Practice of Intravenous Therapy, 6th ed. Philadelphia, PA: Lippincott-Raven, 1997:53, 54.*)

1) Internal jugular vein
- Begins at the cranial base in the posterior compartment of the jugular foramen and descending in the carotid sheath uniting with the subclavian, posterior to the sternal end of the clavicle to form the brachiocephalic vein
- Often used when anomalies of the subclavian vein prevent use or in emergency situations when needed to administer large volumes of fluid quickly
- Use can lead to immediate pulling of air into the venous system as a result of negative pressure within the chest if tubing is accidentally pulled apart

2) External jugular vein
- Easily recognized on the side of the neck; formed by union of the posterior retromandibular and posterior auricular veins near the mandibular angle just below or in the parotid gland, descends to the midclavicle joining the subclavian vein
- Usually preferred over the internal jugular because of easy accessibility, particularly in emergency situations
- Threat of air being pulled into the vascular system if the line is accidentally pulled apart

3) Subclavian vein
- Continuation of the axillary vein extending from outer border of the first rib to medial border of the scalenus anterior muscle, where it joins the internal jugular to form the innominate (brachiocephalic) vein
- Clavicle and subclavius muscle lies anterior to the subclavian vein; subclavian artery lies posterosuperior separated by the scalenus anterior muscle and the phrenic nerve; first rib and pleura lie inferior
- Vein of choice for placement of central venous catheters

4) Femoral vein
- Continuation of the popliteal vein ending posterior to the inguinal ligament at the external iliac, and posterolateral to the femoral artery
- Usually has four to five valves
- Last resort for placement of catheters

g. Scalp veins used for intravenous therapy (Fig. 1.3)
1) Superficial temporal vein
- Begins in a widespread network joined across the scalp to the contralateral vein and to the ipsilateral, supratrochlear, supraorbital, posterior auricular, and occipital veins
- Administration of intravenous therapy in the pediatric patient
- Ease in visualizing; minimal risk

2) Parietal vein
- Branch of superficial temporal vein located in front of ear
- Usually not a vein of choice because of close proximity to ear

3) Occipital vein
- Branch of temporal vein located behind ear

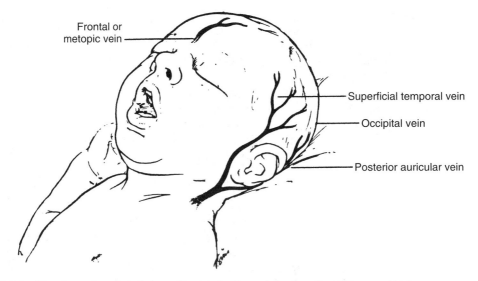

Frontal or
metopic vein

Superficial temporal vein

Occipital vein

Posterior auricular vein

FIGURE 1-3 Sites for scalp vein infusions. (*Reprinted with permission from Terry J, Baranowski L, Lonsway RA, Hedrick C, eds. Intravenous Therapy: Clinical Principles and Practice. Philadelphia, PA: Saunders, 1995.*)

- Usually last choice because of location behind ear
4) Frontal (supratrochlear) vein
   - Originates on the forehead from a venous network connected to the frontal tributaries of the superficial temporal vein; metopic vein forms section of frontal vein that runs down the center of the forehead
   - Most frequently used scalp vein
h. Other veins used for intravenous therapy
   1) Umbilical vein
      - Located within the umbilical cord through umbilicus to liver and ductus venous
      - Frequently used for administering intravenous therapy in newborns
      - Use limited because of high risk of sepsis
   2) Great saphenous vein
      - Runs along medial aspect of leg from ankle upward across knee and thigh to enter femoral ring
      - Lower division above ankle frequently used in infants and toddlers; used frequently for cutdowns
      - Not recommended for use in adults
      - Use requires physician's written order
      - Originates with capillaries of superficial tissues of the foot; can lead to complications when used for intravenous therapy
      - Thrombosis occurs more readily than when veins in upper extremities are used, leading to pulmonary emboli

- More valves present, creating potential for medication to pool behind valves, creating irregular drug absorption
- Patient immobilization potentiates pooling of blood in extremities

5. Capillaries
   a. Minute blood vessels connecting the smallest arteries (arterioles) to the smallest veins (venules)
   b. Exchange of nutrients and oxygen from the blood to the tissues with waste and carbon dioxide from the tissues into the blood (exchange vessels)

II. SKIN ANATOMY AND PHYSIOLOGY

A. Epidermis

1. Outer layer forms a protective covering
2. Thickness varies depending on body part and age
3. Provides support for an intravenous cannula

B. Dermis

1. Connective tissue layer supporting the epidermis
2. Highly vascular, providing nutrition for the epidermis
3. Contains capillaries and nerve fibers that react to temperature, touch, pressure, and pain

III. NERVOUS SYSTEM ANATOMY AND PHYSIOLOGY

A. Central Nervous System: Brain

1. A large mass of nerve tissue filling the cranium
2. Three connective tissue layers called meninges cover the brain and provide protection
   a. Dura mater: outermost double fibrous layer that separates the skull into compartments by its various folds or processes
   b. Arachnoid: middle layer made up of a two-layered fibrous elastic membrane that crosses over the folds and fissures of the brain, creating the spongy arachnoid space
   c. Pia mater: innermost layer rich in small blood vessels supplying the brain with a large volume of blood
3. Anatomically divided into four components: cerebrum, cerebellum, brainstem, and ventricles
4. Cerebrum is the largest portion of the brain
   a. Comprised of gray cells and white matter
   b. Divided into hemispheres or lobes that are named according to overlying cranial bones
      1) Frontal lobe
         - Located in the anterior fossa, extending from anterior portion of each hemisphere to the central sulcus posteriorly

- Controls psychic and higher intellectual functions and higher level centers for autonomic functioning such as cardiovascular responses and gastrointestinal activity

  2) Parietal lobe
     - Located in the middle fossa in the area between the fissure of Rolando and the parieto-occipital fissure
     - Major functions of position, sense, touch, and motor movement
  3) Occipital lobe
     - Pyramidal structure located in the middle fossa behind the parieto-occipital fissure just above the cerebellum
     - Contains the centers for vision
  4) Temporal lobe
     - Located in the middle fossa inferior to the lateral cerebral fissure and extends posteriorly to the parieto-occipital fissure
     - Responsible for primary functions of memory and hearing

5. Cerebellum is approximately one-fifth the size of the cerebrum
   a. Functions primarily in coordinating movement, equilibrium, muscle tone, and position sense
   b. Consists of two lateral hemispheres and a middle portion, the vermis
      1) Lateral hemispheres control movement coordination for the same side of the body
      2) Midbrain connects the cerebellum to the cerebral cortex
6. Brainstem consists of the midbrain, the pons, and the medulla oblongata
   a. Midbrain (mesencephalon)
      1) Forms a junction between diencephalon and pons
      2) Functions to relay stimuli dealing with muscle movement, visual reflexes, and auditory reflexes from the spinal cord, medulla oblongata, and cerebellum to the cerebrum
   b. Pons
      1) Connects the midbrain to the medulla oblongata
      2) Relays impulses to brain centers and to lower spinal centers of the nervous system
      3) Origin for sensory and motor nuclei of the trigeminal, abducens, facial, and acoustic nerves
   c. Medulla oblongata
      1) Contains reflex centers for controlling involuntary functions such as breathing, sneezing, swallowing, coughing, salivation, vomiting, and vasoconstriction
      2) Provides points of origin for the glossopharyngeal, vagus, spinal accessory, and hypoglossal nerves
7. Ventricles are cavities located deep within the brain
   a. Filled with cerebrospinal fluid (CSF), which is produced mostly by lateral ventricles
   b. Connect with each other and with fluid spaces in the spinal cord through small openings
   c. Lateral ventricles serve as a site for placement of Ommaya reservoir

B. Central Nervous System: Spinal Cord

1. Ovoid column of nervous tissue extending through the spinal canal
   a. Originates at the foramen magnum and ends at the superior border of L_2
   b. Tapers in the lower thoracic area into a cone-shaped structure called the conus medullaris
   c. Anchored to the coccyx by the filum terminale, a thin prolongation of the conus medullaris
2. Serves as a center for spinal reflexes and a conducting pathway of impulses to and from the brain
3. Consists of gray (unmyelinated) and white (myelinated) matter
   a. Gray matter integrates the cord reflexes
      1) Has an internal core resembling a butterfly on cross section
      2) Has a pair of projections forming the back wings—posterior or dorsal horns—consisting of multipolar neuron structures that form the motor efferent neurons of the ventral roots or spinal nerves
      3) Contains cell bodies and dendrites of sensory neurons and sensory receptors from the periphery
   b. White matter surrounds gray matter
      1) Consists of long ascending and descending tracts
      2) Serves as pathway between spinal cord and brain for afferent and efferent impulses, which are grouped into anatomical and functional bundles called fasciculi
4. Divided into lateral halves with each lateral half divided into three sections that run the length of the spinal cord
   a. Dorsal
   b. Lateral
   c. Ventral
5. Contains distinct fiber tracts
   a. Ascending fibers bring sensory information to the central nervous system
   b. Descending fibers carry impulses from the brain to motor neurons of the brainstem, spinal cord, and internuncial (association) neurons, which form short ascending and descending tracts that travel between spinal segments
6. Protected by other structures
   a. Vertebral column
      1) Runs from foramen magnum to sacral hiatus, with bony arches of the vertebrae posterior to the vertebral bodies forming a continuum to make up the spinal canal with spaces between the vertebrae being taken up by spinal ligaments
      2) Consists of 7 cervical, 12 thoracic, and 5 lumbar vertebrae with the sacrum and coccyx inferiorly
   b. Spinous processes
      1) Prominence at posterior part of each vertebra
      2) Angulation varies and considered important when inserting needle into epidural space

- Processes almost horizontal in the cervical, lower thoracic, and lumbar regions; may require needle to be inserted at right angles to the sagittal plane
- Processes directly caudal in the midthoracic region with maximal angulation between T_7 and T_8; may require needle to be inserted at varying degrees from the horizontal

  c. Spinal ligaments
  1) Supporting structures that hold vertebrae together posteriorly
  2) Provides access to the spinal canal
  3) Supraspinous ligament runs superficial to tips of spinous processes
  4) Interspinous ligament connects posterior spinous processes
  5) Ligamentum flavum connects laminae of the vertebra
     - Tougher than other ligaments and easily identified by its increased resistance to needle insertion
     - Not present in the sacrum where the laminae are fused together except at the fifth sacral vertebra, which has no laminae and thus forms the sacral hiatus through which the spinal canal may be entered when performing a caudal (sacral) block

  d. Other spinal ligaments
  1) Anterior longitudinal ligament
     - Runs from skull to sacrum
     - Firmly attached to the discs and adjacent margins of vertebral bodies
  2) Posterior longitudinal ligament
     - Connects posterior aspects of the vertebral bodies
     - Forms anterior wall of vertebral column

  e. Meninges (three-layer membrane coverings)
  1) Pia mater: membrane covering, closely attached to spinal cord and spinal nerves
     - Laterally attached to spinal nerve roots, eventually joining arachnoid and dura mater to become the connective tissue surrounding and investing the spinal nerves
     - Separated from arachnoid mater by subarachnoid space, which contains CSF produced by the choroid plexuses in the brain ventricles
  2) Arachnoid mater: thin membrane lying close to the dura mater but separated by the subdural space, which contains lymph
  3) Dura mater
     - Thick band of tissue covering spinal cord and its inner two coverings
     - Space between dura mater and vertebral column called the epidural space contains areolar tissue, fat, and a number of venous plexuses

7. Supplied by numerous blood vessels throughout the epidural space that supply and drain blood from the vertebrae, the spinal cord, its coverings, and the spinal nerves

C. Peripheral Nervous System

1. Cranial nerves form the peripheral nerves of the brain
   a. Divided according to function

        1) Five pairs have only motor fibers

        2) Three pairs have only sensory fibers

        3) Four pairs have both sensory and motor fibers

    b. Correspond to the spinal nerves serving common sensation, voluntary control of muscles, and autonomic functions in the head including the mechanism for the special senses of vision, hearing, smell, and taste

  2. Spinal nerves: 31 pairs arise from different segments of the spinal cord

    a. Each pair is formed by the union of anterior and posterior roots attached to the spinal column

    b. Each pair with its corresponding part of the spinal cord constitutes a spinal segment

        1) Cervical nerves: join at anterior rami to form a complex network of nerve fibers called a plexus

          • Cervical plexus: first four pairs supply sensory and motor impulses to back of head, front of neck, and upper part of shoulder to numerous neck muscles

          • Brachial plexus: latter four pairs supply sensory and motor impulses to scapula and muscles of upper extremities

        2) Thoracic nerves: 12 pairs of spinal nerves with branches running directly to intercostal muscles and skin of thorax

          • Provide both sensory and motor impulses

          • Do not form a plexus

        3) Lumbar nerves: five pairs extend obliquely and inferiorly, making up the lumbosacral plexus

          • Innervate lower extremities

          • Carry both sensory and motor impulses

        4) Sacral nerves: five pairs of spinal nerves

          • Four pairs emerge through the posterior sacral foramina

          • Fifth pair emerges through the sacral hiatus, carrying both sensory and motor impulses

        5) Coccygeal nerves: one pair of spinal nerves

          • Part of the lumbosacral plexus

          • Carries both sensory and motor impulses to the lower extremities

D. Autonomic Nervous System

  1. Part of the peripheral nervous system that regulates the body's internal environment in close conjunction with the endocrine system

  2. Responsible for the unconscious moment-to-moment functions of all internal systems, including visceral organs, involuntary fibers, and glandular functions

  3. Activated by centers in the hypothalamus, brainstem, and spinal cord

    a. Sympathetic nerves

        1) Consists of pre- and postganglionic nerve fibers arising from nerve cells in lateral column of gray matter of spinal cord

2) Transmit impulses that cause an increase in blood pressure and heart rate and vasoconstriction of peripheral blood vessels when external stress situations occur
   - Most frequently termed the flight–fight syndrome
   - Transmitter substance, norepinephrine, secreted by postganglionic nerve terminals
   b. Parasympathetic nerves
   1) Consist of preganglionic fibers arising from cell bodies in cranial nerves III, VII, IX, and X and spinal nerves II through VII
   2) Activated when the body is at rest or relaxed, protects and restores the body's resources

E. Physiological Considerations

1. Epidural anesthesia
   a. Mechanism of action
   1) Mixed spinal nerves in paravertebral space provide only lateral spread of anesthesia to nerve cuffs, playing a minor role in epidural anesthesia
   2) Spinal roots provide initial onset of epidural anesthesia related to inhibition of conduction in spinal roots; anatomical location of spinal nerves favorable because of anatomy of arachnoid membrane in this region, significant uptake of local anesthetics by spinal roots, and correlation between onset of epidural anesthesia and thickness of spinal roots
   3) Spread of epidural anesthetics involves diffusion through the relatively thin dura and arachnoid membranes in the region of the spinal roots near the junction where they form the spinal nerve
      - Agents reaching the CSF penetrate periphery of spinal cord and contribute to degree of nerve blockade
      - Depth of penetration into spinal cord is influenced by the lipid solubility of agent used, the amount of drug taken up by spinal roots and spinal cord, and the physiochemical properties of agent used
   b. Administration of anesthetics
   1) Administration into epidural space in lumbar region; L_1, L_2, L_3, and L_4–L_5 interspaces most commonly used
   2) Lipid solubility is primary determinant of intrinsic anesthetic potency, whereas protein binding determines duration of anesthetic activity
2. Intraspinal analgesia
   a. Mechanism of action
   1) Central nervous system produces endogenous neurotransmitter substance called "P"
      - Released as body reacts to pain stimulus
      - Impulse transmitted to brain with subsequent experience of pain
   2) Endogenous opiates called endorphin and enkephalin capable of blocking "P" by creating a pain inhibition pathway

3) Narcotics mimic the endogenous opiates to produce pain-free state
b. Epidural administration
   1) Application of narcotics next to the spinal cord
   2) Catheter insertion between any vertebral joint
      • Narcotics diffused through a fatty or lipid membrane called the dura with rate of diffusion depending on solubility of narcotic in the lipids
      • The more lipid-soluble the narcotic, the faster its passage through the lipid membrane to relieve pain
c. Intrathecal administration
   1) Application of narcotics inside the spinal cord
   2) Catheter insertion usually between the lumbar vertebrae to minimize risk of danger to spinal cord
   3) Administration of narcotics bypass the dura requiring a reduced dosage (one-tenth of dosage used for epidural analgesia) and increased interval between dosages
d. Intraventricular administration
   1) Direct access to CSF provided with distribution of injected intrathecal medication
   2) Anticancer drugs and analgesics primarily administered
   3) Catheter placed into lateral ventricle

F. Clinical Considerations

1. Epidural anesthesia
  a. Catheter is inserted by a physician
  b. Medications are administered by a physician, or by a nurse in accordance with the state Nurse Practice Act
  c. Anesthetic agents
    1) Low anesthetic potency and short duration of action: procaine and chloroprocaine
    2) Intermediate anesthetic potency and duration of action: lidocaine, mepivacaine, and prilocaine
    3) High anesthetic potency and prolonged duration of action: tetracaine, bupivacaine, and etidocaine
  d. Factors influencing adequacy of epidural blockade
    1) Dose, volume, concentration of agent
    2) Addition of vasoconstrictor to the local anesthetic solution
    3) Site and speed of action
    4) Patient position
    5) Patient age, height, clinical status
  e. Clinical uses and observations
    1) Epidural block in surgery
       • Blocks sensory and motor responses to abdomen, vaginal and perineal areas, kidney, bladder, lower limbs
       • Essential to monitor heart rate, respiratory status, arterial pressure, electrocardiogram (ECG)

       2) Epidural block in obstetrics
- Essential to monitor fetus
- Monitoring of heart rate, arterial pressure, ECG, and breathing necessary

2. Epidural analgesia
   a. Only preservative-free medications used
      1) Morphine: most hydrophilic agent with longest average onset time (35 minutes) and least lipophilic agent with longest duration of action (22 hours)
      2) Methadone: most lipophilic agent with shortest onset time (17 minutes) and shortest duration time (7 hours)
      3) Hydromorphone: intermediate lipophilicity with intermediate onset time (23 minutes) and duration (14 hours)
      4) Fentanyl: extremely lipophilic, inducing sensory analgesia within 10 minutes with a duration of 4 to 6 hours
   b. Optional dosage required for maximal analgesia activity without severe side effects varies widely with the agent used, patient status, and concomitant use of epinephrine
   c. Clinical uses
      1) Acute postoperative pain
      2) Chronic pain syndrome
   d. Nursing considerations
      1) Delivery of medications, maintenance, and care established in organizational policies and procedures in compliance with state Nurse Practice Act
      2) Policies and procedures for obtaining, delivering, administering, documenting, and discarding these medications established in compliance with state and federal regulations because medications are controlled substances
      3) Length of therapy determines type of epidural catheter used
      4) Monitoring and documenting of blood pressure, respiratory rate, depth of respirations, level of consciousness, sedation scale, and side effects essential
      5) Continuous infusions administered by infusion device
      6) Alcohol contraindicated for site preparation and accessing catheter because of potential for migration of alcohol into epidural space and potential to cause nerve damage
      7) 0.2-micron filter without surfactant used for medication administration
      8) Catheter aspirated to ascertain absence of spinal fluid before administration of medication
      9) Ineffective pain control reported to physician; may indicate improperly positioned catheter or need to readjust medication dosage
     10) Naloxone hydrochloride (Narcan) must be readily available
     11) Microbore tubing with Luer-Lok connector and without injection ports essential

        12) Patient monitored for systemic complications including paresthesia, pruritus, nausea, vomiting, urinary retention, respiratory depression, hypotension, and respiratory arrest

        13) Patient assessed for catheter complications including infection, dislodgment, and leaking

        14) Complications documented and reported to physician

    3. Intrathecal analgesia

      a. Only preservative-free medications used

      b. Clinical uses

        1) Chemotherapy

        2) Chronic pain syndrome

        3) Antibiotic therapy

        4) Anesthesia

      c. Modes of delivery

        1) Implantable pump

        2) External pump

        3) Ventricular reservoir

      d. Nursing considerations

        1) Delivery of medications, maintenance, and care established in policies and procedures and in compliance with state Nurse Practice Act

        2) Policies and procedures for obtaining, delivering, administering, documenting, and discarding controlled substances established in compliance with state and federal regulations

        3) Manufacturer's guidelines used to access, fill, and refill ports/pumps

        4) Alcohol contraindicated for site preparation and accessing catheter because of potential for alcohol migration into intrathecal space

        5) 0.2-micron filter without surfactant used for medication administration

        6) Catheter aspirated to ascertain presence of spinal fluid before medication administration; manufacturer's guidelines adhered to when catheter attached to implantable pump

        7) Patient assessed for therapeutic response and complications of therapy; observations dependent on treatment modalities administered

        8) Assessments documented and reported to physician

IV. SKELETAL SYSTEM ANATOMY AND PHYSIOLOGY

A. Functions

    1. Bones collectively form the framework that supports the body; enables it to stand erect

    2. Protects internal organs and other soft tissues

    3. Assists movement by leverage and in coordination with muscles

    4. Manufactures red blood cells (internal marrow)

    5. Provides for storage of minerals, particularly calcium and phosphorus

B. Bone Shapes According to Function

1. Short bones make up wrist and ankle
2. Flat bones make up sternum and scapula
3. Long bones comprise arm and leg
   a. Consist of three parts
      1) Shaft, or long part of bone
      2) Metaphysis, or flared part at the end of the shaft
      3) Epiphysis, or rounded end
   b. Epiphyseal cartilage
      1) Plate of soft tissue between epiphysis and metaphysis
      2) Provides for growth
4. Irregular bones make up vertebrae and patella

C. Intraosseous Infusion

1. Administered as an infusion directly into bone marrow
2. Performed as an emergency short-term procedure when vascular access by the intravenous route cannot be achieved in the pediatric patient
3. Commonly administered into long bones
   a. Distal tibia
      1) Preferred site
      2) No nerve endings
      3) Location behind ankle bone
   b. Proximal tibia
      1) Located one to two fingers below knee inside of leg
      2) Injected away from growth plate
   c. Distal femur
      1) Top third of femur below knee used
      2) Injected away from growth plate
4. Clinical considerations
   a. Inserted upon physician order in accordance with state statutes and state Nurse Practice Acts
   b. Use is established in organizational policies and procedures
   c. Used no longer than 24 hours, while conventional intravenous access is established as soon as the patient is stabilized
   d. Consideration given to use only in patients 6 years of age and younger
   e. Appropriate needles for use
      1) 16 to 18 gauge
      2) Standard sterile hypodermic, spinal, trephine, sternal, or standard bone marrow needles
      3) Consideration given to use of a short shaft to avoid accidental dislodgment
      4) Needle with stylet preferred because stylet prevents bone marrow from entering and occluding needle
      5) Consideration given to use of disposable needles specifically designed for intraosseous access

   f. Insertion
      1) Aseptic technique essential
      2) Sterile gloves with consideration for wearing a gown, mask, and goggles
      3) Site preparation with an antimicrobial solution
      4) Needle placement with confirmation before infusion by aspiration of approximately 5 ml of bone marrow followed by immediate flush of 5 ml 0.9% sodium chloride from a separate syringe
      5) Needle secured with tape to prevent dislodgment or rocking
   g. Discontinuation of infusion
      1) Withdraw needle with a quick straight pull according to established policies and procedures
      2) Site inspection and redressing daily until no drainage observed
5. Contraindications
   a. Fractured or traumatized leg
   b. Areas of infected burns or cellulitis
   c. Osteoporosis
6. Complications
   a. Improper needle placement with a decrease in rate and poor absorption of medications and/or solutions
   b. Needle obstruction with inability to administer medications and/or solutions
   c. Embolus formation caused by fat and bony fragments
7. Nursing responsibilities
   a. Access
   b. Site assessment and maintenance
   c. Evaluation of therapy
   d. Termination of access
   e. Documentation in medical record
   f. Patient and family teaching

PART TWO EQUIPMENT

I. SOLUTION CONTAINERS

A. Material

1. Glass
   a. Necessary for certain solutions that are incompatible with or will leach through plastic
   b. Easily broken when transported if caution is not taken to prevent breakage
   c. Rotation in light necessary before use to detect fine cracks through which microorganisms can enter
2. Plastic
   a. Suitable for most solutions

    b. Easily transported with minimal risk

    c. Squeeze before use to detect punctures as bags are susceptible to punctures that may go undetected and allow microorganisms to enter

B. Sizes

    1. Containers for premixed solutions range from 50 to 1000 ml

    2. Plastic containers for use in preparing solutions are available that will hold up to 4000 ml (frequently used for TPN solutions)

C. Types of Containers

    1. Air-dependent (open system)

      a. Refers to glass or plastic bottles that do not collapse as the solution leaves the bottle

      b. Requires venting (air within system) for the solution to flow

        1) Air must enter solution container through vented administration set or vented spike adapter

        2) Use of needles to vent solution containers is inappropriate because needles allow microorganisms to enter solution and predispose patient to sepsis

    2. Nonair-dependent (closed system)

      a. Refers to plastic bags that collapse as the solution empties

      b. Does not require air for the solution to flow

      c. Reduces risk of air embolism and airborne contamination because of closed system

D. Clinical Considerations

    1. Wash hands before opening and/or spiking solution containers

    2. Inspect bags and bottles before use for cracks, leaks, damaged ports or seals, expiration date, clarity, discoloration, turbidity, and particulate matter; discard if present

    3. Label bags and bottles with date and time the solution container was opened

    4. Cover solutions containing medications that are light-sensitive to prevent degradation of medications

    5. Change solution containers in accordance with the *Intravenous Nursing Standards of Practice,* particularly if a closed system is not maintained, to prevent the potential growth of microorganisms that might have entered the system

    6. Discard solution containers removed from the intravenous system; do not save for later use

II. ADMINISTRATION SETS

A. Types

    1. Vented

      a. Allows air to enter the system through a filtered vent

   b. Necessary for use with bottles
2. Nonvented
   a. Does not allow air to enter the system
   b. Necessary for use with plastic bags

B. Drop Conversion Factor

1. Macrodrip
   a. Set that delivers from 10 to 20 gtts/ml
   b. Used to deliver solutions to the adult patient and when small volumes or critical measurement is not required
2. Microdrip
   a. Set that delivers 60 gtts/ml
   b. Used to deliver solutions to the neonate or pediatric patient and when small volumes or critical measurement is necessary
3. Calculation of flow rates
   a. Determined by the use of a quick, easy formula:

$$\frac{\text{gtts/ml of given set} \times \text{total hourly volume}}{60 \ (\text{minutes in hour})} = \text{gtts/minute}$$

   b. Affected by the height of the solution container, blockage of the cannula, change in position of the cannula, venous spasms, and viscosity of fluids

C. Construction

1. Straight set
   a. Provides for administration of a primary solution
   b. Does not provide measured volumes
   c. May or may not have an injection port
   d. Injection ports do not prevent solutions or medications from flowing back up the tubing and mixing with the primary solution since they do not have a check-valve
2. Check-valve set
   a. Used to administer "piggyback" (secondary) admixtures
   b. Has an in-line check-valve that prevents mixing of primary and secondary solutions, or mixing of primary solution and medications administered through injection ports
      1) Primary solution is lowered on a wire or plastic hanger, creating greater head-height pressure for secondary solution
         • Secondary solution flows and primary solution stops
         • When secondary solution is complete, primary solution flows automatically
      2) Risk of air entering the line between infusion of primary and secondary infusions is eliminated; occlusion without interruption of infusion is prevented
      3) Rate of administration remains the same for both primary and secondary solutions because flow rate is regulated by one clamp

3. Secondary set
   a. Short set used for the administration of "piggyback" medications
   b. Attaches to the primary administration set at the Y-port above the check-valve
      1) Flow-control clamp is an on–off clamp only
      2) Clamp is never used to regulate flow of medication
4. Y-type set
   a. Allows alternate or simultaneous infusion of two solutions
   b. May contain a filter and/or an in-line hand pump for the administration of blood
   c. Use involves a hazard of air embolism because large quantities of air can be sucked into the tubing if one container is allowed to empty
5. Controlled-volume set
   a. Contains a vented, calibrated chamber
   b. May contain a microporous filter to block the passage of air when the chamber empties
   c. Used frequently to measure solutions administered at a microdrip rate
   d. Allows medications to be added directly into the chamber through the medication port
6. Retrograde set
   a. Placed proximal to the infusion site
   b. Allows solution displacement within the set into a syringe as medication is injected into the set
   c. Allows administration of medication proximal to the site, eliminating loss of medication from adherence to the tubing
   d. Used to administer medications to neonates and the pediatric patient
7. Dedicated set
   a. Contains a specific segment that adapts to use with a specific infusion device
   b. Used only with devices for which it is designed
   c. May or may not allow priming outside of the infusion device

D. Internal Tubing Diameter

1. Standard tubing
   a. Allows for infusion flow at a standard rate using a drop size of 10 to 20 gtts/ml
   b. Routinely used for the administration of medications and solutions to the adult patient when small volumes or critical measurement is not necessary
2. Microbore tubing
   a. Uses a reduced drop size to maintain flow at a minimal rate, delivering 60 gtts/ml
   b. Solution viscosity may decrease flow rate
   c. Used for administering infusions to neonates
   d. Considered for use in the pediatric patient and when minimal amounts are infused or a slow rate is desired
3. Macrobore (large-bore) tubing

a. The increased lumen of the tubing and the drop size of the infusion allows for a rapid infusion flow

b. Indicated when large amounts of fluid or blood are needed quickly, as with trauma patients

E. Clamps

1. Device on a tubing that allows the user to affect the flow rate of the solution by increasing or decreasing the diameter of the tubing
2. Roller clamp
   a. Uses a plastic roller to adjust tubing diameter by applying pressure on the tubing, allowing regulation of flow rate
   b. Used on most administration sets
   c. Requires time-consuming adjustments to establish and maintain the rate because changes in drop rate invariably occur after the rate has been regulated
3. Screw clamp
   a. Uses a plastic screw to adjust the tubing diameter by applying pressure on the tubing
   b. Frequently difficult to regulate the infusion rate
   c. Requires time-consuming adjustments to establish and maintain the rate because changes in the drop rate invariably occur after the rate has been regulated
4. Slide clamp
   a. Clamp that slides across the tubing to open or close the tubing
   b. On–off clamp only
   c. Not used to regulate flow

F. Injection Ports

1. Location
   a. Distal to drip chamber
   b. Proximal to distal end of set
2. Number: varies with set and purpose of set
3. Configuration may vary
4. Purpose
   a. To allow for the infusion of solutions and/or medications "piggyback"
   b. To administer medications proximal to the site as with an "IV push" or bolus medication

G. Connection Mechanisms

1. Luer slip
   a. Allows connection of the tubing with an add-on set or cannula by inserting the male luer of the administration set into the female luer of an add-on device or cannula with a twisting motion
   b. Can be easily pulled apart, opening the system to airborne contaminants and possible free flow of blood externally

2. Luer-Lok
   a. Allows connection of the tubing with an add-on set or cannula by insert-ing the male luer of the administration set into the female luer with a locking clasp using a screwlike mechanism
   b. Prevents leaking at connections and accidental disconnections that place the patient at risk of infection, air embolus, and/or loss of blood through the cannula

H. Considerations When Using Administration Sets

1. Assess product and package integrity before use; do not use if violated
2. Change the peripheral and central primary sets used in accordance with the *Intravenous Nursing Standards of Practice*
3. Change sets at the time of the peripheral cannula change or when a new solution container is initiated
4. Change peripheral and central secondary sets in accordance with the *Intravenous Nursing Standards of Practice*
5. Consider and treat secondary sets detached from a primary set as primary intermittent administration sets
6. Change primary intermittent sets in accordance with the *Intravenous Nursing Standards of Practice*
7. Remove needles attached to primary intermittent sets immediately after use and replace with a sterile needle using aseptic technique
8. Change sets used for TPN administration in accordance with the *Intravenous Nursing Standards of Practice*
9. Discard sets used to administer lipid emulsions after each unit unless addi-tional units are administered consecutively, and immediately if contamina-tion is suspected or product integrity is compromised; change sets used to administer consecutive units every 24 hours
10. Change sets used to administer blood and blood products after each unit or at the end of 4 hours, whichever comes first, and immediately if conta-mination is suspected or product integrity is compromised
11. Change hemodynamic and arterial pressure monitoring sets, including the dome in accordance with the *Intravenous Nursing Standards of Practice*
12. Label sets with the date and time of initiation
13. Maintain sets as closed systems whenever possible
14. Disinfect injection ports before use
15. Never flush or irrigate sets to improve flow rate
16. Change administration and secondary sets with the cannula and solution if phlebitis, thrombophlebitis, cellulitis, or intravenous-related bacteremia is suspected
17. Consider using a needleless system when accessing intravenous tubing to prevent transmission of bloodborne pathogens to the healthcare worker

III. ADD-ON DEVICES

A. Extension Sets

1. Features
   a. Used to add length to tubing or to provide additional entry into system
   b. May or may not have an on–off clamp
   c. May or may not have one or more Y-ports for use when administering medications and/or solutions
2. Types
   a. Straight extension set
      1) Frequently used to add tubing length
      2) Less risk of contamination than Y-extension set or multi-entry set because of fewer entry points for bacteria to enter system
   b. Y-type extension set
      1) Forms a "Y"
      2) Provides two entry points into system
      3) Usually has a clamp on both segments of the "Y," allowing solutions to run simultaneously or separately
      4) May have injection ports or check-valves in one or both segments to prevent solution backflow into either segment
   c. Multi-entry extension set
      1) Set with three or more "pigtails," allowing three or more entries into system
      2) May have clamps, additional ports, or check-valves in one, two, or all of the segments
3. Considerations
   a. Use only when definite need exists because each entry into the system provides an opportunity for bacteria to enter the system
   b. Provide Luer-Lok connections
   c. Change at the same time device to which they are attached is changed, and if contamination is suspected

B. Stopcocks

1. Features
   a. Used to provide multiple entries into infusion system when additional access is needed or to provide an alternate entry into the system if an emergency arises
   b. Available with or without an extension set
   c. Available with varying types of ports, including needleless ports
2. Considerations
   a. Potential mechanism for transmission of bacteria
   b. Frequently assess latex ports for integrity because multiple injections into the latex port may cause leakage

    c. Consider port cover contaminated once removed; replace with a new sterile cover

    d. Change at time device to which it is attached is changed, and if contamination is suspected

C. Connectors

1. Device used to connect tubings and/or cannula
2. Types
    a. Y-connector
      1) In the shape of a "Y"
      2) Usually used to administer two infusions simultaneously
    b. T-connector
      1) In the shape of a "T"
      2) Usually connected to a short extension set
        • Short arm of the "T" provides a male luer for connection to cannula
        • Second short arm serves as an injection port
        • Long arm as an extension set
      3) Frequently used in neonates, infants, and small children to attach an administration set to a cannula and to provide an injection port proximal to the site to allow for immediate administration of medications without medication loss within the tubing
    c. J-connector
      1) Shaped like a "J"
      2) Frequently used to connect an administration set to a cannula or with an injection cap to make an intermittent device
    d. U-connector
      1) In the shape of a "U"
      2) Usually used to connect tubing and cannula to prevent kinks in the tubing
3. Considerations
    a. Use according to established policies and procedures
    b. Know that use increases the potential for infection because of the increased opportunity for manipulation and/or risk of separation
    c. Change when the device to which it is attached is changed, and if contamination is suspected

D. Latex Injection Ports

1. Resealable rubber cap designed to accommodate needles or plastic cannula (as with some needleless systems) for administering medications and/or solutions into the vascular system
2. Disinfection
    a. Established in policies and procedures
    b. Cleanse with a single-unit antimicrobial-approved solution, such as tincture of iodine 2%, 10% povidone-iodine, 70% isopropyl alcohol, or chlorhexidine

     c. Cleanse immediately before use to prevent the entry of microorganisms into the vascular system

  3. Access

     a. Established in policies and procedures

     b. Use needles of 25- to 21-gauge that do not exceed 1 inch in length

     c. Needles smaller than 25-gauge are not recommended because they may break and enter the system

     d. Port integrity is confirmed before and immediately after use

  4. Change requirements

     a. Established in policies and procedures

     b. Replace when tubing is changed if it is an integral part of the tubing

     c. Latex injection ports attached to a peripheral cannula are replaced when the cannula is changed, and immediately if contamination is suspected or product integrity is compromised

     d. Latex injection ports attached to central venous catheters are changed at least every 7 days, and immediately if contamination is suspected or product integrity is compromised

E. Solid Caps

  1. Closed plastic caps used to cover the end of syringes filled with medications

  2. Aseptic technique used for removal before administering medication

  3. Single use only; discarded once medication is administered

F. Vented Spike Adapters

  1. Adapters applied to nonvented tubing to allow air to enter the system through a filtered port

  2. Treated as part of the administration set to which it is attached

  3. Replace at time of tubing change or immediately if contamination is suspected

G. Transducers and Domes

  1. Used for hemodynamic and arterial pressure monitoring

  2. Consider a closed system along with the administration set, the continuous flush device, and the flush solution

  3. Change every 96 hours at the time of set and bag change, and immediately if contamination is suspected or product integrity is compromised

IV. FILTERS

A. Features

  1. Device that prevents the passage of undesired substances

  2. Product design determines the size of the substances retained

  3. Characteristics vary with the filter used; optimal characteristics include:

     a. Retention of particulates, bacteria, fungi, and endotoxin

     b. Removal of air from system and vents to atmosphere

   c. Nonbinding ability with drugs, allowing dosage to pass
   d. Allowance for high gravity flow rates
   e. Pressure tolerance to withstand pounds per square inch (PSI) of an electronic infusion device

B. Types

1. In-line filter (filter that forms an integral part of the administration set)
   a. Advantages
      1) Associated with less risk of contamination because filter is integral part of tubing design
      2) No risk of separation
   b. Disadvantages
      1) Usually in upper part of administration set instead of at distal end, retaining only those substances that enter the line above the filter
      2) Entire set must be changed if filter becomes clogged
2. Add-on filter (filter added to an administration set)
   a. Advantages
      1) Easily changed when filter becomes clogged or defective without removing entire tubing
      2) Placed at distal end of tubing, removing all substances that enter the line above the filter
   b. Disadvantages
      1) May be accidentally separated from infusion line or cannula, potentiating the risk of infection and/or possible hemorrhage
3. Filter needle (needle that retains particulates from 1 to 5 microns)
   a. Frequently used when preparing intravenous medications
   b. Recommended when withdrawing medications from ampules or multi-dose vials, particularly if the medication is to be administered as a bolus and cannot be administered through a bacteria-retentive filter

C. Structural Configuration

1. Depth filter: consists of fibers or fragmented material that has been bonded or pressed to form a tortuous maze
   a. Cannot be given an absolute rating because pore size is not uniform; assigned a nominal rating, the particle size above which 98% of the contaminants will be retained
   b. Removes particulates only; does not remove air
2. Membrane filter: screen-type with uniformly sized pores that provide an absolute rating, retaining all particles on the membrane greater than its size
   a. May retain bacteria, fungus, and air depending on pore size
   b. May have a unique membrane that removes endotoxins, microbial contaminants, particulate matter, and air; bacteria retained may break down

after 24 hours and release bacterial toxin confined within the body of a bacterium

3. Hollow fiber filter: contains fibers that trap undesired substances
   a. Provides a large filtering area that makes for easy priming and prevents clogging and binding of medications
   b. Withstands pressures up to 45 PSI

D. Surface Area

1. Refers to area with which the solution and/or medication comes in contact
2. Impacts flow rate
   a. The larger the surface area, the greater the area through which fluid or medication can flow, increasing the flow rate
   b. The smaller the area, the slower the rate

E. Pressure Limitations

1. Amount of pressure that can be exerted on the filter membrane without rupturing the filter
2. Rated according to the PSI
3. Varies with the device being used
4. Consideration necessary before applying flow control devices

F. Indications For Use

1. Intravenous solutions: available in a variety of pore sizes, forms, and materials; pore size determines what substances are retained
   a. 0.2-micron filter: absolute bacteria-retentive, air-eliminating filter that removes particulates of 0.2 microns or larger
      1) Recommended for routine delivery of intravenous therapy because filter decreases potential for air emboli; use with certain infusions such as TPN solutions and intermittent antibiotics
      2) Contraindicated for administration of blood/blood components; lipid emulsions; low-dose (< 5 µg/ml), low-volume medications (total amount < 5 mg over 24 hours); IV push medications; medications in which the pharmacological properties are altered by the filter membrane and in medications that bind to the filter membrane
      3) Air venting filters automatically vent air through a nonwettable (hydrophobic) membrane and permit uniform high gravity flow rates through large wettable (hydrophilic) membranes, preventing air block and plugged cannulas
      4) Should be an integral part of infusion system
      5) Place as close to cannula site as possible to achieve final filtration
      6) Requires PSI of the filter exceeding that of the infusion device used
      7) Should comply with manufacturer's guidelines
   b. 1.0-micron filter: removes particulates greater than 1.0 microns; often termed a particulate matter filter

1) May be designed as an integral part of the administration set, as a membrane filter in a burette chamber, as an add-on device, or as a needle
2) May be air-retentive
3) Recommended use
   - Administration of infusions that contain medications with a pore size greater than 1.0 micron
   - Preparation and/or administration of solutions and/or medications to remove particulates that have the potential for obstructing vascular and/or pulmonary systems

c. 1.2-micron filter: recommended for administering TPN solutions that contain lipid emulsions because fat molecules are larger than 1.2 microns
   1) Should be changed every 24 hours at time of tubing change, and immediately if contamination is suspected or product integrity is compromised
   2) Usually air-retentive

d. 5-micron filter: particulate matter filter removing particles larger than 5 microns
   1) May be designed as part of an administration set, as a filter needle, or as a filter straw
   2) Recommended for use when infusing or admixing medications and/or solutions with a pore size greater than 5 microns

2. Blood/blood products: usage should be established in policies and procedures
   a. Used to remove particulate matter from blood/blood components
   b. Single-use only (for one unit of blood) because it would be difficult to identify the unit of blood responsible for a transfusion reaction when more than one unit is infused through a filter
   c. Integral part of the administration set
   d. Used in compliance with manufacturer's guidelines
   e. Routine use is not necessary for infusion of commercially prepared plasma products such as albumin; manufacturer's guidelines should be consulted
   f. Filtering capacity
      1) Standard blood filters
         - Range from 170 to 260 microns
         - Trap blood clots
      2) Microaggregate blood filters
         - Range from 20 to 40 microns
         - Recommended for administration of whole blood and/or packed red blood cells stored for 5 or more days because filters trap microaggregates (degenerating platelets, white cells, and fibrin strands that form in stored blood); routinely used during cardiopulmonary bypass
         - Not routinely used in settings requiring rapid transfusion because use will impede flow rates

3) Leukocyte-poor blood filters
- Remove leukocytes from red blood cells
- Classified according to efficiency level, not micron size, removing up to 99% of the leukocytes from red blood cells

4) Leukocyte-poor platelet filters
- Remove leukocytes from platelets
- Classified according to efficiency level, not micron size, removing 95 to 99.9% of the leukocytes from platelet units

g. Surface area
1) Amount of area through which the blood flows
2) The greater the area, the faster the flow rate
3) The smaller the area, the slower the flow rate

V. CANNULAS

A. Description

1. Term used to refer to a hollow tube made of plastic or metal that is used for accessing the vascular system
2. Varies in gauge, length, composition, and design

B. Peripheral Cannula (cannula less than 3 inches long)

1. Types
   a. Stainless steel needle: hollow tube made of stainless steel, usually 1 inch long and attached to plastic wings to aid insertion
      1) For short-term intravenous therapy, such as single-dose medications and drawing of blood samples
      2) Less thrombogenic than catheters as a result of decreased formation of fibrin sheath around needle
      3) Increased risk of infiltration, a concern if administering medications and/or solutions with vesicant potential
   b. Over-the-needle cannula: catheter with an internal needle stylet to promote venipuncture
      1) Catheter pushed off stylet once venipuncture is made and threaded into the vessel; stylet is removed and discarded
      2) Catheter of choice for peripheral intravenous therapy and for home intravenous antibiotic therapy of 7 or fewer days
   c. Through-the-needle cannula: catheter threaded through a needle until the desired length is in the vein
      1) Needle usually removed once catheter is threaded
      2) Not recommended for therapy because of risk of puncture or shearing of catheter
   d. Double-lumen catheter
      1) Provides two separate lumens, one through which the needle stylet resides
         - Second port appears as a side port with a short extension, which al-

lows exit of solution and/or medication through an outlet or "eye" above the end of the catheter
- Two entries into system with one venipuncture
2) Each port provides independent flow of medications and/or solutions, never mixing while infusing through the catheter
3) Consideration must be given to compatibility of solutions and/or medications being administered because distance between distal and proximal ports are minimal; manufacturer's guidelines should be consulted
e. Midline catheter: catheter designed for intermediate-term therapies of 2 or more weeks
1) Catheter length greater than 3 inches
- Tip resides below axilla
- Insertion site no more than 1.5 inches above or below antecubital fossa
2) Inserted through basilic, cephalic, or median veins in antecubital region with the tip residing in the larger vessels of upper arm, providing greater hemodilution
2. Composition
a. Made of Teflon, polyvinylchloride, polyurethane, or silicone
b. Vary as to thrombogenicity or potential for producing vein inflammation
1) Teflon considered most thrombogenic
2) Silicone considered least thrombogenic
c. Available impregnated with heparin to decrease thrombogenicity
3. Properties
a. Only radiopaque catheters should be used so that in the event of a fragmented catheter, the catheter fragment can be visualized by radiography
b. May be entirely radiopaque or may be clear with a radiopaque strip; radiopaque strips are considered to promote insertion because of visibility of blood flow when the vein has been entered
4. Gauge and length
a. Gauge refers to the actual lumen size or interior space of the catheter
b. The smallest gauge, shortest length of cannula that will accommodate the prescribed therapy is used to minimize complications associated with therapy
5. Cannula change
a. Peripheral venous cannulas should be changed in accordance with the *Intravenous Nursing Standards of Practice*
b. A cannula should be removed immediately if a cannula-related complication is suspected; consideration should be given to culturing the cannula
c. Midline catheters should be removed immediately if contamination is suspected, if product integrity is compromised, or when therapy is discontinued
1) The maximum dwell time should be limited to 2 to 4 weeks
2) Longer periods for dwell time should be based on nurse's professional

judgment after considering length of therapy remaining, patient's peripheral venous status, patient's condition, vein condition of catheter placement, and skin integrity

C. Central Venous Catheters

1. Types
   a. Percutaneous catheter: catheter inserted percutaneously through a needle or introducer, or over a guidewire that has been threaded through the needle or introducer
      1) Risk of catheter puncture or shearing when inserting catheter directly into vein through a needle; catheter should never be retracted through needle at any time during procedure
      2) Selection of catheters dependent on length needed and patient need
      3) Use for continuous or intermittent infusions of short duration (less than 60 days)
      4) Includes peripherally inserted central catheter (PICC)
      5) Multilumen configuration available
      6) Cannula removal
         • Removed immediately if contamination is suspected, if product integrity is compromised, and if therapy is discontinued
         • Removed by a registered nurse (RN) in accordance with established policies and procedures and the state Nurse Practice Act
   b. Tunneled cannula: catheter surgically placed by a physician by tunneling the catheter under the skin from the vein entry point to an exit point on the chest wall
      1) Venous status of patient, catheter preference, length of therapy, and patient's ability to care for the catheter considered
      2) Multilumen configurations available to accommodate multiple therapeutic and diagnostic procedures
      3) 0.9% sodium chloride for flushing before and after each use followed by heparin as recommended by manufacturer's guidelines
      4) Long-term catheter use (1 to 2 years)
      5) Silastic material composition
      6) Dacron cuff encircling catheter provides security and serves as a barrier to prevent infection
      7) Cannula removal
         • Optimal time interval for removal unknown
         • Medical act requiring removal by physician
   c. Implanted vascular access device: small plastic, stainless steel or titanium housing attached to a catheter surgically implanted under the skin by a physician
      1) Catheter insertion sites: jugular or subclavian vein, threaded into the superior vena cava
      2) Considerations

- Available venous access
- Duration of therapy
- Patient preference and ability to care for catheter
- Catheter of choice by many patients due to need for minimal care since it is implanted under skin

3) Flush with heparin solution monthly according to established policies and procedures when not in use
4) Long-term catheter use (1 to 2 years)
5) Removal
- Optimal dwell time is unknown
- Medical act requiring removal by physician

2. Lumens
   a. Single lumen catheters: provide only one port of entry into the vascular system
      1) Less risk of contamination because of decrease in manipulation with single lumen
      2) Use restrictive because there is only one entry point
   b. Multilumen catheters: provide two or more catheter lumens for multiple entries into the vascular system
      1) Accommodate multiple therapeutic or diagnostic procedures
      2) Associated with higher infection rates because of multiple manipulations associated with each port

3. Composition
   a. Made of Teflon, polyvinylchloride, polyurethane, or silicone
   b. Vary as to thrombogenicity or potential for producing vein inflammation
      1) Teflon considered most thrombogenic
      2) Polyurethane less thrombogenic than Teflon or polyvinylchloride
      3) Silicone considered least thrombogenic and most preferred

4. Properties
   a. Should be radiopaque so that catheter tip placement can be verified by radiography
   b. May have a Dacron cuff to provide a barrier against infection and to promote catheter stability

5. Gauge and length
   a. Dependent on catheter type and insertion site
   b. Catheter tip should be in the superior vena cava

6. Insertion techniques
   a. Direct venipuncture: associated with insertion of central catheters directly into the vein, usually subclavian or jugular
   b. Tunneled: associated with tunneling of the catheter from the entry point into the vein to an exit point on the chest wall
   c. Implanted: associated with port implantation under the skin, usually on the chest wall, with the catheter being placed in the subclavian vein
   d. Peripherally inserted: insertion of a catheter usually into the basilic or cephalic vein at the antecubital fossa, with threading of the catheter into the superior vena cava

D. Therapy-specific

1. Venous
   a. Choice of cannula depends on vein accessibility, type and duration of therapy
   b. Radiopaque over-the-needle catheters are considered state of the art; consider using these catheters for routine intravenous therapy
   c. Assess patient's vasculature and estimate blood flow around the cannula to prevent potential injury
   d. Use smallest gauge, shortest length cannula that will accommodate prescribed therapy
2. Arterial
   a. Choice of cannula is established in the intravenous policies and procedures
   b. Cannula choice is critical because of potential complications associated with arterial puncture
   c. Stainless steel needles are used for intermittent arterial blood sampling; they are never used for indwelling access
   d. Radiopaque catheters routinely are used for indwelling, continuous arterial access
   e. Use smallest gauge and shortest length that will accommodate prescribed therapy
   f. Remove every 96 hours, and immediately if contamination is suspected
3. Epidural
   a. Catheter specifically designed to deliver medications into the epidural space adjacent to the spinal cord
   b. Three different systems are available
      1) Externally threaded catheter
         • Tunneled subcutaneously from the epidural space to an abdominal exit site
         • Connected to an injection cap and a 0.2-micron filter with an extension set through which medication can be administered intermittently or continuously
         • Use possibly as a temporary or permanent catheter
      2) Total internal system
         • Catheter connected to a reservoir placed in the abdomen
         • Slow, continuous administration of medication provided
         • Placement permanent and usually for long-term pain management
      3) Catheter attached to a portal chamber
         • Placed beneath the skin over a bony surface and anchored to muscle tissue; tunneled subcutaneously and then threaded into epidural space at the desired level, usually L_1 or L_2
         • Permanently placed and usually used for long-term pain management
         • Inserted between vertebrae joints and passed through ligamentum flavum

4. Intrathecal
   a. Specifically designed catheter to deliver narcotics inside the spinal cord (intraspinal)
   b. Usually inserted between the lumbar vertebrae
5. Intraosseous
   a. Uses standard sterile hypodermic spinal, trephine, sternal, and standard bone marrow needles
      1) Needle with stylet preferred because stylet prevents bone marrow from occluding needle during placement
      2) Consideration given to use of a needle with a short shaft to avoid accidental dislodgment
      3) Consideration given to use of disposable needles specifically designed for intraosseous access
   b. Must be 16 to 18 gauge
6. Ventricular reservoir
   a. A receptacle attached to a catheter surgically placed in the lateral ventricle of the brain with the catheter threaded into the spinal space
   b. Access provided to the brain and/or the cerebrospinal fluid (CSF)
   c. Access obtained by penetrating the reservoir dome with a 25-gauge or smaller needle; CSF may be withdrawn or other fluid may be injected into the reservoir
   d. Gentle pumping of the reservoir distributes the medication into the CSF
   e. Strict aseptic technique is required when accessing the reservoir
   f. Advantages
      1) Allows immediate access to CSF and ventricles
      2) Eliminates repeated lumbar punctures
      3) Available for use with a wide range of drugs
      4) Permits better drug distribution
      5) Allows family to be taught use of system
   g. Disadvantages
      1) Infection is most common complication
      2) Sterile technique required for accessing
      3) Malfunction caused by clogging
      4) Possible misplacement as a result of slippage of catheter

VI. INFUSION DEVICES

A. Electronic Infusion Devices

1. Controller: electronically controlled device that delivers solutions with the aid of gravity
   a. Regulates flow rate by counting the drops and transmitting the rate to the device that controls the tubing pressure, increasing or decreasing the tubing diameter to deliver the rate set on the controller
   b. Has alarms that are activated when established flow rates are violated or when resistance is detected; useful for detecting infiltrations

    c. Requires solution container be placed approximately 36 inches above the intravenous site to overcome venous resistance and operate properly

    d. Reduces potential for "runaways" and empty bottles and for repeated venipunctures associated with gravity feed systems

    e. Maintains constant, accurate flow rate without pressure infusion

2. Positive-pressure infusion pump: infusion device that exerts pressure to overcome vascular resistance to administer medications and/or solutions

    a. PSI used to describe the measurement of pressure exerted

    b. Average pressure is 5 to 10 PSI

    c. Pumps with pressures greater than 10 to 12 PSI should be used with extreme caution

    d. Used to deliver high volumes, in high acuity situations, and with complex therapies

    e. With infusion resistance, the incidence of nuisance alarms is reduced

    f. Delivers accurately as programmed

    g. Features vary with pump

B. Mechanical Infusion Devices

1. Elastomere balloon: balloon safely encapsulated inside a rigid, transparent container that varies in shape and size

    a. Made of soft, rubberized material capable of being inflated to a predetermined volume, with a solution of relatively small volume and a specific infusion time

    b. Provides a tamper-proof port for injection of medication into the balloon, preventing accidental opening and contamination

    c. Provides an outlet port with preattached tubing or a hub to which kink-resistant tubing can be attached; tubing should be Luer-Lok with minimal priming volume

    d. Used primarily for the administration of antibiotics; can be used for the delivery of small-volume parenteral therapies

    e. Used for infusion home therapies

2. Spring-coil piston syringes: piston syringe powered by a spring-coil to deliver medication and/or solution

    a. Incapable of sensitivity to change or interference, such as increased resistance from infiltration

    b. Syringes may be prefilled and frozen depending on medication

3. Spring-coil container: uses a combination of a spring-coil and a collapsible, flattened disk to deliver medication

    a. May be a multi-use, small-volume administration device

    b. Used for home infusion therapy

C. Implantable Pumps

1. Surgically implanted, usually in the abdomen, to deliver medication continuously

2. Ideal for home use because it requires little care
3. Refills are necessary at specific intervals depending on the volume of the reservoir and on the rate of administration

D. Mechanisms of Delivery

1. Volumetric pump: calculates solution delivery by measuring the solution volume as it is displaced into a reservoir attached to the administration set
   a. Types of action
      1) Syringe: piston withdraws and pushes solution through tubing
      2) Linear peristaltic: peristaltic fingers compress tubing in a wavelike motion, pushing solution through tubing
      3) Filling and emptying of microreservoirs: filled and emptied in sequence and measured in hundredths of a milliliter
   b. Measures solution delivery to the nearest milliliter of the amount that is emptied out of the reservoir; measures to the nearest tenth of a milliliter with micropumps
2. Syringe pump: syringe driven by a piston to deliver solutions
   a. Rate set to deliver solution continuously, intermittently, or continuously and intermittently simultaneously
   b. For patient-controlled analgesia or intermittent medication delivery, such as antibiotics
   c. Delivery of minute amounts (as little as .01 ml/hour) of medications and/or solutions; ideal for use with infants and for maintaining patency of arterial lines
   d. Volume is limited to the size of the syringe used in the device, usually a 60 ml syringe, but can be as small as 5 ml
   e. Rate is controlled by the drive speed of the piston attached to the syringe plunger
3. Piston pump: piston action to control the flow of solution
   a. Usually requires a special dedicated administration set
   b. Allows rates to be set to deliver fluids continuously, intermittently, or continuously and intermittently simultaneously
   c. May operate by battery or electricity; compact and portable
4. Drop sensor: device used with an infusion device designed to count drops as they fall and thus calculate the volume of solution being administered
   a. Confirms the presence or absence of flow only
   b. Variation in the drop size may cause flow rate errors

E. Indications for Use

1. Critical drug dosing
   a. Antiarrhythmics
   b. Antihypertensives
   c. Bronchogenics
   d. Heparin (continuous)
   e. Insulin (continuous)
   f. Oxytocin

    g. Vasopressors

    h. Narcotics

2. Anesthetics

3. Arterial drug delivery

4. Electrolyte infusion

    a. Potassium chloride in 250 ml or less

    b. Magnesium sulfate solutions

5. Patients requiring severe fluid restriction

6. High-volume infusions

7. Administration of TPN solutions

8. Continuous antineoplastic therapy

9. Neonatal use and consideration in pediatric patients based on age, therapy, diagnosis, and condition

F. Features

1. Alarms: mechanisms designed to help prevent air emboli, circulatory overload, and occlusion by alerting the user to air-in-line, empty container, or an occlusion

    a. Other alarms may include machine malfunction, secondary medication infused, pressure limits met, door open, and low battery

    b. Alarm will continue to sound until condition is corrected appropriately; some alarms can be silenced while being corrected

2. Controls: buttons or pads that can be pressed to turn the power on, set parameters, lower alarm sound, set occlusion detection limits, and/or silence alarms

3. Electronic operation: operated by electricity or by an inner battery pack

    a. Usually large in size as a result of having an inner battery pack that allows battery time when pump is not plugged in

    b. Inner battery pack life is variable as to operation time and how battery is recharged; depends on pump used

    c. Most pumps have an alarm system to indicate when the battery is low and when the pump needs to be plugged in to electricity

4. Battery operated: operated by batteries that provide varied lengths of time depending on rate of infusion, type of battery used, and number of programs

    a. Various sizes and weights; usually of transistor radio size and weight

    b. Ideal for use with ambulatory patients and individuals receiving intravenous therapy outside the institutional setting

    c. Alarms alert user when batteries need to be replaced; appropriate battery replacement for operations necessary

    d. Use is increasing as a result of an increase in ambulatory services and outpatient services

5. Pressure considerations

    a. Pumps provide pressure to deliver programmed infusion rates

    b. Should not exceed the pressure of the filter in use as the filter may rupture, allowing all particulates and bacteria on the membrane to empty into the vascular system

c. Must be high enough to overcome the arterial pressure if being used on an arterial line

d. May allow variable pressure adjustments

G. Considerations

1. Vary as to the type of therapy being administered, patient age, needs, mobility, and setting in which device is used
2. Selection of device
   a. Safety features: prime consideration
      1) Audible alarms
      2) Appropriate grounding to prevent electrical hazards and interference from other electrical equipment
      3) Automatic anti-free flow when door is opened and/or administration set is removed
      4) Adequate features to minimize tampering
      5) Delivery rate within plus or minus 3 to 5% accuracy
   b. Type of therapy being administered
   c. Patient mobility
   d. Patient setting: in a homecare setting, the size, safety, cost, mobility, and type of venous access are critical when selecting a device
3. Selection of administration set
   a. Universal set: one that can be used with any infusion device
      1) Standard set that can be used with or without the device as a gravity system
      2) Ability to be primed with solution independent of infusion device
      3) Generally cheaper and use reflects a cost savings
      4) Free flow may not be prevented when removed from the device
   b. Device-specific: set that is designed to be used with a specific infusion device
      1) May or may not be primed and used independent of pump
      2) Usually more expensive because of design
      3) Usually provides feature that prevents free flow when set is removed from infusion device
4. Preventive maintenance
   a. Established in policies and procedures
   b. Frequency should comply with manufacturer's guidelines, those established by the Joint Commission on Accreditation of Healthcare Organizations (JCAHO), and those of the Association for the Advancement of Medical Instrumentation (AAMI)
5. Clinical considerations
   a. User knowledge includes but is not limited to indications for use, mechanical operation, troubleshooting, PSI rating, and safe use
   b. Controllers or nonpressure devices are considered the instruments of choice for administering vesicant medications

    c. Electronic infusion devices are recommended for use on all central lines

    d. Electronic infusion devices are considered an adjunct to nursing care and are not intended to alleviate responsibility for monitoring and ensuring the ordered flow rate

    e. Electronic infusion devices may be used to administer transfusion therapy

      1) Ensure that hemolysis does not occur

      2) Consult manufacturer's guidelines before transfusing RBCs with an infusion pump designed for use with crystalloid or colloid solutions

VII. BLOOD/FLUID EQUIPMENT

A. Blood/Fluid Warmer

1. Device that warms solutions or blood to body temperature
   a. Uses electronically heated plates or a warm water bath
   b. Heating blood under hot water faucets, in incubators, or in microwave ovens is not acceptable practice because of possible hemolysis of red blood cells
2. Indications for use
   a. Transfusion therapy
      1) Patients with potent cold agglutinins, unexpected antibodies that react at temperatures below 20°C
      2) Exchange transfusions in neonates and children
      3) Massive rapid transfusions produce a hypothermic effect, lowering the temperature of the sinoatrial node to below 30°C, at which point ventricular arrhythmias with cardiac arrest can occur
   b. Fluid therapy
      1) Patients with extensive hypothermia
      2) Rapid administration of refrigerated fluids
3. Blood warmer features
   a. Provides a constant temperature between 32 and 37°C
   b. Includes safety mechanisms such as thermostats and alarms for closely monitoring the blood temperature because overheating of blood/fluid may cause hemolysis (American Association of Blood Banks (AABB) states that blood warmers should not be used without an audible alarm that will sound before temperatures reach 42°C)

B. Blood Administration Pressure Cuff

1. Device used for increasing the flow rate of a transfusion
2. Uses a sleeve that fits snugly around a blood bag
3. Cuff is filled by a pressure manometer, causing blood to drip at a rapid rate
4. Use based on established policies and procedures

PART THREE EDUCATION OF PATIENT/SIGNIFICANT OTHER

I. PATIENT EDUCATION

A. Overview

1. Educating the patient and family or significant other is essential to administering the prescribed therapy
2. Patients and their support systems are more amiable to those delivering care and more likely to provide support for the prescribed therapy if they understand the who, what, when, and how of their therapy

B. Teaching Protocols

1. Vary depending on:
   a. Setting where patient receives therapy
   b. Ordered therapy
2. Role of patient and family
   a. Initiation of therapy
   b. Delivery of therapy
   c. Maintenance of therapy

II. EDUCATIONAL PROCESS

A. Assessment of the Learner

1. Assessment parameters
   a. Needs
   b. Level of comprehension
   c. Readiness and motivation to learn
   d. Maturation level and age
   e. Cultural, social, religious, and economical factors
2. Sources of information
   a. Interviews with patient, family, and other caregivers
   b. Review of patient's medical record
   c. Discussions with other healthcare team members involved in patient's care
   d. Patient observation
   e. Restatement of information by the patient
   f. Patient choice of instructional methods

B. Assessment of the Teacher

1. Energy level
2. Attitude
3. Knowledge
4. Skill

C. Development of a Teaching Plan

1. Foundation
   a. Individualized to meet the needs of the patient, with input from the patient

   b. Based on patient goals, objectives, and desired outcomes
      1) Written in behavioral terms
      2) Clear and concise
2. Identification of the learner
   a. Patient
   b. Family
   c. Other
3. Identification of the material to be covered
   a. Ordered therapy
   b. Rationale for therapy: why is it being administered?
   c. Benefits of therapy: what is the purpose, what will hopefully be accomplished by the therapy?
   d. Initiation and maintenance of therapy: role of caregiver, patient, and support personnel
   e. Infusion system: cannula, administration set(s), and infusion device
   f. Side effects of therapy: prevention, intervention, and treatment
4. Determination of material sequence
5. Selection of teaching methods
   a. Verbal instructions
   b. Audiovisuals
   c. Written instructions
   d. Demonstration
   e. Return demonstration
6. Environmental considerations: environment that promotes learning
   a. Seating
   b. Visibility
   c. Temperature
   d. Limited number of persons in attendance
   e. Adequate audiovisuals
   f. Adequate space for supplies and equipment
   g. Limited distractions from television, radio, and others

D. Implementation

1. Establish a rapport to reduce anxiety and fear
2. Incorporate a variety of teaching methods to reinforce concepts
3. Use language the learner can understand
4. Present information in small parts grouped together
   a. Promotes learning
   b. Prevents learner overload
5. Present the most important information first
6. Ask questions frequently and encourage feedback to ensure comprehension
7. Offer verbal praise to reward learning
8. Express concern for the patient through voice and body language
9. Adjust learning goals as necessary
10. Frequently summarize teaching

III. EVALUATION

A. Ongoing

1. Throughout implementation
2. At completion of each teaching session
3. Areas to address
   a. Discussions of information learned
   b. Responses of learner
   c. Return demonstrations
   d. Written evaluations
   e. Observations relative to compliance and lifestyle changes

B. Patient Outcomes (identified as indicators for measuring patient/learner education)

1. Verbalization of understanding of instructions and provided information
2. Return demonstration of learned procedures
3. Improved adherence to the therapeutic regimen
4. Increased patient satisfaction
5. Enhanced patient recovery

C. Revisions in Teaching Plan (as necessary based on evaluations)

IV. DOCUMENTATION

A. Patient's Ongoing Medical Record (as established in agency protocol)

1. Narrative form
2. Checklist

B. Criteria

1. Assessment of patient/learner knowledge deficit and readiness to learn
2. Learning objectives
3. Implementation of teaching plan
4. Patient/learner skills demonstrated
5. Patient and/or learner response to teaching
6. Evaluation of overall teaching process
7. Patient outcomes

PART FOUR INITIATION OF INTRAVENOUS THERAPY

I. INITIATION OF THERAPY

A. Indications (for therapeutic and/or diagnostic purposes)

1. Maintain or replace body stores of water, electrolytes, vitamins, proteins, calories, and/or nitrogen in the patient who cannot maintain an adequate intake by mouth

2. Restore acid-base balance
3. Replenish blood volume and/or administer blood components
4. Administer continuous or intermittent medications
5. Administer intravenous anesthetics
6. Administer diagnostic reagents
7. Monitor hemodynamic function
8. Maintain patent vascular access in case of an emergency
9. Assist in pain management

B. Physician's Order (necessary to initiate intravenous therapy)

1. Verification of information
   a. Solution: type, volume, rate, and medications including dosage and route (must be specified; cannot assume intravenous administration)
   b. Medications: type, dosage, rate, frequency, and route
2. Clarification of information: legible, complete, clear, and appropriate for patient
3. Compatibility of medications/solutions: compatibility of all medications with primary and secondary solutions must be verified before administration

II. PATIENT ASSESSMENT

A. Patient's History (to determine past conditions that might result in an adverse effect on the patient and/or the ordered therapy)

1. Diagnosis, primary as well as secondary
2. Conditions that may be affected by ordered therapy
3. Previous side effects of therapy and/or allergic conditions
4. Previous problems associated with fluid and electrolyte imbalances
5. Transfusion history, if transfusion ordered
6. History of coagulation problems
7. History of respiratory problems

B. Laboratory Data (to determine patient's present clinical status and provide a baseline for monitoring reactions and responses to therapy)

1. Renal function
   a. Blood urea nitrogen (BUN)
   b. Serum creatinine
   c. BUN:creatinine ratio
   d. Serum osmolality (also indicates electrolyte levels)
   e. Urine specific gravity
   f. Urine osmolality
2. Electrolyte levels
   a. Sodium
   b. Potassium
   c. Calcium
   d. Magnesium

  e. Chloride

  f. Phosphorus

3. Hemoconcentration and hemodilution

  a. Complete blood count

  b. Evaluation of total leukocytes, myelocytes, band neutrophils (bands), segmented neutrophils (segs), lymphocytes, monocytes, eosinophils, and basophils

4. Coagulation problems

  a. Platelet level

  b. Clotting time

  c. Prothrombin time

  d. Partial thromboplastin time

  e. Plasma thrombin time

5. Respiratory status, if necessary, by drawing arterial blood gases (ABGs)

  a. pH

  b. $PaCO_2$

  c. PaO_2

  d. Bicarbonate

  e. Base excess

C. Physical Assessment (to determine patient's present clinical status and provide a baseline for monitoring reactions and responses to therapy)

1. Vital signs

  a. Temperature: changes in body temperature can indicate an infectious process or a fluid and electrolyte imbalance

    1) Dehydration: associated with elevated body temperature, a fluid-volume deficit complicated by infection (probably resulting from decreased metabolism)

    2) Elevated body temperature: possible fluid imbalance if extra fluids not supplied as indicated

      • Elevation of 101 to 103°F increases 24-hour fluid requirements by at least 500 ml

      • Elevation above 103°F increases 24-hour fluid requirements by at least 1000 ml

  b. Pulse rate

    1) Weak, low-volume pulse: indicates fluid-volume deficit

    2) Bounding full-volume pulse: indicates fluid-volume excess

    3) Irregular pulse rate: associated with potassium imbalances and magnesium deficits

  c. Respirations

    1) Deep, rapid respirations: may be a compensatory mechanism for metabolic acidosis or may indicate a primary disorder causing respiratory alkalosis

    2) Slow, shallow respirations: may be a compensatory mechanism for

metabolic alkalosis or may indicate a primary disorder causing respiratory acidosis

    3) Moist rales in absence of cardiopulmonary disease: indicate fluid-volume excess

  d. Blood pressure

    1) Postural hypotension (fall in systolic pressure exceeding 10 mm Hg from lying to standing): can indicate fluid-volume deficit or magnesium excess

    2) Hypertension: can occur with fluid-volume excess and with magnesium deficit

2. Intake and output

  a. Comparison of measurements and determination of kidney function

    1) Intake: all fluids (intravenous, oral, and tube feedings)

    2) Output: urine, vomitus, diarrhea, and drainage from suction apparatus; drainage from wounds, lesions, or ulcers (estimate volume); important to note fluid loss through perspiration and prolonged hyperventilation

  b. Important to note the time of day and the type of fluid loss and gain

  c. Normal urinary output

    1) 1 ml/kg of body weight per hour

    2) Adult patient: usually 1500 ml/24 hr or 40 to 80 ml/hour

3. Skin turgor (skin elasticity)

  a. Best measured by pinching skin over sternum or forehead

  b. Abdominal area or medial aspects of the thighs are preferred by some when testing turgor in children

  c. Normal person: pinched skin immediately falls back to its normal position when released

  d. Fluid-volume deficit: pinched skin remains slightly elevated for many seconds

  e. Children: turgor diminishes after 3 to 5% of body weight is lost

  f. Infants: poor turgor can be caused by severe malnutrition without fluid depletion; can be deceptive in obese infants and lead to failure to recognize a fluid-volume deficit

  g. Older adults (55 years of age and older): reduced turgor common as a result of decrease in skin elasticity; skin on sternum and inner aspects of thighs best for determining turgor

4. Tongue turgor

  a. Normal person: one longitudinal furrow on the tongue

  b. Fluid-volume deficit: smaller tongue with additional longitudinal furrows

  c. Sodium excess: the tongue is red and swollen

5. Moisture in oral cavity

  a. Fluid-volume deficit: dry mouth, if not related to mouth breathing

  b. True fluid-volume deficit: dryness in the area where the cheek meets the gum (this area is normally moist from mouth breathing)

   c. Sodium excess: dry, sticky mucous membranes; oral cavity feels like "fly paper"
6. Thirst
   a. Subjective sensory symptom
   b. Prominent in patients with increased water loss, as in hyperglycemia, high fever, or diarrhea
7. Tearing and salivation
   a. Absence is a sign of fluid-volume deficit in a child; obvious with 5% or greater loss in the total body weight
   b. Absence may be a symptom of other problems within the adult and older population, not relative to infusion therapy
8. Appearance of skin
   a. Metabolic acidosis: warm, flushed skin as a result of peripheral vasodilation
   b. Severe fluid-volume deficit: skin pale and cool because of peripheral vasoconstriction
9. Facial appearance
   a. Drawn facial expression can indicate a fluid-volume deficit
   b. Sunken eyes indicate a fluid-volume deficit
10. Edema
   a. Presence of excessive interstitial fluid (fluid between the cells) resulting from the increase in total body sodium content
      1) Pitting edema: manifested by a small depression that remains after pressing a finger into an edematous area and then removing
      2) Dependent edema: refers to flow of excess fluid by gravity to most dependent portions of body (feet and ankles, if standing; back and buttocks, if lying)
   b. Usually not apparent in the adult until 5 to 10 pounds of excess fluid have been retained
11. Body weight
   a. Possible indication of fluid balance problems if the baseline weight is taken before initiating therapy
   b. Rapid loss indications
      1) 2% of total body weight: indicates mild fluid-volume deficit
      2) 5% of total body weight: indicates moderate deficit
      3) 8% of total body weight: indicates severe deficit
   c. Rapid gain or loss of 1 kg (2.2 lb): equivalent to the gain or loss of 1 liter of fluid
12. Neck veins
   a. Distended neck veins: indicate elevated venous pressure with the possibility of fluid-volume overload
   b. Flat neck veins: can indicate decreased plasma volume

D. Psychological Assessment
1. Assess patient's ability to comprehend and understand therapy
2. Assess patient's ability to maintain therapy

E. Assessment of Appropriateness of Therapy

1. Ordered therapy evaluated in relation to the patient's history, lab values, clinical findings, and psychological assessment
2. Initiation of therapy is delayed and the physician notified if therapy appears inappropriate based on nursing assessment; nurses are not protected from liability for implementing orders when they know the orders are inappropriate

III. PATIENT PREPARATION

A. Explanation of Procedure

1. Patient response directly affected by the nurse's approach
   a. Undesirable response possible in which the patient refuses therapy
   b. Reassurance and support are helpful in overcoming fears
   c. Patient has the right to refuse therapy; therapy is not initiated if the patient refuses and is of sound mind
2. Preconceived ideas
   a. Rumors
   b. Association with critical illness and/or death
3. Vasovagal reactions
   a. Triggering of associated autonomic nervous system responses by an exaggerated response to fear
   b. Syncope is a possible manifestation
   c. Sympathetic reaction is possible following syncope, resulting in vasoconstriction with peripheral collapse, limiting vein availability
   d. Prevention is possible if the nurse appears confident and reassures the patient
   e. Patient instruction to lessen extreme anxiety
      1) Inhale and exhale slowly
      2) Avoid looking at the site and initiation of therapy
      3) Focus on a pleasant image or past experience
4. Repeated venipunctures
   a. Increase patient frustration
   b. Possible causative factor in patients who refuse therapy
   c. Insertion only by those persons experienced in venipuncture technique reduces multiple attempts

B. Identification of Patient

1. An essential requirement before the administration of ordered therapy to the appropriate patient
2. Confirmed by following established procedures
   a. Call the patient by name and ask him/her to respond, if able
   b. Check the patient identification bracelet
   c. Check with another person who knows the patient
   d. Confirm a patient's identity with another nurse/significant other if the patient cannot respond or if the identification bracelet is absent

IV. SITE SELECTION

A. General Principles

1. Choose most appropriate vascular delivery access site for the prescribed therapy
2. Determine risk of complications before initiating therapy

B. Assessment Relative to Therapy

1. Patient's condition, age, and diagnosis
   a. Skin condition and its ability to support a cannula
      1) Skin in an elderly patient may be too thin to support a peripheral cannula
      2) Cannula should not be placed in areas where lesions, cellulitis, or weeping tissues are located
   b. Potential for bleeding disorders
      1) Patients with bleeding disorders may bleed around cannula entry site
      2) Tourniquet use may cause excessive bleeding into interstitial tissues
   c. Patients with a diagnosis of mastectomy and/or axillary dissection
      1) Veins within involved extremities are avoided, if possible
      2) Veins are used only after assessing patient for lymphedema, determining length of time since surgery, and obtaining an order for use from the physician
2. Condition, size, and location of vessel
   a. Peripheral therapy through a peripheral vein
      1) Vein should be palpated to determine condition and size
      2) Avoid injured or sclerosed veins
      3) Avoid areas of flexion unless no other access available
         • Extremity should be immobilized using appropriate protocols if a vein is used in an area of flexion
         • Veins in the antecubital fossa should be reserved for peripherally inserted central catheter (PICC) and for drawing blood samples
      4) Veins in lower extremities of the adult patient should be avoided
         • Small veins in the lower extremities communicate with multiple venous networks and are located distal to the heart, predisposing the vessels to congestion of blood with pooling and subsequent inflammation leading to the formation of emboli and thrombophlebitis
         • Site is changed as soon as an appropriate site can be established if it is absolutely necessary to use the veins of the lower extremities
         • Policies and procedures should dictate the use of veins within the lower extremities
      5) Site selection should be routinely initiated in the distal areas of the upper extremities with subsequent cannulations made proximal to the previous cannulated site
         • Cannulation should not be performed in the involved extremity if unable to place the cannula proximal to the previous site

- Assurance that bifurcations or articulations do not exist between two veins with the possibility of subsequent infiltration/extravasation can only be made by fluoroscopy
- Use of the opposite extremity is advisable after the infiltration of a vesicant
- Execution of an extravasation protocol does not ensure future viability of veins
- Protocol executed only to neutralize the vesicant and to prevent further damage to tissues

    6) Vein chosen to accommodate the cannula gauge and length required to deliver the prescribed therapy

    7) Appropriate veins for use include metacarpal, cephalic, basilic, and median veins

b. Central therapy through a peripheral vein

    1) Antecubital fossa usual site for insertion

    2) Cephalic and basilic veins most appropriate for use

    3) Veins differentiated from arteries by palpation

    4) Injured or sclerosed veins avoided

    5) Vein should accommodate gauge of catheter

    6) Anatomical measurements taken to determine catheter length required to ensure full advancement of catheter with tip in superior vena cava

    7) Avoid veins in the arm of a patient who has undergone a mastectomy and/or axillary dissection, if possible

c. Central therapy through a central vein

    1) Medical act requiring insertion by a physician

    2) Internal jugular and subclavian veins most appropriate for use; catheter tip located in the superior vena cava

    3) Femoral vein may be used; catheter tip located in inferior vena cava

d. Arterial therapy through an artery

    1) Pulse presence should be palpated before performing an arterial puncture

    2) Radial artery most commonly used and considered site of choice

    3) Brachial and femoral arteries also appropriate

    4) Extremity assessed for circulation distal to site; Allen's test used to determine circulation if brachial or radial arteries used

3. Type and duration of therapy

  a. Peripheral therapy through a peripheral vein

    1) Short-term intravenous therapy that can be maintained by the peripheral route

    2) Intravenous administration of medications and solutions

    3) Consideration given to arteriovenous (AV) fistulas or grafts before using intravenous therapy; may be indicated for dialysis use only

  b. Central therapy through a peripheral vein

    1) Used in hospital and alternate-care settings to provide intravenous therapy for a term shorter than 2 to 3 months and longer than 2 weeks

2) Short-term therapy when venous access is poor or when cephalic or basilic veins at antecubital fossa provide the only access
3) Provides central route with peripheral insertion, allowing insertion by a registered nurse as determined by state Nurse Practice Act
    c. Central therapy through a central vein
1) Provides a route for therapies that must be administered into a central vein
2) Allows for continuous or intermittent use for an indefinite period of time depending on type of catheter used (percutaneously inserted, tunneled, or implanted)
    d. Therapy through an artery
1) Hemodynamic monitoring and drawing arterial samples such as ABGs
2) Prohibition of medication administration because of possible arterial spasm closing off the blood supply to the involved extremity
3) 0.9% sodium chloride is the preferred solution for arterial pressure monitoring

V. CANNULA SELECTION
A. General Principles
1. Provide the most appropriate vascular access device that will deliver the prescribed therapy
2. Minimize potential complications associated with infusion therapy

B. Length of Therapy
1. Stainless steel needles limited to short-term (less than 8 hours), single-dose administration, and drawing of ABGs
2. Peripheral catheters used for intravenous therapy of less than 4 weeks
3. Subclavian single- and multilumen catheters used for intravenous therapy of less than 60 days; used most frequently in hospital settings because of an increased risk of infection
4. Right atrial catheters, central venous catheters with a three-position valve and closed distal tip and implanted ports used to maintain therapy for 1 to 2 years

C. Type of Therapy
1. Peripheral cannulas (used for most intravenous therapies)
    a. Smallest gauge and shortest length catheter that will accommodate the prescribed therapy: used to decrease patient discomfort (infused solution and/or medication is hemodiluted, decreasing venous irritation and subsequent vein inflammation)
    b. Larger cannula is used in delivering viscous solutions and/or medications as smaller gauge results in decreased rates
2. Central venous catheters

a. Critically ill patients

b. Administration of all types of intravenous therapy

   1) Chemotherapy

   2) Parenteral nutrition

   3) Antimicrobial agents

   4) Blood component therapy

c. Blood sampling

3. Arterial cannulas

a. Continuous hemodynamic pressure monitoring and for frequent drawing of ABGs

b. Use of steel needles (frequently) to draw ABGs

D. Venous Accessibility

1. Causes of limited venous access

a. Previous therapy resulting in injured or sclerosed veins

b. Use of veins for AV fistulas or grafts

c. Prolonged therapy without allowing sufficient venous healing time

d. Injury, amputation, cellulitis, open draining wound, surgery, or burns of extremity

e. Mastectomy and/or total axillary dissection

f. Superior vena cava syndrome

2. Considerations for clotting disorders

a. Patients with hemophilia and other clotting disorders frequently bleed at the catheter insertion site

b. Placement of a central catheter decreases the risk of bleeding from catheter site changes

c. Low platelet counts may preclude placement of a PICC

VI. CANNULA SITE PREPARATION

A. Requirements

1. Prepare site aseptically

2. Reduce the potential for microorganisms to enter the vascular system

B. Peripheral Catheter Through a Peripheral Vein

1. Before site preparation

a. Hands should be washed

b. Gloves should be worn to perform venipuncture

c. Protective equipment (goggles and gown) should be worn if splash is anticipated

2. Site preparation

a. Excess hair is removed by clipping; shaving is not recommended because of potential for causing microabrasions

b. If skin is unusually dirty, site should be cleansed with soap and water before applying an antimicrobial solution

  c. An approved antimicrobial solution should be used to prepare the cannula site; approved antimicrobials include tincture of iodine 2%, 10% povidone-iodine, 70% isopropyl alcohol, and chlorhexidine
   1) If patient is allergic to iodine, chlorhexidine or 70% isopropyl alcohol should be used to cleanse the site; should be applied with friction for at least 30 seconds or until final application is visually clean
   2) Single-unit-use antimicrobial should be considered for use
  d. Solution should be applied in a circular motion starting at the intended site and working outward
   1) Surface area for prepping is dependent on size of extremity
   2) Area of 2 to 3 inches in diameter is usually cleansed in the adult patient
  e. Excess solution at the site is not blotted; solution is allowed to completely air dry
  f. Povidone-iodine is not removed with 70% isopropyl alcohol because alcohol has the ability to negate the effect of the iodine

C. PICCs (usually require surgical preparation, particularly if catheter is not enclosed in a sterile protective cover)

 1. Before catheter insertion
  a. Hands should be washed, completing a 5-minute scrub from hands to elbows using an iodine-based or chlorhexidine solution
  b. Mask, cap, sterile gown, and gloves should be donned before prepping the patient
  c. Talc-containing gloves should be rinsed with sterile water after donning to avoid powder adherence; gloves should be changed after preparation and draping
  d. Consideration should be given to wearing goggles
  e. Patient should be positioned with the head to the opposite side
 2. Site preparation
  a. Site should be cleansed with an iodine-based solution applied in a circular motion starting at the intended site and working outward
  b. Sterile drapes and towels should be applied

D. Percutaneously Inserted Central Lines

 1. Before catheter insertion
  a. Patient should be placed in the Trendelenburg position (head lower than the feet) or supine to facilitate venous distention and to decrease risk of potential complications during insertion
  b. Surgical scrub should be performed
  c. Mask, sterile gloves, and gown should be worn
  d. Site should be draped with sterile towels
 2. Site preparation for central catheters surgically placed is in accordance with operating room policies and procedures

VII. CANNULA PLACEMENT

A. Considerations

1. Most appropriate cannula is used
2. Most appropriate vein for delivery is selected

B. Peripheral (insertion of cannula into either a peripheral vein or an artery)

1. Place for a definite therapeutic and/or diagnostic indication
2. Place using aseptic technique
   a. Cannula should be considered contaminated if aseptic technique is compromised, as in an emergency situation
   b. Cannula should be removed and replaced as soon as the patient stabilizes, within 24 hours
3. Maximum number of attempts at venipuncture in non-life-threatening situations is two
4. Cannula is inspected for product integrity before use and discarded if defective or if product integrity is compromised
5. Stylets, needles, and/or guidewires are used with caution
   a. Stylets should never be reinserted into a catheter or a catheter withdrawn through a needle because of the potential for severing and/or puncturing the catheter
6. Only one cannula should be used for each cannulation attempt
7. Adherence to Standard Precautions
   a. Gloves should be worn when performing venipunctures
   b. Impervious gowns and goggles should be worn if splashing of blood is suspected
   c. Needles, stylets, and guidewires should be discarded after use into a needle container that meets Occupational Safety and Health Administration (OSHA) guidelines
8. Use of a tourniquet
   a. Need for a tourniquet should be assessed
      1) May not need a tourniquet on certain patients with large veins
      2) May cause bleeding into tissues of certain patients, preventing venipuncture, such as in the elderly patient with poor skin turgor or the patient with a clotting disorder
   b. Should be applied 4 to 6 inches above the site to impede venous but not arterial flow
   c. Discard or disinfect after each procedure because of the potential for cross contamination; consider using disposable tourniquets
   d. Tourniquets used in isolation rooms are left in the room and discarded after the patient is removed from isolation
9. Alternative vein dilation techniques are evaluated to provide the most appropriate technique for the patient
   a. Opening and closing of the fist forces blood into veins, causing veins to distend

  b. Lightly tapping vein helps to dilate the vessel
  c. Holding the extremity in a dependent position below the level of the heart increases the blood supply within the veins
  d. Heat application causes vasodilation
     1) Apply to the entire extremity for 10 to 20 minutes
     2) Maintain until venipuncture performed
10. Venipuncture techniques
  a. Direct or one-step method
     1) Thrust cannula through the skin and directly into the vein with one quick motion
     2) Excellent for use with large veins
     3) Possible formation of hematoma if used in small veins
  b. Indirect method
     1) Two complete motions
     2) Insertion of cannula through the skin below point where vein is visible and relocation of vein with entry into vein
  c. Bevel-up technique
     1) Insertion of cannula with bevel facing up
     2) Produces less trauma to skin and vein
  d. Bevel-down technique
     1) Insertion of cannula with bevel down, facing site
     2) Often necessary in small veins to prevent extravasation
     3) Any readjustments of the cannula are made before releasing the tourniquet to prevent puncturing the vein and producing a hematoma

C. PICC

1. Inserted into a peripheral vessel and threaded into the superior vena cava
2. Inserted when a definite therapeutic indication exists
3. Use aseptic technique; mask, cap, sterile gloves, and gown are worn during insertion, with consideration given to wearing goggles
4. Catheter is not withdrawn through the needle during placement because of the potential for shearing of the catheter
5. Catheter tip placement is confirmed before initiating therapy

D. Central Insertion

1. Placement is a medical act
2. Nurse's role in assisting the physician should be established in policies and procedures and includes but is not limited to:
  a. Assessment of product integrity
  b. Awareness of the insertion procedure using aseptic technique
  c. Position the patient in the Trendelenburg position or supine with a towel roll placed along the spine between the clavicles to ease insertion, increase venous distention, and reduce potential for complications

   d. Instruct patient to use Valsalva maneuver to reduce the risk of an air embolism
3. Sterile gloves, mask, and gown should be used for the insertion
4. Catheter tip placement should be confirmed before initiating therapy
   a. Appropriate catheter tip location through the subclavian vein is in the superior vena cava
   b. Appropriate catheter tip location through the femoral vein is in the inferior vena cava

VIII. FOLLOW-UP

A. Dressing

1. Aseptic application is followed to minimize the potential for microorganisms to breed under the dressing
2. Sterile gauze dressing
   a. Use should be established in policies and procedures
   b. All edges should be secured with tape
   c. Use of roller bandages is not recommended because of the potential for impaired circulation
3. Transparent semipermeable membrane (TSM)
   a. Use should be established in policies and procedures
   b. Dressing is applied according to manufacturer's recommendations
   c. Tape over the TSM dressing may compromise dressing properties and interfere with visual inspection of the skin-cannula junction site

B. Labeling

1. Site
   a. Includes date of insertion, gauge and length of cannula, and initials of the professional inserting the cannula
   b. Provides a quick reference of the device gauge in an emergency situation and promotes change of device as established in agency policies and procedures
2. Tubing
   a. Placed on tubing below drip chamber
   b. Provides a quick reference of the date the tubing was hung and/or the date the tubing must be changed

C. Documentation

1. Date and time therapy is initiated
2. Type and amount of solution
3. Additives and dosages
4. Flow rate
5. Gauge, length, and type of venipuncture device or catheter used
6. Insertion site
7. Patient's response to the procedure

8. Any problems or difficulties encountered with the procedure
9. Name and title of the professional inserting the cannula
10. Name and title of the professional making an entry in the medical record if different from the professional inserting the cannula (such as cannula inserted by a physician)

PART FIVE ROUTINE CARE AND MAINTENANCE

I. PATIENT CARE

A. Assessment

1. Use of the nursing process to monitor patient, therapy, and system used to deliver therapy
2. Ongoing process designed to achieve desired patient outcomes and determine appropriateness of therapy
   a. Observation of patient's current status
   b. Observation of response
      1) Effectiveness of therapy
      2) Signs and symptoms of adverse reactions
   c. Monitoring
      1) Patient need for and response to therapy
      2) Appropriateness of therapy
      3) Infusion system including cannula site, flow rate, and appropriateness of system
      4) Frequency should be established in policies and procedures

B. Diagnosis

1. Evaluation of data from assessment
2. Determination of interventions
3. Possible changes due to a change in patient's clinical condition

C. Outcome Identification

1. Identifies expected outcome of therapy
2. May relate to patient diagnosis or to intervention diagnosis, such as outcome related to treatment of an infiltration

D. Plan of Care

1. Establish interventions to attain expected outcomes
   a. Individualized to patient's needs
   b. Establish within 24 hours of initial nursing assessment or immediately if intervention is necessary because of an identified complication
2. Revise as patient's clinical status changes
3. Should reflect both long-term and short-term planning
4. Develop with patient, significant others, and healthcare providers when appropriate, such as for home intravenous care

E. Implementation

1. Implement interventions as identified in the care plan
2. Change as the plan of care changes
3. Document in the patient's medical record

F. Evaluation

1. Patient's progress toward attainment of identified outcomes
2. Reflection on appropriateness of the care plan

II. CANNULA SITE CARE

A. Site Inspection

1. Observe and evaluate skin-cannula junction, surrounding tissues, and dressing
2. Assess site and surrounding area for signs of local complications
   a. Local complications appear at or near the infusion site
      1) Infiltration
      2) Extravasation
      3) Phlebitis
      4) Ecchymosis
      5) Hematoma
      6) Thrombosis
      7) Thrombophlebitis
      8) Fragmented/broken cannula
      9) Occluded cannula
   b. Should be observed for visual signs/symptoms and palpated for swelling, warmth, tenderness, and drainage
3. Assess dressing for dryness and occlusiveness
4. Frequency of inspection is determined by type of infusion therapy, patient condition and age, and practice setting
   a. Adult patient
      1) Site should be inspected in hospital setting every 2 to 4 hours as established in policies and procedures
      2) Site should be inspected by patient and/or significant other in home-care setting every 2 to 4 hours or more frequently as trained by home-care nurse
   b. Pediatric patient
      1) Site should be inspected in hospital setting every 1 to 2 hours or more frequently as established in policies and procedures
      2) Site should be inspected by parent or significant other in homecare setting every 1 to 2 hours or more frequently as trained by homecare nurse

B. Cannula Site Care

1. Observe and evaluate skin-cannula junction and surrounding tissue
   a. Defined as aseptically cleansing the skin-cannula junction with an approved antimicrobial solution and applying a sterile dressing

b. Coincides with a change in dressing
2. Is a measure to control infection
3. Because application of an antimicrobial ointment is controversial, its use should be defined in organizational policies and procedures

III. DRESSING CHANGE

A. Gauze

1. Change in accordance with the *Intravenous Nursing Standards of Practice*
2. Considerations
   a. Sterile gloves and mask should be worn when changing the dressing at a central venous catheter site
   b. An occlusive dressing is maintained using an adhesive material to cover the entire dressing
   c. Gauze dressing covered with a transparent semipermeable membrane (TSM) dressing should be considered and treated as a gauze dressing

B. Transparent Semipermeable Membrane Dressing

1. Change in accordance with the *Intravenous Nursing Standards of Practice*
2. Considerations
   a. Sterile gloves and mask should be worn when changing the dressing at a central venous catheter site
   b. Tape is not applied over TSM dressing because it could compromise the dressing properties
   c. Change in accordance with the manufacturer's guidelines

IV. ADMINISTRATION SETS

A. Primary Administration Sets

1. Product integrity is checked before use
2. Peripheral and central primary sets should be changed in accordance with the *Intravenous Nursing Standards of Practice*
3. Change at the time the peripheral cannula is changed or at the time a new solution container is initiated
4. Sets used with central venous catheters should be changed in coordination with the initiation of a new solution container

B. Sets Used to Administer TPN Solutions

1. Change in accordance with the *Intravenous Nursing Standards of Practice*
2. Change at the time of bag changes
3. Filters and add-on devices are changed at the time the administration set is changed

C. Sets Used to Administer Fat Emulsions

1. Check fat emulsions for separation of oil before spiking with a set; pharmacy is consulted if oil is present
2. Discard after each unit unless additional units are administered consecutively, immediately if contamination is suspected or product integrity is compromised
3. Change every 24 hours if additional units are administered consecutively

D. Secondary Administration Sets

1. Product integrity is checked before use
2. Secondary sets are changed on both peripheral and central lines in accordance with the *Intravenous Nursing Standards of Practice*
3. Change coincides with primary administration set change and initiation of a new solution container

E. Intermittent Therapy Sets

1. Product integrity is checked before use
2. Intermittent sets are changed in accordance with the *Intravenous Nursing Standards of Practice*
3. Needles attached to these sets are removed immediately after use, and a new sterile needle is applied
4. Consideration is given to the use of recessed needles, plastic cannulas, or other needleless systems to prevent accidental needlestick injuries; these devices are changed when the set to which they are attached is changed

F. Blood/Blood Component Sets

1. Type used is dependent on the component being administered and organizational policies and procedures
2. Change after each unit or at the end of 4 hours, whichever comes first, and immediately if contamination is suspected or product integrity is compromised

G. Hemodynamic and Arterial Pressure Monitoring Sets

1. Administration set, dome, and pressure tubing are included
2. Change in accordance with the *Intravenous Nursing Standards of Practice*
3. Change at the same time a new solution container is initiated

H. Add-on Sets

1. Stopcocks, extension sets, manifold sets, extension loops, and any other device added to the administration set are included
2. Use only when there is a definite need and when not provided as an integral part of the administration set

3. Change coincides with the change of the set to which it is attached, and immediately if contamination is suspected or product integrity is compromised

I. Latex Injection Ports

1. Disinfect before use with an antimicrobial solution such as tincture of iodine 2%, 10% povidone-iodine, 70% isopropyl alcohol, or chlorhexidine
2. Access using a 25- to 21-gauge needle that does not exceed 1 inch in length
   a. Smaller needles have the potential for breaking and entering the system
   b. Larger needles penetrate the port and may cause leaking of the port
3. Check for integrity before each use
4. Change depending on the site and if removable latex injection caps are used
   a. Peripheral lines: change when cannula is changed, and immediately if contamination is suspected or product integrity is compromised
   b. Central lines: change in accordance with the *Intravenous Nursing Standards of Practice*
   c. Discard when removed from the system; do not reuse
   d. Only Luer-Lok caps are used

V. SOLUTION CONTAINER

A. Pre-Use Inspection

1. Squeeze to detect leaks
2. Hold bottles in the light and rotate to detect cracks
3. Check expiration date

B. Frequency of Change

1. Bags and bottles should be changed in accordance with the *Intravenous Nursing Standards of Practice*
2. Change more frequently if contamination is suspected or product integrity is compromised
3. Discard before 24 hours if removed from the system

VI. DOCUMENTATION

A. Date and Time

B. Observations

1. Objective: those visualized or palpated, including complications
2. Subjective: those stated by the patient/family
3. Cardinal: diagnostic studies relative to therapy, such as laboratory work

C. Procedures Performed

D. Flow Rate

E. Interventions (such as changes in prescribed therapy if indicated)

F. Patient Response to Therapy and Procedure(s)

G. Name and Title of Professional Performing the Procedure(s)

I. COMPLICATIONS

A. Overview

1. Potential for complications is always present
2. Are not always preventable
3. With frequent monitoring and appropriate interventions, the severity can be diminished

B. Effects of Complications

1. Increase length of hospital stay and/or length of therapy
2. Increase nursing responsibilities
3. Can be painful to the patient
4. Place the patient at risk for other medical problems
5. Increase the costs associated with care and treatment

II. LOCAL COMPLICATIONS

A. Overview

1. Usually seen at or near the site as a result of trauma to the vessel wall or as a result of mechanical failure
2. May be easily corrected
3. Usually associated with no serious problems when appropriate interventions are initiated
4. Serious complications are possible if left untreated or unrecognized

B. Mechanical Complications

1. Intravenous system fails to adequately deliver therapy at the prescribed rate
2. Treatment consists of identifying and correcting the problem
3. Frequent observation can lead to early recognition and correction of a potential problem
   a. Site: check for swelling above, over, and below insertion site to rule out site-related problems, such as infiltration/extravasation
   b. Cannula: observe in relation to fluid flow
      1) Cannula against vessel wall: causes fluid flow to decrease or stop
         • Pulling back slightly on cannula can eliminate problem

- Taping cannula to prevent movement of cannula within vessel may prevent problems
2) Kinked or bent cannula: causes fluid flow to decrease or stop
   - Remove cannula to prevent possible cannula breakage and subsequent catheter embolus
   - Appropriate taping helps to prevent bending or kinking of cannula
3) Cannula in flexion area: may cause fluid flow rate to increase or decrease as a result of movement of the involved extremity
   - Flexion and extension of extremity after insertion of cannula can aid in detection of a positional cannula (fluid flow increases and decreases with flexion and extension)
   - Repositioning extremity and applying an arm board according to organization immobilization protocol helps to prevent changes in flow rate
   - Avoid cannula sites in areas of flexion
4) Defective cannula: may leak at the hub-cannula junction, creating a wet dressing, or cannula may be obstructed as a result of the manufacturing process
   - Remove cannula; save cannula along with the package; manufacturer should be notified
   - Some manufacturers require the cannula be returned so they can check for defects; others require only the lot number be saved
   - Lot number should be noted and cannula placed in a puncture-resistant container that meets the standards of the Occupational Safety and Health Administration (OSHA)
c. Solution container: check for appropriate volume
   1) Empty container: solution cannot flow from an empty container
      - Hanging a full container easily corrects problem
      - Time-taping solution containers is helpful in noting when a container should be empty
   2) Lack of adequate gravity flow: maintain solutions at a level to promote optimal flow
      - Hang solution at least 30 inches above level of heart for adequate gravity flow
      - Solutions hanging less than 30 inches below this level will not flow well; flow may cease, creating an occluded cannula
      - Increase the height of viscous solutions to obtain adequate flow rates as necessary
   3) Air vent: some solution containers (most bottles) require air for adequate flow
      - Vented administration set or vented adapter allows exchange of air and fluid, permitting solution flow
      - Bags do not require venting because they collapse as solution flows from bag
      - Needles are inappropriate to use as a vent because they provide a potential site for microorganisms to enter into the vascular system

4) Bag-entry ports: solution cannot pass through an obstructed port or an administration set spike that has not penetrated the port seal

5) Solution temperature: administration of cold solutions may produce vasospasm, causing vasoconstriction with a decrease in solution flow; solutions other than blood and blood components should be removed from the refrigerator and allowed to reach room temperature before administering

   d. Tubing

      1) Pinched, kinked, or crimped tubing
- Creates an inaccurate flow rate or stops solution flow
- Loop and tape tubing to avoid pinching or crimping

      2) Occluded filter: may decrease or stop flow rate
- As particulates are removed from solutions and/or medications, the filter may occlude
- Change filter when this occurs

      3) Patient's involved extremity: checked for anything that might act as a tourniquet and impede solution flow, such as constrictive clothing, identification bracelet, jewelry, or immobilization device

C. Ecchymosis/Hematoma

1. Description
   a. Blood infiltrates into the tissues
   b. Ecchymosis occurs when blood spreads out across the tissues; may result in the formation of a hematoma
   c. Both ecchymosis and a hematoma limit the use of the venous system
      1) Damage tissues
      2) May limit use of the extremity

2. Signs and symptoms
   a. Tissue discoloration from blood infiltrating the area
   b. Swelling as hematoma is formed
   c. Onset immediate or slow depending on the amount of subcutaneous tissue between the vein and epidermis

3. Contributing factors
   a. Venipuncture by unskilled professionals
   b. Use of fragile veins for venipuncture
   c. Application of a tourniquet to fragile skin
   d. Multiple entries into a vein
   e. Attempts made into poorly visible or impalpable veins
   f. Venipunctures in patients with a blood dyscrasia or in those who bruise easily
   g. Use of steroids or anticoagulants

4. Interventions
   a. Ecchymosis (occurs during venipuncture from bleeding around the cannula as the vein is penetrated or as the cannula penetrates the opposite wall of the vein)
      1) Remove cannula and apply light pressure dressing

        2) Do not apply heavy pressure because it may rupture fragile vessels within the area and increase bleeding

        3) Area usually feels sore but is rarely painful unless a hematoma has formed

        4) Area appears unsightly, but this usually disappears in 1 to 2 weeks

    b. Hematoma

        1) Remove cannula immediately and apply direct pressure to the area

        2) Elevate involved extremity until bleeding ceases

        3) Apply a dry, sterile dressing to the site

        4) Apply ice to the area to prevent hematoma enlargement

        5) Monitor the site for break-through bleeding

        6) Monitor the extremity for circulatory, neurological, and motor function

  5. Documentation

    a. Not necessary to document every incidence

    b. Severe ecchymosis and/or hematoma with excessive bleeding or hematoma requiring medical intervention should be documented

  6. Preventive measures

    a. Hematomas are not always preventable, but the severity can be minimized by the performance of venipuncture by highly skilled professionals

    b. Performance of venipunctures on fragile veins without a tourniquet

D. Infiltration

  1. Description

    a. Inadvertent administration of a nonvesicant solution and/or medication into surrounding tissues

    b. Usually caused by a dislodged cannula

  2. Signs and symptoms

    a. The skin feels tight at venipuncture site

        1) Difficult to flex or extend involved extremity

        2) Skin becomes taut and stretched as more solution accumulates in the interstitial tissues

    b. Blanching and coolness occur as more solution gathers within the tissues

    c. Tenderness or discomfort at the area of infiltration may occur

    d. Degree of infiltration is determined by the volume and type of solution within the tissues; isotonic solutions generally do not produce much discomfort, while solutions with an acidic or alkaline pH are more irritating

  3. Differential diagnosis

    a. Complete assessment with an evaluation of the patient, site, and involved extremity is essential to determining an infiltration

    b. Infusion rate usually remains unchanged with an infiltration

    c. Involved extremity should be compared with the opposite extremity

    d. Patient's medical status should be evaluated

        1) Patients with hemodynamic problems, heart failure, toxic conditions,

compromised kidney function, hypothermia, and vascular insufficiency are prone to vascular edema

    2) Patients with muscular weakness or extremity paralysis may experience edema of an extremity

  e. Applying pressure over the vein above the cannula tip will decrease or stop the flow rate if the cannula is in the vein; if an infiltration is present, the rate will remain unchanged

  f. Best method to determine an infiltration is to apply a tourniquet proximal to the entry site tightly enough to restrict venous flow; if the infusion continues, an infiltration has occurred

  g. Checking for blood flow is an unreliable method for determining an infiltration; blood may flow freely with seepage of solution around the cannula-vein entry point

4. Complications

  a. Patient is deprived of solutions and/or medications

  b. Use of extremity is limited

  c. Patient may experience unnecessary discomfort

  d. Tissue damage may be extensive, exposing the patient to infection and the need for advanced treatment, such as skin grafts

  e. Veins are limited for future access

5. Interventions

  a. Remove cannula immediately and apply sterile dressing to site

  b. Warm compresses, such as warm moist towels, should be applied to the infiltrated area if the infiltrated solution is isotonic and has a normal pH; heat promotes absorption of the infiltrated solution by increasing circulation to the area

  c. Cold compresses should be applied to the area if the infiltrated solution is hypertonic or has an elevated pH, such as potassium chloride; warm compresses promote displacement of solution into the tissues with the potential for necrosis and sloughing

6. Documentation

  a. Date and time

  b. Presence of infiltration with signs and symptoms according to the *Intravenous Nursing Standards of Practice*

  c. Use scale according to the *Intravenous Nursing Standards of Practice* for noting degree of infiltration

  d. Unusual results associated with infiltration, such as blisters or solution leaking through the skin

  e. Nursing interventions with patient response

  f. Monitoring the site until resolution of the infiltration

7. Monitoring statistics

  a. Maintained on an ongoing basis using a standard infiltration scale

  b. Infiltration rate is calculated according to a standard formula:

$$\frac{\text{Number of Infiltration Incidents}}{\text{Total Number of IV Peripheral Lines}} \times 100 = \% \text{ Peripheral Infiltrations}$$

8. Preventive measures and/or minimizing the severity
   a. Avoid flexion areas for venipunctures
   b. Tape the cannula securely to prevent an in-and-out movement of the cannula with movement of the extremity
   c. Avoid excessive movement or pressure over the site by using an arm board or other immobilization device
      1) Immobilization devices should be applied only when absolutely necessary and according to agency protocols in compliance with guidelines established by the Joint Commission on Accreditation of Healthcare Organizations (JCAHO)
      2) Immobilization devices should be well padded and positioned so they do not cause nerve damage, constrict circulation, or pressure areas
      3) Immobilization devices should be removed at frequent intervals and the involved extremity given range-of-motion exercises
   d. Patient education is a key factor in the prevention and early recognition of signs and symptoms
      1) Care of the infusion
      2) Recognition of potential problems and immediate interventions minimize complications

E. Extravasation

1. Description
   a. Inadvertent administration of a vesicant solution and/or medication into the surrounding tissues as a result of a dislodged cannula
   b. Vesicant solution: a solution and/or medication causing the formation of blisters and the subsequent sloughing of tissues
      1) Presence of a vesicant within tissues coupled with blistering causes tissue death or necrosis and may involve underlying connective tissues, muscles, tendons, and bone, necessitating surgical intervention
      2) Severity of damage is directly related to the type, concentration, and volume of infiltrated solution
         • Most harmful vesicants are antineoplastic agents
         • Other medications that act as vesicants: dopamine hydrochloride (Intropin), norepinephrine (Levophed), potassium chloride in high doses, amphotericin B (Fungizone), calcium preparations, and sodium bicarbonate in high concentrations
2. Signs and symptoms
   a. Feeling of skin tightness above, below, or at the cannula site making it difficult to flex or extend the involved extremity (skin becomes taut and stretched as more solution accumulates into the interstitial tissues)
   b. Increasing edema is dependent on the infusion rate, how tight or loose the patient's tissues are, the location of the extravasation in relation to the cannula tip, and extent to which the cannula has penetrated the vessel
   c. Blanching and coolness occurs as more solution gathers
   d. Tenderness or discomfort depends on the amount of fluid within the tissues

      e. Solution flow rate usually decreases as more solution collects within the area

  3. Differential diagnosis

      a. Early diagnosis with intervention is essential to prevent extensive tissue damage

      b. Complete assessment is necessary

          1) Evaluate site and involved extremity before and frequently during administration of vesicant agents

          2) Involved site and extremity are compared with same area of the opposite extremity

      c. Best method to determine an extravasation is to apply a tourniquet proximal to the entry site tightly enough to restrict venous flow; if the infusion continues, an extravasation has occurred

      d. Checking for blood flow is an unreliable method to determine an extravasation since solution can seep into the tissues from a previous puncture site or from around the vein infusion site

  4. Interventions

      a. Stop infusate immediately

      b. Carry out established protocols for extravasations immediately

          1) Cannula usually is left in place until residual medication and blood are aspirated

          2) Antidote specific to the vesicant is instilled into the tissues (see Chapter 7, Antineoplastic Therapy)

      c. Apply sterile dressing to the site after removal of the cannula

      d. Apply cold compresses to an extravasation of an alkylating and antibiotic vesicant, and warm compresses to an extravasation of the vinca alkaloids

      e. Elevate extremity regularly and observe for pain, erythema, induration, and necrosis

      f. Establish a new access site in the opposite extremity, if possible

          1) Choose a site above and away from extravasated site if use of opposite extremity is contraindicated

          2) Consider using a central venous catheter

      g. Notify the physician and frequently report condition of the site and surrounding tissue

      h. Instruct the patient to monitor the site for several weeks after an extravasation occurs

          1) Tissue necrosis may not develop for 1 to 4 weeks

          2) Surgical intervention may become necessary if tissue necrosis is severe

  5. Documentation

      a. Date and time

      b. Insertion site

      c. Cannula type and gauge

      d. Medication and approximate volume extravasated

      e. Signs, symptoms, and severity of each

      f. Nursing, medical, and surgical interventions with patient response

  6. Monitoring statistics

    a. Maintain on ongoing basis

    b. Always rated a Grade 4 when using the recommended *Intravenous Nursing Standards of Practice* infiltration scale

    c. Rate calculated using the same formula as for infiltration

7. Preventive measures and/or minimizing the severity

    a. Administration of vesicants should be performed only by those qualified and trained in venipuncture and administration of vesicant medications

       1) Route and time frame in which medications were administered

       2) Early signs and symptoms

       3) Preventive measures

       4) Associated treatment protocols

    b. Intravenous site should be assessed for patency before, during, and after administration of a vesicant: vein patency can be determined by the infusion of 5 to 10 ml of 0.9% sodium chloride while observing the site and surrounding area before vesicant administration

    c. Blood should be withdrawn into a syringe every 3 to 5 ml when administering a vesicant directly into a vein

       1) Good blood return does not guarantee an extravasation has not occurred

       2) Any change in blood flow return could indicate the need to investigate the possibility of an extravasation

    d. Vesicants should be administered through a side port of a free-flowing infusion because the severity of tissue damage is related to the amount and concentration of the vesicant

    e. Taping the cannula to prevent an in-and-out movement may prevent the possible enlargement of the vein cannula entry site, decreasing the potential for the vesicant to seep into the interstitial tissues

    f. Vesicants should not be administered in flexion areas

    g. Venipuncture sites in the hands should be avoided for vesicant administration because of the close network of tendons and nerves that might be destroyed if an extravasation occurs

    h. Sites may be protected from excessive movement with the use of immobilization devices in accordance with established organizational policies and procedures

    i. Knowledge of previous venipuncture locations and when last used can prevent use of areas that potentiate an extravasation because vesicants have been known to seep into the tissues at the vein entry site of a previous infusion

    j. Gravity and heat should be used to distend small fragile veins, especially those that have been used repeatedly for administering antineoplastic agents; venipunctures should be performed without a tourniquet or with a loosely applied tourniquet to decrease the potential for an extravasation in these patients

    k. Before a vesicant is administered, consideration should be given to change the site preferably to the opposite extremity, when the cannula has been in place longer than 24 hours

   l. Consideration to the placement of a central venous access system
      1) Limited peripheral veins
      2) Therapy longer than 2 weeks
      3) Use of continuous vesicant infusion
  m. Use of a central venous catheter should not provide false assurance that an extravasation cannot occur because extravasations have been documented as a result of catheter rupture, catheter leakage, and separation of ports
   n. Patient education is a key factor in the prevention and early recognition of signs and symptoms
      1) Care of the infusion
      2) Recognition of potential problems and immediate interventions minimize the consequences associated with an extravasation

F. Phlebitis

  1. Description
    a. Commonly reported complication in which the vein intima becomes inflamed
  2. Signs and symptoms
    a. Pain and/or tenderness at the catheter site or along the course of the vein
      1) Skin should be palpated at tip of cannula along the vein course, using slight pressure to check for tenderness
      2) Pain around cannula site is usually a precursor to phlebitis
      3) Pain alone, however, does not constitute a phlebitis
    b. Erythema or redness results from vein inflammation as a result of capillary congestion from the dilation of the superficial capillaries
    c. Inflammatory swelling with a feeling of warmth at the site is the best indicator for phlebitis
  3. Measure according to the *Intravenous Nursing Standards of Practice* phlebitis scale
  4. Chemical phlebitis
    a. Associated with administration of an irritating medication or solution resulting in venous irritation and subsequent inflammation from trauma to the endothelial vein lining
    b. Contributing factors
      1) Solution pH
        • pH refers to the hydrogen ion concentration and is measured as acid or alkaline; the more acidic an intravenous solution, the greater the risk of phlebitis
        • Solutions with a high pH or osmolality, such as 3% sodium chloride, predispose the vein walls to trauma
        • Admixing of medications to solutions can alter the pH of a solution
      2) Solution osmolality
        • Osmolality refers to the measure of solute concentration
        • Parenteral solutions are classified according to the tonicity of the solution in relation to normal blood plasma: blood plasma osmolality is

290 mOsm/liter; solutions approximating 290 mOsm/liter are considered isotonic; those with an osmolality significantly higher are considered hypertonic, while those with an osmolality significantly lower are considered hypotonic
- Vein walls become traumatized by the administration of hyperosmolar solutions (solutions having an osmolality higher than 300 mOsm/liter), especially if they are administered at a rapid rate or through a small vessel
- Isotonic or nearly isotonic solutions may become hyperosmolar when mixed with certain medications, such as electrolytes, antibiotics, and nutrients

3) Infusion rate
- Slow rates create less venous irritation than do rapid rates because they provide absorption time with hemodilution of smaller amounts of solutions and/or medications
- Rapid rates, although getting through the vessels quicker, do not allow for hemodilution and irritate the vessel walls by providing a larger concentration of solution that hits the vessel walls much like a bolus

4) Improperly mixed or diluted medications
- Medication incompatibilities or interactions render the medication and/or solution ineffective, creating a physical change in which crystals are formed that traumatize the vein walls
- Reaction may or may not be visible

5) Particulate matter
- Usually forms as a result of medication particles not fully dissolved during mixing
- Creates a potential for vein irritation and/or embolus formation

6) Cannula
- Certain catheter materials can predispose the vein to inflammation
- Steel needles are the least thrombogenic but rarely used because of increased potential for infiltration
- Incidence of phlebitis increases progressively with the increasing period of cannulation

c. Preventive measures
1) Use of filters
- A 1 to 5-micron particulate matter filter during admixture eliminates most particulates from an admixed solution
- A 0.2-micron filter is considered a bacterial, particulate-retentive, air-eliminating filter and may decrease the potential for microorganisms to be delivered into the vascular system by removing those that enter the system above the filter

2) Use recommended solutions when mixing medications and/or solutions
3) Dilute known irritating medications to the greatest extent possible
4) Administer medications and/or solutions at the recommended rate

     5) Administer IV push medications through a port of a compatible free-flowing infusion

     6) Rotate infusion sites immediately on suspected contamination or complication and in accordance with the *Intravenous Nursing Standards of Practice*

     7) Use of large veins for the administration of hypertonic or acidic solutions to promote hemodilution

     8) Use of the smallest-gauge cannula that will adequately deliver the required infusion

5. Mechanical phlebitis
   a. Associated with cannula placement
   b. Contributing factors
      1) Cannulas placed in flexion areas, creating venous irritation with resultant injury to the vein intima as the involved extremity is moved
      2) Cannula gauge larger than vein lumen in which it is placed, creating inflammation
      3) Poorly taped cannulas that move in and out of vein, causing catheter tip to irritate vein wall
      4) Cannulas placed by unskilled professionals
   c. Preventive measures
      1) Avoid flexion areas when placing cannula
      2) Avoid placing cannula in lower extremities because of increased potential for phlebitis formation
      3) Use cannula smaller than vessel in resting state
      4) Tape cannula appropriately to prevent in-and-out movement of cannula within vein
      5) Cannula placement by highly skilled professional; in comparative trials, the availability of an intravenous therapy team of highly experienced nurses who insert intravenous catheters and provide close surveillance of infusions resulted in a two-fold lower rate of infusion-related phlebitis and an even greater reduction in catheter-related sepsis

6. Bacterial phlebitis
   a. Occurs from inflammation of the vein wall associated with a bacterial organism
   b. Less frequent than chemical or mechanical phlebitis with far more serious complications, predisposes the patient to septicemia
   c. Contributing factors
      1) Poor hand-washing techniques
      2) Lack of aseptic technique in preparation of intravenous site and/or intravenous system
      3) Failure to check equipment for compromised integrity before use
      4) Poorly taped cannula allowing in-and-out movement of cannula with skin contaminants being carried into the vascular system
      5) Poor venipuncture insertion technique
      6) Extended cannula dwell time

7) Site not observed frequently, with a failure to recognize early signs of phlebitis

d. Preventive measures

1) Hand washing is single most important procedure for preventing a nosocomial infection
   - Hands should be washed before and after initiation of therapy
   - Standard Precautions dictate that healthcare providers wear gloves when performing venipunctures; hands should be washed before gloves are donned to minimize potential for contaminants to be carried into the vascular system from their transfer to the gloves

2) Equipment should be checked for expiration date, cracks, leaks, cloudiness, particulate matter, and signs of contamination
   - Squeeze bags to detect punctures
   - Hold bottles up to the light and rotate to detect fine cracks

3) Shaving surrounding site is not recommended because of potential for causing microabrasions, which can allow microorganisms to enter the vascular system

4) Insertion site should be cleaned to reduce potential for carrying microorganisms into the vascular system from the skin
   - Skin should be washed first with soap and water if extremely dirty, then cleansed with antimicrobial solution such as tincture of iodine 2%, 10% povidone-iodine, 70% isopropyl alcohol, or chlorhexidine
   - Antimicrobials should be applied in a circular motion, starting at intended site for puncture and working outward to prevent contaminants from being carried from an unclean to a clean area
   - Antimicrobials should be allowed to completely air dry; do not blot excess solution

5) Aseptic technique should be maintained during cannula insertion; maintain sterility of cannula by not laying cannula on the skin during insertion or touching cannula with fingertips

6) Only one cannula should be used per venipuncture attempt; cannulas that have penetrated the skin should be considered contaminated

7) Sterile tape and dressings should be used over cannula insertion site

8) Cannula should be taped to prevent an in-and-out movement, which creates potential for skin microorganisms to be drawn into the vascular system

9) Cannula sites should be rotated in accordance with the *Intravenous Nursing Standards of Practice*

10) Cannula dressings should be changed in accordance with the *Intravenous Nursing Standards of Practice*

11) Sites should be checked frequently and changed at the first sign of tenderness, redness, or inflammation

7. Interventions

a. Cannulas should be removed at the first sign of tenderness, redness, or inflammation

   b. Cannula should be cultured using the semi-quantitative culture techniques if an infection is suspected: the surrounding skin is cleaned with 70% isopropyl alcohol and allowed to air dry before culture; purulent drainage is cultured before cleansing the skin
   c. Consideration should be given to obtaining blood cultures to determine proliferation of cannula-related infections
   d. Cannula should be relocated to the opposite extremity if possible or to a vein in which the phlebitic vein does not empty
   e. Application of warm moist compresses will promote healing and patient comfort
 8. Documentation
   a. Date and time
   b. Location of phlebitis and severity using the standard scale
   c. Medication and/or solution being infused
   d. Catheter gauge and dwell time
   e. Nursing interventions with patient response

G. Postinfusion Phlebitis

 1. Description
   a. Commonly reported complication associated with inflammation of the vein that is not evident until after the cannula is removed
   b. Usually evident within 48 hours of cannula removal
   c. Possible precursor to infection
 2. Signs and symptoms
   a. Consistent with those of phlebitis
 3. Phlebitis measurement according to the same uniform phlebitis scale used for phlebitis
 4. Contributing factors
   a. Cannula insertion technique
   b. Patient condition
   c. Type, compatibility, and pH of solutions and/or medications being infused
   d. Ineffective filtration
   e. Gauge, size, length, and cannula material
   f. Cannula dwell time
 5. Interventions
   a. Hot or cold compresses are applied once a postinfusion phlebitis is detected
   b. Site and area are observed for further signs and symptoms of increasing phlebitis, and the patient is monitored for signs of septicemia
   c. Medical interventions may be necessary, depending on the degree of postinfusion phlebitis
 6. Documentation
   a. Date and time symptoms are noted
   b. Signs, symptoms, and severity as noted on the phlebitis scale
 7. Preventive measures

a. Cannula replacement by highly skilled professionals
b. Maintain aseptic technique when using or manipulating the intravenous system
c. Determine compatibility of solutions and/or medications before use
d. Use final filters
e. Use cannula smaller than vein in the resting state to promote hemodilution of infusions
f. Add a buffer to known irritating medications and/or solutions and to those solutions with a different pH than normally found within the vascular system
g. Use large veins for administering hypertonic or acidic solutions to promote hemodilution
h. Rotate infusion sites and change dressings and tubings according to the *Intravenous Nursing Standards of Practice*
i. Change solution containers every 24 hours when the system is not maintained as a closed system
j. Change latex injection ports on peripheral intermittent devices at the time of cannula change and when the integrity of the port is compromised

H. Thrombosis

1. Description
   a. Formation of a blood clot within a blood vessel caused by an injury that breaks the integrity of the endothelial lining of the venous wall
   b. Usually occurs at the point at which the cannula touches the vein intima
   c. Platelet adherence to the injured wall creates a thrombus
2. Signs and symptoms
   a. Decreasing solution flow rate as a result of narrowing of vein lumen as thrombus forms
   b. Swelling of an extremity and surrounding area resulting from circulatory involvement
   c. Tenderness with erythema of the area
   d. Possible circulatory impairment of extremity
3. Contributing factors
   a. Venipuncture by an unskilled professional
   b. Multiple venipuncture attempts
   c. Use of a cannula larger than the vein lumen at a resting state
   d. Poor circulation with venous stasis
   e. Administration of incompatible medications and/or solutions
   f. Administration of medications and/or solutions with a high pH or tonicity
   g. Ineffective filtration
   h. Use of thrombogenic catheter materials
4. Interventions
   a. Discontinue infusion immediately
   b. Relocate site to the opposite extremity, if possible
   c. Initially, apply cold compresses to the site to decrease the flow of blood to the area

 d. Notify physician
 e. Monitor site to determine need for surgical intervention
 f. Observe extremity frequently for circulation impairment and tissue damage
 g. Monitor patient for signs of potential pulmonary embolus and/or septicemia
5. Documentation
 a. Date and time symptoms were first noted
 b. Signs, symptoms, and severity of each
 c. Interventions with patient response
6. Preventive measures
 a. Cannula placement by highly skilled professionals
 b. Avoid lower extremities when performing venipunctures in an adult
 c. Use smallest gauge and shortest cannula possible to deliver the prescribed therapy to decrease potential injury to the endothelial lining
 d. Avoid areas of flexion when placing cannula
 e. Anchor cannula securely with tape to avoid in-and-out movements
 f. Consider placement of central venous catheter when venous access is poor

I. Thrombophlebitis

1. Description
 a. Condition denoting a twofold injury: the occurrence of inflammation and the presence of a clot
 b. Most frequent in patients with a history of medication addiction
2. Signs and symptoms
 a. Inflammation along the vein line, characterized by erythema as the first symptom noted
 b. Edema, pain at the site, and a feeling of warmth along the vein line follows
 c. Vein becomes hard and tortuous as vein becomes thrombosed
 d. Marked erythema, increased edema, marked pain along the vein, and aching of the extremity occur if the condition is allowed to continue
 e. Patient's temperature may be elevated
3. Measurement
 a. Measured in accordance with the *Intravenous Nursing Standards of Practice* phlebitis scale
4. Contributing factors
 a. Any irritation to the vein intima predisposing the vein to inflammation with clot formation
 b. Incidence and degree of inflammation increases with the duration of the infusion
 c. Other causative factors as previously discussed under "Phlebitis" and "Thrombosis"
5. Interventions
 a. Observe intravenous site and vein line at frequent intervals for signs and symptoms consistent with thrombophlebitis

b. Discontinue infusion immediately and notify the physician if any symptoms are observed
c. Culture cannula using a semi-quantitative culture technique if infection is suspected
   1) Skin surrounding cannula is cleansed with 70% isopropyl alcohol and allowed to air dry before cannula is removed for culture
   2) Culture any purulent drainage before skin is cleansed
d. Establish new site using a new cannula, tubing, and solution container in the opposite extremity if continuation of therapy is necessary; if unable to use the opposite extremity, a separate vein that does not form a tributary to the traumatized vein should be used
e. Initially apply cold compresses to the site to decrease flow of blood to the area, follow with warm compresses
f. Evaluate extremity
g. Caution patient against rubbing or massaging the area, which could cause an embolus to be released into circulation
h. Monitor patient and extremity for the possibility of embolus formation and/or septicemia
6. Preventive measures
   a. See "Phlebitis" and "Thrombosis"

J. Occluded Peripheral Cannula

1. Description
   a. Condition in which the cannula is filled with blood and/or a precipitant, prevents solution flow
2. Signs and symptoms
   a. Inaccurate flow rate is first sign of a partially occluded cannula
      1) Infusion rate decreases
      2) Changing flow control clamp does not increase flow rate
   b. Infusion ceases as cannula becomes more occluded, or resistance met if attempts made to flush cannula
3. Contributing factors
   a. Solution container is allowed to become completely empty
   b. Positional cannula placement
      1) Cannula promotes increase or decrease of solution flow as the involved extremity is flexed and/or extended
      2) Usually related to cannula being placed in a flexion area
   c. Inappropriate administration of flush solutions when administering medications, drawing blood from a cannula, or using an intermittent device
   d. Administration of incompatible medications and/or solutions with precipitant formation
   e. Kinked catheter or pinched tubing
4. Interventions
   a. Do not flush an occluded cannula because of the potential of pushing an embolus into the circulation

    b. Remove cannula and examine for integrity

    c. Apply dry, sterile dressings to the site

    d. Place a new cannula in another vein if therapy is to be continued

5. Documentation

    a. Date and time noted

    b. Nursing diagnosis of occlusion

    c. Interventions with patient response

6. Preventive measures

    a. Change solution containers when there is less than 100 ml of solution remaining in the container; time-taping solution containers is helpful in noting when a container should be empty

    b. Check solutions and medications for incompatibilities before mixing

    c. Develop policies and procedures for flushing intermittent devices

        1) Manufacturer's recommendations should be used in the establishment of polices and procedures for flushing all cannulas because not all are flushed with heparin

        2) American Society of Healthcare Pharmacists (ASHP) recommends the use of 0.9% sodium chloride to maintain patency of a peripheral intermittent device

        3) Heparinized saline should be used for flushing most central venous catheters; the lowest possible concentration of heparin should be used and the amount and frequency of flush should be used such that the patient's clotting factors are not altered

        4) Cannula should be flushed with 0.9% sodium chloride before and after administration of medications incompatible with heparin

        5) Cannula should be flushed after administration of medications and blood/blood products, blood withdrawal, when converting a continuous infusion to an intermittent device, and every 8 to 12 hours when the cannula is not used

        6) Consideration should be given to maintenance of positive pressure in the cannula to prevent blood reflux into catheter tip after flushing

           • Maintain positive pressure by clamping the tubing while infusing the last 0.2 ml of flush solution

           • Remove the flush syringe while instilling the last 0.2 ml of flush solution

    d. Instruct patient in the care of the cannula/tubing and early recognition of potential problems, such as kinked or pinched tubing and decreased flow rates

K. Local Infection

1. Description

    a. An infection that occurs usually at the cannula-skin entry point as a result of being a point of entry into the vascular system

    b. Can occur in the absence of phlebitis

2. Signs and symptoms

    a. Pain, swelling, and inflammation at the cannula entry point

    b. Discolored tissue of the surrounding area and purulent drainage may be present

    c. May occur while cannula is in place or after cannula has been removed

  3. Contributing factors

    a. Break in aseptic technique at the time of cannula insertion, during cannula care, or at cannula removal

    b. Lack of dressing and/or cannula care at established intervals in accordance with the *Intravenous Nursing Standards of Practice*

    c. Use of contaminated equipment

    d. Inadequate hand washing before administering site care

    e. Site contamination from the patient tampering with the dressing

    f. Use of flexion areas for cannula insertion or inappropriate taping of the cannula with subsequent in-and-out movements of the cannula within the vein, allowing contaminants to be carried into the venipuncture site

  4. Interventions

    a. Remove cannula and culture it to make sure it is not the source of the infection; drainage should be cultured before cleaning the skin with 70% isopropyl alcohol

    b. Notify physician; an antibiotic ointment with sterile dressing changes may be ordered

    c. Systemic antibiotic therapy may be necessary; occasionally, surgical intervention is necessary

    d. Monitor site until infection is resolved

  5. Documentation

    a. Note date and time

    b. Signs, symptoms, and severity of each

    c. Interventions, monitoring, and patient response

  6. Preventive measures

    a. Use good hand washing techniques

    b. Maintain aseptic techniques during cannula insertion, site care, dressing change, and cannula removal

    c. Assess cannula, tubing, and dressing for integrity before use

    d. Immediately change any equipment suspected of being contaminated

    e. Avoid areas of flexion for cannula insertion

    f. Tape cannula appropriately to prevent in-and-out movement in the vein

    g. Cannula dressings should be changed in accordance with the *Intravenous Nursing Standards of Practice*

    h. Educate patient relative to site and dressing care

L. Arterial or Venous Spasm

  1. Description

    a. Sudden involuntary contraction of an artery or vein (vasoconstriction)

    b. Results in temporary cessation of blood flow through the vessel

  2. Signs and symptoms

    a. Feeling of numbness in the involved extremity, with cramping or pain above the infusion site; the first symptom recognized by the patient

b. Pain may not be felt until tissue damage occurs

c. Loss of pulse with localized blanching usually indicates an arterial spasm with loss of blood flow to the areas supplied by the artery

3. Differential diagnosis

   a. Arterial spasms

      1) More serious than venous spasms because arteries supply circulation to large areas of the body

      2) Arterial damage resulting in loss of blood supply to the surrounding area with tissue necrosis and gangrene

   b. Venous spasms

      1) Multiple veins return blood to the heart from all areas of the body

      2) Collateral circulation occurs when a vein is injured causing the blood supply to the area to decrease, usually not to a great extent

4. Contributing factors

   a. Administration of cold medications and/or solutions

   b. Administration of irritating medications and/or solutions

   c. Inadvertent puncture of an artery for a vein

5. Interventions

   a. Arterial

      1) Remove cannula immediately

      2) Apply pressure to the site for approximately 5 minutes or until bleeding has stopped

      3) Apply sterile dressing

   b. Venous

      1) Cannula is usually not discontinued

      2) Identify cause of the spasm and give appropriate treatment

         • Decrease infusion rate and/or further dilute medication if cause is related to administration of an irritating medication and/or solution

         • Apply warm compresses above the site to promote vasodilation and increase blood supply; will aid in the elimination of spasms from the administration of cold medications and/or solutions

         • 0.25 ml of lidocaine 1% may be given to alleviate pain associated with spasms, according to agency policies and procedures; should be given only with a physician's order after an allergy history has been obtained

6. Documentation

   a. Only when there is a need for interventions and/or the potential for tissue damage exists

   b. Date and time of incidence

   c. Signs, symptoms, and severity of each

   d. Interventions with patient response

7. Preventive measures

   a. Cannula placement by highly skilled professionals

   b. Dilute medications

   c. Remove solution containers from the refrigerator in a timely manner to allow solutions to reach room temperature before use

    d. Use fluid warmers for the administration of cold solutions and in patients with hypothermia

    e. Use blood warmers for the administration of rapid transfusions in patient with potent cold agglutinins, for exchange transfusions in neonates, and in patients with hypothermia

III. SYSTEMIC COMPLICATIONS

A. Overview

1. Complications occurring in circulation
2. Potential to affect all body systems
3. Usually serious, requiring immediate intervention

B. Septicemia

1. Description
   a. Pathological state or pyrogenic reaction
   b. Usually accompanied by a systemic illness occurring when a pathogenic bacteria invades the bloodstream
2. Signs and symptoms
   a. Chills, fever, general malaise, and headache are first symptoms noted
   b. Increased pulse rate and prostration as fever increases
   c. Flushed face, backache, nausea, vomiting, and hypotension are possible
   d. Symptoms become severe with cyanosis, increased respirations, and hyperventilation if condition goes undetected or untreated
   e. Vascular collapse, shock, and death as organisms overcome the system
3. Contributing factors
   a. Solution containers
      1) Possible focal point for not only contamination but microbial growth
      2) Solutions may be contaminated during the manufacturing process, storage, setup, or while in use as a result of manipulation or improper handling
         • Organisms associated with contamination during the manufacturing process include gram-negative organisms, *Klebsiella, Serratia,* and *Enterobacter* species
         • Organisms associated with sepsis from contaminated infusates while in use include *Enterobacter cloacae, Enterobacter agglomerans,* and *Pseudomonas cepacia*
      3) Infusate composition promotes growth of certain microorganisms
         • 5% dextrose in water solutions show rapid growth of *Klebsiella, Enterobacter, Serratia,* and *Pseudomonas cepacia* within 24 hours
         • Blood products are excellent sources for growth of *Klebsiella* microorganisms
         • TPN solutions support growth of *Candida* species
      4) Hypertonic solutions or solutions containing large amount of particulates

- Tend to irritate the vascular intima
- Cause an inflammatory reaction predisposing the vessel to thrombus formation, providing a nidus for infection

5) Solution containers in use longer than 24 hours can potentiate septicemia because bacteria proliferate in solution containers after 24 hours at room temperature

b. Equipment can become contaminated at the factory, on route from the factory, during storage, and at the time of use

c. Stopcocks are a frequent source of microorganisms entering the intravenous system because of frequent manipulation

d. Catheter structure (gauge and catheter rigidity) can promote potential for sepsis

1) Large catheters come in contact with greater skin area and produce a large hole in the skin and vessel, increasing potential for bacterial entry

2) Large catheters often used for purposes requiring more frequent entries into the system increase potential for bacterial entry; studies show the use of multilumen catheters increases risk of infections by as much as 12.8% because of increased number of entries into the vascular system

3) Rigid catheters increase risk of infection by promoting thrombogenesis and an inflammatory response that may facilitate colonization

4) More flexible catheters (silicone, elastomer, and polyurethane) are much less thrombogenic than catheters made of other materials

e. Catheter materials can promote the adherence of microorganisms more readily than do others

1) *Candida* species shown to adhere to polyvinylchloride catheters more than to polytetrafluoroethylene catheters

2) Potential for fibrin sheath formation

- Although some catheter materials are less thrombogenic than others, most authorities believe all catheters become encased in a fibrin sheath within several hours of insertion
- Whether sheath represents an asset or a liability is unclear
- Some materials appear to promote adherence of certain pathogenic strains of microorganisms; with the use of these catheters, the fibrin sheath may be relatively protective
- Conversely, other catheter materials do not promote microbial adherence; in these materials, the fibrin sheath may represent a nidus for infection

f. Experience, knowledge, and techniques of the practitioner directly impact the risk for sepsis; good aseptic insertion techniques lower the risks associated with infection

g. Insertion site is the primary route by which microorganisms gain access to the vascular system along the catheter insertion site

1) Skin organisms gain access to transcutaneous tract (space between catheter and subcutaneous tissue) at the time catheter is inserted and

migrate along tract to bloodstream, where bacteremia or fungemia is produced

   2) Intravenous cannulas can be contaminated during insertion as a result of microorganisms on the practitioner's hands or on the patient's skin

h. Hematogenous seeding occurs when microorganisms are carried from a remote site or another source of infection, such as the urinary tract or a surgical wound, and seed on to the catheter

   1) Most vascular access yeast infections appear to be the result of hematogenous dissemination from another site

   2) Hematogenous seeding can occur if a catheter is inserted into a patient who has a high-grade bacteremia or candidemia

   3) Factors affecting catheter seeding: causative pathogen, degree and duration of bacteremia, patient's clinical status, and catheter dwell time

   4) Patients with gut translocation are susceptible to sepsis
      • Increase in gram-negative rod and *Candida* sepsis
      • Patients usually extremely ill, have not been fed enterally for a long time, and receive TPN through a central venous catheter, causing bacterial cecal count to increase and secretory immunoglobulin to decrease, preventing bacteria from attaching to intestinal wall
      • Bacteria, mainly *Escherichia coli* and *Candida,* move across cell membrane to mesenteric lymph nodes, spleen, liver, and the blood and can be carried to the intravascular cannula with seeding and sepsis, or sepsis may occur once organism enters the blood

i. Manipulation of the delivery system provides a potential for microorganisms to enter the intravascular system; frequent manipulations of the cannula or the intravenous system greatly increase the risk of sepsis

j. Catheter dwell time and catheter length increase risks for vascular access infection

   1) Risk associated with catheter infections increases with length of time catheter is in place

   2) Catheters should not be left in place longer than absolutely necessary

k. Pressure monitoring devices are associated with epidemic and endemic nosocomial intravascular infections

   1) Common pathway for microorganisms to enter bloodstream with these devices
      • Fluid column in the tubing between patient's intravascular catheter and pressure monitoring apparatus
      • Microorganisms in a fluid-filled system moving from pressure monitoring apparatus to patient, or from patient to pressure monitoring system

   2) Contaminated infusates introduce microorganisms into system from contaminated disinfectant used on the domes; contaminated monitoring system related to blind, stagnant columns of fluid between transducer and infusion system

4. Interventions
   a. Assessment and evaluation are required for early symptoms with a differentiation of possible causes
      1) In the absence of other causes such as kidney, respiratory, or wound infection, the intravenous system should be considered as the source of infection
      2) Fever in a person with a central venous catheter should be attributed to the catheter until proven otherwise
   b. Monitor vital signs, and if sepsis is suspected, notify the physician immediately
   c. Remove the cannula and culture cannula using the semi-quantitative method, only after the skin around the cannula has been cleaned with 70% isopropyl alcohol and allowed to dry
   d. Exceptions for cannula removal may include patients with limited sites for central venous access, patients at risk for mechanical complications, or the presence of *Candida* or other fungal infections
   e. Draw blood cultures to determine the causative organisms
   f. Antibiotic therapy may be ordered
5. Documentation
   a. Date and time of symptoms noted
   b. Signs, symptoms, and severity of each
   c. Interventions and patient response
   d. Monitoring and further development of signs and symptoms
6. Preventive measures
   a. Wash, rinse, and dry hands thoroughly before initiating an infusion and before handling any part of the intravenous system
   b. Check all solution containers before use for clarity, cracks, and presence of a vacuum
   c. Cleanse site for cannula placement with an antimicrobial solution that is applied with friction, working outward from the center to the periphery and allow to air dry; acceptable antimicrobials include tincture of iodine 2%, 10% povidone-iodine, 70% isopropyl alcohol, and chlorhexidine
   d. Clip excessive hair over the venipuncture site; the area should not be shaved because bacteria could cause microabrasions
   e. Tape cannula to prevent in-and-out movement that could allow micro-organisms to enter into the vascular system
   f. Apply sterile dressings to the cannula site using aseptic technique and change in accordance with the *Intravenous Nursing Standards of Practice*
   g. Tubing used for continuous therapy should not be taken apart to allow patients to ambulate or to change gowns
   h. Use aseptic technique when initiating therapy or when manipulating the system
   i. Do not touch cannula at any time during insertion; those placed in emergency situations should be replaced at the earliest opportunity
   j. Cannula sites should be changed in accordance with the *Intravenous Nursing Standards of Practice*

    k. Solution containers used for intravenous therapy should be changed in accordance with the *Intravenous Nursing Standards of Practice*

    l. Use Luer-Lok connections when possible; other connections should be secured with connecting devices to avoid accidental separation

    m. Limit use of add-on devices to situations in which an absolute need exists as the addition of these devices allow opportunities for bacteria to enter the system; change at the same time the administration set is changed

    n. Disinfect injection ports with an antimicrobial solution (tincture of iodine 2%, 10% povidone-iodine, 70% isopropyl alcohol, or chlorhexidine) before use

    o. Change latex injection caps on peripheral lines in accordance with the *Intravenous Nursing Standards of Practice*

    p. Change needles on secondary medication administration sets with each use

    q. Check product integrity before use; if integrity is compromised do not use product

    r. Check intravenous sites periodically as established in agency policies and procedures and change immediately at first sign of complications

    s. Access injection ports according to manufacturer's recommendations; use only 1-inch, 25- to 21-gauge needles with injection ports

    t. Consider use of a needleless system when accessing intravenous tubing as a measure to prevent transmission of bloodborne pathogens to the healthcare worker

C. Pulmonary Embolism

  1. Description

    a. Condition that occurs when a mass of undissolved matter becomes free-floating and is carried by venous circulation to the right side of the heart, occluding a pulmonary vessel

    b. Matter may be solid, liquid, or gaseous; may consist of bits of tissue, tumor cells, fat globules, air bubbles, or clumps of bacteria or foreign bodies such as catheter fragments, hair, or glass

  2. Signs and symptoms

    a. Cardiac disturbances if the embolus obstructs the pulmonary artery

    b. Pulmonary hypertension with right-sided heart failure if multiple emboli are passed into pulmonary circulation

    c. Dyspnea

    d. Pleuritic pain or discomfort

    e. Apprehension and restlessness

    f. Cough and unexplained hemoptysis

    g. Sweats

    h. Tachypnea

    i. Tachycardia

    j. Cyanosis

k. Possible low-grade fever

l. Possible pleural friction rub on lung auscultation

3. Interventions

a. Place patient in semi-Fowler's position if a pulmonary embolism suspected

b. Take and monitor vital signs

c. Notify physician; orders may include:

   1) Oxygen to maintain blood gas levels

   2) Complete blood count (CBC) and partial thromboplastin time (PTT) as a baseline for heparin administration

   3) Heparin infusion, usually preceded by heparin bolus administration

   4) Radiographic lung scan to verify pulmonary embolism

4. Preventive measures

a. Use filter to remove particulates from intravenous solution and/or medications

b. Use filter designed to retain blood clots and other debris during the administration of blood and blood components

   1) Standard blood filters with a pore size of 170 to 260 microns routinely used to trap large blood clots

   2) Microaggregate blood filters of 20 to 40 microns used to administer whole blood and packed red cells that are stored 5 or more days and used during cardiopulmonary bypass surgery

c. Avoid veins in lower extremities

   1) Blood pooling easily in the small network of veins in the feet creating venous gorging

   2) Subsequent damage to vein walls may result in a clot released into circulation

d. Use good judgment when flushing intravenous lines

   1) Lines should not be irrigated or flushed to improve flow rates because of the potential for releasing a clot

   2) Force should not be applied when flushing an intermittent device or intravenous tubing because of the potential of forcing a small clot into circulation

e. Use measures that prevent injuries to the endothelial lining of the veins

   1) Cannula placement by highly skilled professionals

   2) Use smallest cannula possible to deliver the required therapy

   3) Use large veins when administering irritating solutions and/or medications to promote hemodilution of infusates

   4) Use proper taping techniques to prevent cannula movement

f. Before venipuncture, cleanse area and clip hair to eliminate the possibility of severing cannula after insertion

D. Air Embolism

1. Description

a. Condition that occurs when a bolus of air is allowed to enter the vascular system

b. Small bubbles form tenacious bubbles that block pulmonary capillaries, causing distress
2. Signs and symptoms (generally rapid and acute)
   a. Chest pain
   b. Shortness of breath
   c. Shoulder or low back pain (depending on location of air embolism)
   d. Cyanosis
   e. Hypotension
   f. Weak, rapid pulse
   g. Continuous churning sound over the precordium on auscultation
   h. Faint feeling or loss of consciousness
   i. Shock with cardiac arrest if condition is unrecognized or untreated
3. Contributing factors
   a. Open port or leak in the infusion system, allowing air to enter the system
   b. Tubing change without clamping the tubing appropriately or failure to ask patient to perform the Valsalva maneuver while tubing is changed on a central catheter
      1) Inhalation creates a negative pressure within the chest cavity, pulling air into the vascular system when a central line is opened
      2) Exhalation creates a positive pressure, preventing air from being drawn into the vascular system
   c. Allowing solution containers to run dry without the use of a filter
   d. Lack of Luer-Lok connections predisposing the system to separation
   e. Failure to remove air from the system before use
   f. Failure to remove air from syringes before the administration of medications or flush solutions
4. Interventions
   a. Replace leaking or open infusion systems immediately with a new set filled with solution to prevent air from being drawn into the system
   b. Immediately place patient on the left side with the head lower than the heart
   c. Assess vital signs
   d. Notify physician; oxygen is usually ordered and administered
   e. Continuously monitor vital signs
   f. Carry out emergency measures as necessary
5. Preventive measures
   a. Clamp infusion tubings and extension sets before tubing change
   b. Have patient exhale to prevent air from being drawn into the system before tubing changed on central lines, if clamps are not provided on the central line extension ports
   c. Change solution containers while solution remains in container; many manufacturers provide an overfill in each container to allow for changes before container is completely empty
   d. Use air-eliminating filters to prevent passage of air into the vascular system
   e. Change leaking sets immediately to prevent air from being drawn into the system

    f. Place patient in Trendelenburg position before insertion of a central ve
       nous catheter

    g. Use Luer-Lok connections to prevent separation of infusion lines

    h. Remove air from infusion systems, including Y-injection ports, before use

    i. Remove air from syringes before the administration of medications and
      flush solutions

    j. Instruct patient in the care and maintenance of the infusion system

    k. Do not flush or irrigate cannulas to improve flow rates because an
      embolus may be released into the vascular system

E. Catheter Embolism

1. Description
   a. Condition that occurs when a piece of catheter is severed and enters
      circulation
2. Causative factors
   a. Defective catheter
   b. Shearing of catheter during insertion
   c. Catheter rupture from a forced injection
   d. Inappropriate clamping of a silastic catheter
   e. Withdrawal of the catheter after insertion of a through-the-needle catheter,
      with resultant catheter shearing (most common cause)
3. Signs and symptoms
   a. Local
      1) Cannula and hub separation
      2) Severed cannula noted on withdrawal
   b. Systemic
      1) Cyanosis
      2) Hypotension
      3) Increased central venous pressure
      4) Tachycardia
      5) Weak, rapid pulse
      6) Fainting and/or loss of consciousness
      7) Arrhythmias, perforation of the heart, or endocarditis if embolus
         lodges in the heart
      8) Cardiac arrest
      9) Pulmonary thrombosis if embolus passes through the heart and lodges
         in lung
   c. Severity
      1) Depends on location of embolism
      2) Severe symptoms appear suddenly at the time of injury because of
         proximity of the subclavian vein to the heart
      3) Catheter fragment may lodge in heart without any symptoms
4. Interventions
   a. Place tourniquet on arm above the venipuncture site and place patient on
      strict bed rest
   b. Notify physician, implement orders

          1) Radiographic studies to determine location of catheter fragment

          2) Surgical intervention as determined by physician once complete assessment of catheter fragment location and patient condition is made

      c. Monitor patient and assess for further distress

    5. Documentation

      a. Date and time of symptoms noted

      b. Signs, symptoms, and severity of each

      c. Cause, if known

      d. Interventions with patient response

      e. Continued monitoring of the patient's condition

    6. Preventive measures

      a. Check catheter for product integrity before use

      b. Avoid pulling through-the-needle catheters back through the needle during insertion

      c. Withdraw over-the-needle catheter stylets only when venipuncture is complete (do not withdraw and reinsert once the catheter has been partially or fully threaded)

      d. Do not exert positive pressure when a flush solution or medication is administered through a silicone catheter

      e. Use 10-ml syringes or greater when medications or flush solutions are administered through a silicone catheter

F. Pulmonary Edema

    1. Description

      a. Condition precipitated by the presence of more fluid volume than the circulatory system can manage, causing an increase in venous pressure with the possibility of cardiac dilation

      b. Danger of heart failure, shock, and cardiac arrest if unrecognized or untreated

    2. Signs and symptoms

      a. Early signs

         1) Restlessness

         2) Slow increase in pulse rate

         3) Headache

         4) Shortness of breath

         5) Cough

         6) Possible flushing

      b. With continued fluid build-up

         1) Hypertension

         2) Severe dyspnea with gurgling respirations

         3) Productive cough

      c. Progressive symptoms

         1) Engorged neck veins

         2) Elevated wedge pressure

         3) Moist rales on auscultation

         4) Puffy eyelids

    d. Weight gain of more than 1 pound per day may suggest pending pulmonary edema, particularly if the patient is receiving TPN

3. Interventions (include measures to decrease the heart's workload)
    a. Decrease infusion rate to a slow drip
    b. Place patient in a high Fowler's position
    c. Assess vital signs and fluid balance
    d. Notify physician
    e. Administer oxygen
    f. Follow physician's orders, which may include:
        1) Administration of morphine sulfate
          • Decreases preload through peripheral venous vasodilation
          • Decreases afterload by decreasing arterial blood pressure
          • Decreases myocardial workload
        2) Therapeutic phlebotomy to relieve workload of heart and reduce venous pressure
        3) Administration of diuretics intravenously to produce rapid diuresis
        4) Administration of an intravenous vasodilator such as sodium nitroprusside to decrease afterload

4. Preventive measures
    a. Assess patient before initiation of therapy
        1) History of problems associated with having received intravenous therapy
        2) History of cardiac and respiratory problems
        3) Evaluation of present status for ability to tolerate fluid volume
    b. Monitor patient for tolerance to volume of fluids and/or medications administered
    c. Maintain infusion rates as ordered unless such rates would compromise the patient's well-being; rates are not increased to allow for administration of solutions whose rates have gotten behind
    d. Use metered-volume chamber sets, infusion devices, or both when solutions or medications are administered requiring accurate measurement, and when administered to the neonate, pediatric patient, elderly patient, or the patient whose condition warrants critical management to prevent fluid overload

G. Speed Shock

1. Description
    a. Systemic reaction occurring when a substance foreign to the body is rapidly introduced into circulation
    b. Frequently confused with pulmonary edema because of rapid infusion (differentiated by volume)
        1) Speed shock results from flooding heart and brain, rich in blood supply, with a medication in toxic proportions
        2) Increased volume not necessary to precipitate the condition

2. Signs and symptoms
    a. Early symptoms

        1) Dizziness
        2) Facial flushing
        3) Headache
        4) Symptoms associated with medication administration
     b. Progressive symptoms
        1) Chest tightness
        2) Hypotension
        3) Irregular pulse
        4) Anaphylactic shock
  3. Contributing factors
     a. Rapid uncontrolled infusion of a medication
     b. Medication administration at a rate that exceeds recommended practice
  4. Interventions
     a. Discontinue infusion immediately
     b. Maintain patent intravenous line for emergency use
     c. Administer emergency measures as necessary
     d. Notify physician and carry out interventions as ordered
  5. Preventive measures
     a. Administer medications by individuals with knowledge of the medication being administered
     b. Administer medications at the recommended rate or at a decreased rate based on an assessment of the patient's condition
     c. Monitor gravity infusion systems to ensure medications are administered at the appropriate rate
     d. Use metered-volume chamber sets and/or electronic infusion devices to deliver solutions and/or medications that have the potential for producing speed shock

H. Allergic Reaction

  1. Description (see Chapter 6, Transfusion Therapy for allergic reactions related to the administration of blood and blood components)
     a. Involves the immediate or delayed response from the administration of a medication or solution to which the patient is sensitive
     b. May occur from the passive transfer of sensitivity to the patient from a blood donor, or patient sensitivity to substances normally present in the blood, as in a transfusion reaction
  2. Signs and symptoms (depend on internal response to an allergen)
     a. Chills and fever with or without urticaria, erythema, and itching
     b. Shortness of breath with or without wheezing
  3. Interventions
     a. Make patient comfortable as possible
     b. Notify physician and carry out interventions as ordered
     c. Administer medications as ordered; may include antihistamines, epinephrine, cortisone, or aminophylline
  4. Preventive measures

a. Note admission assessment of known allergies to medications, latex, or iodine in the medical record and on pharmacy profile
b. Check allergy bracelet before the administration of all medications
c. Individual administering medications should have knowledge of medication classifications and related medications
d. Adequate screening of donor and recipient blood

IV. COMPLICATIONS ASSOCIATED WITH CENTRAL VENOUS CATHETERS

A. Overview

1. Central venous catheter use has risen greatly over the past few years and will continue to grow
   a. As new treatment modalities are invented
   b. As patients continue to be placed on long-term therapies
   c. As patients are treated within alternate care settings
2. The availability of different catheter types contributes to various complications, with some being specific to certain catheters

B. Insertion-related Complications: Pneumothorax

1. Description
   a. Air entering the pleural space and visceral pleura
   b. Results from a puncture of the pleural covering of the lung during catheter insertion
      1) Usually due to the anatomical proximity of lungs to the subclavian veins
      2) Lung may be punctured with danger of an air embolism from puncture of the vein with surgical emphysema
2. Signs and symptoms (dependent on size of pneumothorax)
   a. Sudden onset of chest pain or shortness of breath during catheter insertion
   b. May be asymptomatic if the pneumothorax is not discovered until radiographic confirmation of catheter tip placement
   c. Crunching sound is usually heard on auscultation as a result of mediastinal air accumulation
   d. Marked dyspnea if the pneumothorax is severe
3. Interventions
   a. If the pneumothorax is not diagnosed until radiographic confirmation of catheter tip placement, notify physician
   b. Remove catheter immediately
   c. Turn patient to the affected side and instruct to raise arm above head
   d. Monitor vital signs and for signs of pleural effusion and shock
   e. Administer oxygen
   f. Prepare patient for placement of a chest tube, if necessary; small pneumothoraces often resolve spontaneously with no need for chest tubes

4. Documentation
   a. Date and time of symptoms noted, or report made of radiographic studies of catheter tip placement, if the patient is asymptomatic
   b. Interventions and patient response
   c. Monitoring and further interventions with responses
5. Preventive measures
   a. Insertion of central venous catheters by highly skilled professionals
   b. Place patient in the Trendelenburg position before catheter insertion, with a rolled towel placed between the shoulders to elevate the subclavian vein and ease insertion

C. Insertion-related Complications: Hemothorax

1. Description
   a. Blood entering the pleural cavity
   b. Result of trauma or transection of a vein during insertion of a central venous catheter
2. Signs and symptoms
   a. Sudden onset of chest pain with dyspnea during catheter insertion
   b. Patient may be asymptomatic and undiagnosed until radiographic confirmation of catheter tip placement
3. Interventions
   a. Condition noted during catheter insertion
      1) Remove insertion needle and catheter
      2) Apply pressure to site
      3) Monitor and evaluate vital signs
      4) Administer oxygen
      5) Chest tubes may be inserted
   b. Condition noted during radiographic confirmation of catheter tip placement
      1) Notify physician
      2) Remove catheter and apply pressure to site
      3) Administer oxygen
      4) Monitor patient for development of further complications
      5) Chest tubes may be inserted depending on amount of blood within thoracic cavity
4. Documentation
   a. Date and time of symptoms noted, or radiographic studies confirming hemothorax
   b. Patient assessment noting signs, symptoms, and severity of each
   c. Interventions and patient response
   d. Continued monitoring
5. Preventive measures
   a. Insertion of central venous catheters by highly skilled professionals
   b. Place patient in Trendelenburg position with rolled towel placed between the shoulders to lift the anatomical position of the subclavian catheter during catheter insertion

D. Insertion-related Complications: Hydrothorax

1. Description
   a. Intravenous solutions are infused directly into the thoracic cavity
   b. Results from transection of the subclavian vein and placement of the catheter into the thorax
2. Signs and symptoms
   a. Chest pain
   b. Dyspnea
   c. Absence of vesicular breath sounds
   d. Murmur with a flat sound over location of fluid
3. Interventions
   a. Remove catheter
   b. Fluids may need to be aspirated from the pleural space
   c. Chest tubes may need to be inserted
   d. Monitor patient and assess vital signs
4. Preventive measures
   a. Insertion of central venous catheters by highly skilled professionals
   b. Obtain radiographic confirmation of catheter tip location before administering fluids and/or medications

E. Insertion-related Complications: Brachial Plexus Injury

1. Description
   a. Injury that occurs when one of the brachial plexus (network of lower cervical and upper dorsal spinal nerves supplying the arm, forearm, and hand) is accidentally punctured during insertion of a central venous catheter
2. Signs and symptoms
   a. Tingling sensations in fingers
   b. Pain shooting down arm
   c. Paralysis in involved extremity
3. Interventions
   a. Notify physician
   b. Administer pain medication as ordered
   c. Physical therapy is usually ordered
   d. Monitor patient for resolution of symptoms
   e. Treatment is palliative and does not always resolve injury
4. Preventive measure
   a. Insertion of central venous catheter by highly skilled professional

F. Insertion-related Complications: Inadvertent Arterial Puncture

1. Description
   a. Unintended puncture of an artery while attempting to place a central venous catheter
   b. Usually not a serious problem if symptoms are noted at the time of insertion, catheter is removed, and pressure is applied to the area
2. Signs and symptoms

    a. Bright red blood withdrawn via insertion needle
    b. Hematoma formation with tracheal compression and/or respiratory distress, if symptoms not noted immediately
    c. Central neurological deficit if air or debris enters the artery and embolizes to the brain
  3. Interventions
    a. Apply pressure (if possible) to the arterial puncture site for at least 5 minutes, longer if the patient has a history of bleeding or a platelet disorder
    b. Pressure cannot be applied to the insertion site of all arteries, particularly if the site is under bone as is sometimes seen with the subclavian vein under the clavicle
    c. Monitor patient for signs of bleeding
  4. Preventive measures
    a. Not always preventable
    b. Placement of central venous catheter by highly skilled professional

G. Insertion-related Complications: Extravascular Malposition

  1. Description
    a. Central venous catheter is placed with the tip of the catheter outside the vascular system
    b. Catheter or introducer slips out of the vein during the process of threading the catheter
    c. Hydromediastinum results if the catheter tip is placed in the mediastinum and medication is infused into the space where the heart and great vessels are located
  2. Signs and symptoms
    a. Consistent with those associated with pneumothorax if the pleural covering of the lung or the lung is punctured
    b. Consistent with those associated with hemothorax if blood enters the pleural system
    c. Symptoms possibly not experienced until an infusion is administered if the vein has been punctured and the catheter tip has been placed in the neck or chest area outside the pleural cavity
    d. As solution enters the chest, possible chest, arm, or neck swelling of the adjacent area
  3. Interventions
    a. Notify physician if the condition is not noted during insertion
    b. Remove catheter immediately
    c. Assess patient's condition and monitor for the development of further complications and/or resolution of the condition
    d. Treat each complication (pneumothorax, hemothorax, hydrothorax) as necessary
  4. Preventive measures
    a. Placement of the catheter by a highly skilled professional
    b. Condition is not always preventable; radiographic confirmation of

catheter tip before use can minimize more serious complications associated with the use of a catheter

H. Insertion-related Complications: Intravascular Malposition

1. Description
   a. Misplacement of the catheter tip within the intravascular system
   b. Optimal position for the central venous catheter tip is the superior vena cava (SVC)
   c. Usual sites for misplacement include the internal jugular vein instead of the subclavian as a result of the anatomical location of the internal jugular and subclavian veins
   d. Documented misplacement sites include the contralateral innominate vein, the azygos vein, the right and left internal thoracic veins, the superior intercostal veins, and the accessory hemizygous veins
   e. Most common misplacement occurs with the antecubital approach into the internal jugular vein
   f. Most common malposition by the cephalic vein is the axillary vein
2. Signs and symptoms (frequently noted with catheter use)
   a. Difficulty with aspiration or infusion through the catheter
   b. Discomfort or pain in the shoulder, neck, or arm
   c. Edema in the neck or shoulder area
   d. "Ear gurgling" sound: often described as a "running stream" rushing past the ear (associated with the infusion of solutions through a catheter aberrantly place in the internal jugular vein)
   e. Undesired neurological effects
      1) Caused by infusion of medications through a catheter located in internal jugular vein
      2) Result of retrograde perfusion into intracranial venous sinuses and tributary vein
3. Interventions
   a. Studies indicate that misplaced central venous catheters can be safely and effectively repositioned without subjecting the patient to the potential morbidity associated with repeated percutaneous cannulation
      1) Rapid flush technique: most misplaced silastic catheters can be repositioned by rapidly flushing catheter with 20 ml of 0.9% sodium chloride at 4 to 5 ml/second
      2) Catheters that loop back into the axillary or peripheral veins in the axilla: lower rate of being repositioned
      3) Rapid flushing technique: unsuccessful with double- or triple-lumen catheters or with rigid or semirigid single-lumen catheters because of the inflexibility of the catheters
      4) Catheter rupture: has occurred during use of rapid flush technique when a silastic catheter is obstructed; technique should be performed only when there is no resistance to injection and patient exhibits no signs of venous occlusion

   b. Repositioning the patient is helpful when repositioning a malpositioned catheter and before flushing the catheter
      1) Misplaced into jugular vein: place patient in Fowler's position
      2) Misplaced in contralateral vein: place patient in ipsilateral position with head of bed slightly raised
      3) Misplaced in axillary vein: place patient in contralateral position with head of bed slightly raised
      4) Simple looping of catheter into subclavian, innominate, or internal jugular veins: place patient in one of the previously mentioned positions to allow gravity and blood flow to reposition the catheter overnight
   c. Malpositioned catheters with the tip in the subclavian, internal jugular, or innominate veins: reposition into the appropriate vein by guidewire exchange
   d. Catheters malpositioned beyond the SVC into the right atrium or ventricle: partially withdraw provided the catheter is not an inflexible catheter with memory looped in the great vein
   e. Most reliable and safest method of repositioning a central venous catheter: direct fluoroscopic visualization by a team of radiologists
4. Preventive measures
   a. Not always possible to prevent central venous catheter misplacement during insertion
   b. Helpful measures include:
      1) Insertion of catheters by highly skilled professionals
      2) Use soft catheters such as silicone elastomer
         • Softer catheter materials enhance blood's ability to carry catheter tip
         • Allow catheter to readily follow contour of veins
      3) Measure distance from the proposed insertion site to the right atrium to prevent catheter malposition with peripherally inserted central catheter placement; distance measured from the proposed site on the skin along the presumptive anatomical vein course to the right chondrosternal junction, or to one-third the way down the suprasternal notch to the xiphoid process
      4) Properly position patient before catheter insertion
         • Place patient in Trendelenburg position with a rolled towel between the scapulae; facilitates catheter placement into the SVC
         • Turn patient's head toward side of insertion to make angle between subclavian and internal jugular veins; facilitates placement of catheter through the basilic vein into the subclavian vein
      5) Catheter advancement under fluoroscopy can prevent a malpositioned catheter
      6) Radiographic confirmation of tip placement frequently prevents complications associated with the use of a malpositioned catheter
         • Difficult to determine correct position of catheter placed in left side of mediastinum because of the close proximity of the internal thoracic vein to the SVC when the area is viewed in a frontal chest radiograph

• Location confirmed by obtaining lateral chest x-ray and injecting a contrast medium

I. Insertion-related Complications: Pericardial Tamponade

1. Description
   a. Condition caused by penetration of the atrium by a centrally placed catheter
2. Signs and symptoms
   a. Cardiovascular collapse with neck vein distention, a narrow pulse pressure, and hypotension with or without symptoms of heart failure
   b. Usually delayed because blood or solution must leak into the pericardial space and compress the heart to cause pericardial tamponade
3. Interventions
   a. Emergency intervention by a physician is essential; the pericardial sac should be aspirated from just below the xiphoid process of the sternum
   b. Catheter should be removed and replaced after resuscitative measures are complete
4. Preventive measures
   a. Insertion of central venous catheters by a highly skilled professional
   b. Use soft catheters, such as those made of silicone

J. Indwelling Central Venous Catheter Complications: Dislodgment and Twiddler's Syndrome

1. Description
   a. Dislodgment: displacement of a catheter or port after insertion; ports frequently become freely movable, migrating from one area to another
   b. Twiddler's syndrome: displacement of a port resulting from the nervous habit of a patient "twiddling" with his port
2. Signs and symptoms
   a. Noticeable movement of the port when accessed
   b. Catheter pulled out or its external length is longer than usual
   c. Noticeable coiling of the catheter under the skin (tunneled catheters or ports)
   d. Exposure of Dacron cuff
   e. Difficulty with flow rate or aspiration from the catheter
   f. Leaking of solution from catheter exit site or around needle inserted into a port
   g. Edema of shoulder and/or arm of the involved side
   h. Burning sensation or pain when solution is infused
3. Assessment
   a. Measure length of the external catheter
      1) Long external catheter may indicate the catheter tip is not at the original placement point
      2) Radiographic reconfirmation of tip placement may be necessary
   b. Palpate exit site and catheter line

1) Coiling may indicate catheter tip is not at the original placement point
2) Radiographic reconfirmation of tip placement may be necessary

4. Interventions
   a. Catheter pulled out
      1) Apply sterile occlusive pressure dressing, such as Vaseline gauze or Telfa, covered with an antibiotic ointment to the site; dressing can usually be removed within 24 to 72 hours
      2) Notify physician
      3) Place new catheter with new tubing and solution container if continued therapy is necessary; secure catheter with sutures
      4) Instruct patient in care and maintenance of catheter, particularly if patient tampering created the problem
   b. Catheter not pulled out, or suspected displacement of tunneled or implanted port
      1) Notify physician
      2) Perform radiographic studies to determine catheter tip placement
      3) Catheter may need to be repositioned or removed depending on radiographic studies
      4) Place new catheter with new tubing and solution container if continued therapy is necessary; secure catheter with sutures
      5) Instruct patient regarding care and maintenance of catheter

5. Preventive measures
   a. Suture external catheter at the skin-exit site
   b. Use occlusive dressing
   c. Loop and tape catheter to prevent pulling on catheter at skin-exit site
   d. Educate patient on catheter care and the dangers associated with manipulating the catheter or port

K. Indwelling Central Venous Catheter Complications: Catheter Migration

1. Description
   a. Movement of the catheter tip from one position to another
   b. Catheter tip often migrates into the right atrium or into the internal jugular vein on insertion
   c. May migrate into axillary vein
   d. Spontaneous migration of the catheter tip is frequently reported

2. Causative factors
   a. Forceful flushing of catheter or changes in intrathoracic pressure associated with coughing or sneezing
   b. Reduced blood flow and dilated vessels associated with congestive heart failure
   c. Displacement by invading tissue (tumor) or venous thrombosis

3. Signs and symptoms
   a. Change in functional capability
   b. Inability to inject solutions
   c. Arrhythmias from migration into the right atrium or ventricle

      d. Ear gurgling sound from migration into the internal jugular vein (palpation of the catheter in the internal jugular can confirm migration)

   4. Interventions

      a. Discontinue infusion

      b. Notify physician

      c. Perform radiographic studies to verify catheter tip location

      d. Reposition catheter under fluoroscopy or remove

      e. Place new catheter with a new solution container and tubing if continued therapy is necessary

   5. Preventive measures

      a. Not always preventable

      b. Avoid trauma to catheter site

      c. Avoid placement of catheter near the site of local disease

      d. Suture catheter

L. Indwelling Central Venous Catheter Complications: Fibrin Formation with Occlusion

   1. Description

      a. Formation of fibrin on catheter tip or along catheter line where catheter touches the vessel, creating a clot that occludes the catheter

   2. Causative factors

      a. Inadequate heparinization

      b. Pump malfunction

      c. Break in catheter system

      d. Patient hypercoagulability

      e. Administration of incompatible medications with precipitant formation; most common precipitates are calcium, diazepam, and phenytoin sodium

      f. Pinching of catheter between clavicle and first rib

      g. Multilumen catheter outlets lying against the vessel wall, as in a one-way obstruction

         1) Aspiration causes the venous wall to be sucked into the catheter, blocking blood withdrawal

         2) Infusion forces the wall away from the outlet and restores patency

      h. Fibrin "flap" on the catheter tip

         1) Allows infusion flow

         2) Prevents blood aspiration

   3. Signs and symptoms

      a. Partially occluded catheter

         1) Discomfort, pain, or edema in shoulder, neck, arm, or at insertion site

         2) Resistance when solution, flush, or medication is instilled

         3) Sluggish infusion

         4) Bubbles in tubing (blood is foamy on aspiration)

         5) Leaking of solution from insertion site as solution tracks back along a fibrin sheath

      b. Occluded catheter

         1) Inability to draw blood from catheter

2) Complete resistance when catheter is used
4. Interventions
   a. Assess catheter or port for occlusion
   b. Evaluate causative factors
   c. Reposition patient: sit up, lie down, raise the arm above the head and cough
   d. "One-way" catheter obstruction: created by catheter opening lying against the vein wall requires catheter be flushed with 0.9% sodium chloride or an infusion be initiated to force catheter from catheter opening
   e. With suspected catheter occlusion, attempt to flush catheter using light pressure and a 10-ml syringe
      1) Resistance to flush or to establish fluid flow: attempt to aspirate occlusion using a gentle push–pull technique with 0.9% sodium chloride
      2) Inability to aspirate blood and infuse solution (a two-way obstruction exists): causative factors should be determined (precipitant or clot formation)
   f. With precipitant occlusion, remove catheter or use ethanol, hydrochloric acid, or sodium bicarbonate
   g. With a suspected clotted port, remove needle, reaccess port with a new needle, and evaulate patency
      1) Frequently, needles accidentally pull out of the septum
      2) Needle should not be pushed back into portal because microorganisms can be carried into portal housing
   h. For certain catheters and ports, use of a thrombolytic agent should be considered to lyse a clot or fibrin
      1) Urokinase (Abbokinase Open-Cath) is preferred medication for declotting central venous catheters because of the decreased risks associated with an allergic reaction; recommended concentration is 5000 IU/ml, using a volume equal to the volume of the catheter
      2) Notify physician and obtain order to declot catheter
      3) Establish policies and procedures for thrombolytic agent use, specifying which catheters can be declotted because all catheters do not expand and cannot support the addition of even a small amount of medication when occluded
5. Preventive measures
   a. Comply with established policies and procedures for maintenance of patency
   b. Maintain positive pressure when lines are flushed: clamping or removing syringe during instillation of last 0.2 ml of heparin or 0.9% sodium chloride when flushing
   c. Use infusion pumps when indicated to alert the nurse of an empty solution container
   d. Monitor infusion system and catheter frequently for mechanical problems, such as an empty solution container or kinked tubing
   e. Mix medications and/or solutions appropriately before and during administration to prevent precipitant formation
   f. Educate patient in the care and maintenance of catheter or port

g. Use low-dose anticoagulant therapy, especially with patients who have hypercoagulability problems

M. Indwelling Central Venous Catheter Complications: Vessel Thrombosis (catheter-related thrombosis)

1. Description
   a. Formation of a blood clot in a vessel within the neck, chest, or arm that occurs as a result of placement of a central venous catheter
   b. Pathophysiology is identified as a triad of thromboses
      1) Stasis: result of the effect of intrapulmonary or mediastinal disease
      2) Vessel wall injury: attributed to aggregation of platelets on catheter surface
         • Mechanical irritation of vessel intima by catheter tip
         • Catheter's entry into vein
         • Catheter infection
         • Exposure of vessel wall to TPN solutions or chemotherapeutic agents
      3) Hypercoagulability: frequently associated with malignancy
   c. Related to suboptimal internal catheter tip location and left-sided catheter placement with tunneled catheters
2. Signs and symptoms
   a. Chest pain
   b. Earache
   c. Jaw pain
   d. Edema of the neck, supraclavicular area, or extremities
   e. Other conditions may be noted that relate to other complications, such as:
      1) Pulmonary embolism
      2) Cerebral anoxia
      3) Laryngeal edema
      4) Bronchial obstruction
      5) Death
3. Interventions
   a. Notify physician immediately when a thrombosis is suspected
   b. Radiographic studies using dye (venography) are usually performed to verify catheter placement
   c. Patient is usually placed on anticoagulant therapy
   d. Evaluation of clot size and area of impaired circulation may indicate the need to lyse the clot; lysis is performed by imbedding a peripheral catheter into the clot with fluoroscopic guidance while infusing a thrombolytic agent
4. Preventive measures
   a. Use low-dose anticoagulant therapy for patients at high risk for clotting disorders
   b. Insertion of catheter by a highly skilled professional
   c. Place catheter into the right subclavian vein

N. Indwelling Central Venous Catheter Complications: Damaged Catheter

1. Description
   a. Damage to catheter such as rupture, pinholes, shearing, or cutting, making the catheter unusable

2. Causative factors
   a. Use of scissors at or near the catheter during a dressing change
   b. Inappropriate use of needles, creating pinholes in the catheter; catheters are made of nonresealable materials and do not accommodate the use of needles directly into them
   c. Catheter rupture from exertion of force or when using a syringe smaller than 10 ml to flush the catheter
   d. Cracking with a rupture of catheter caused by repeated pinching from the anatomical location of the subclavian vein and the clavicle
   e. Damage from failure to use the clamping sleeve with certain catheters
3. Signs and symptoms
   a. Wet dressing or leaking at the insertion site during an infusion or when flushing catheter
   b. Solution leaking through pinholes or tears
   c. Observable separation of the catheter, or pinholes or tears in the catheter
   d. Swelling in the chest area or arm
4. Interventions
   a. Apply nonserrated clamp proximal to the damaged part of catheter
   b. Repair damaged catheter, if possible
   c. Remove catheter immediately to prevent more serious complications, if repair is not possible
      1) Any opening in catheter serves as a portal for bacteria and predisposes patient to septicemia
      2) Air may be drawn into the system from negative pressure created within the heart, and the patient could experience an air embolism
5. Preventive measures
   a. Clamp the reinforced area provided on silicone catheters
   b. Use a nonserrated clamp if there is a need to clamp the catheter at another point
   c. Avoid use of scissors or other sharp objects around the catheter
   d. Use small-bore needles, 25- to 21-gauge, 1 inch or less in length when accessing latex injection ports on catheters
   e. Administer medications and flush solutions without using force
   f. Consider using a 10-ml syringe when administering medications through a silicone catheter
   g. Educate patient/significant other about the potential problems associated with "twiddling" ports and playing with external catheters

O. Indwelling Central Venous Catheter Complications: Superior Vena Cava (SVC) Syndrome

1. Description
   a. Occlusion or compression of the SVC, making the passage of blood impossible
   b. Usually the result of blood clot, fibrin, or both creating an occlusion
   c. May be result of a tumor or enlarged lymph nodes compressing the SVC

2. Signs and symptoms
   a. Progressive shortness of breath, dyspnea, and/or cough
   b. Sensation of skin tightness in the area
   c. Unilateral edema
   d. Cyanosis of the face, neck, shoulder, and arms
   e. Extensive edema of the upper body without edema of lower body parts, often called "short cap edema"
   f. Possible edema and cyanosis of the mucous membranes of the mouth, pharynx, larynx, thorax, and, occasionally, hydropericardium
   g. Engorged, distended jugular, temporal, and arm veins
   h. Prominent vein pattern over the chest from dilated thoracic vessels
   i. Headache, visual disturbances, and altered mental status from increased intracranial pressure if the condition goes unnoticed and untreated
   j. Cerebral anoxia, bronchial obstruction, and death if the condition is allowed to persist
3. Interventions
   a. Place patient in the semi-Fowler's position
   b. Administer oxygen
   c. Provide emotional support because patients often become anxious and fear suffocation
   d. Notify physician immediately
   e. Confirm diagnosis by radiographic studies
   f. Ability to start an alternate route is dependent on the severity of symptoms and on the type of catheter in place
   g. Anticoagulant therapy is usually initiated, and symptoms treated
   h. Monitor patient's cardiovascular, neurological, and fluid volume status to minimize further edema
4. Preventive measures
   a. Condition is rare
   b. Insertion of a central venous catheter by a well-trained, experienced professional
   c. Anticoagulant therapy, particularly with the use of long-term catheters in patients at high risk for the development of clotting problems

P. Indwelling Central Venous Catheter Complications: Site Infection

1. Description
   a. Infection at the catheter exit site with or without sepsis
2. Signs and symptoms
   a. Redness, edema, and/or drainage at the catheter exit site
   b. Tenderness or pain around the catheter
3. Interventions
   a. Notify physician immediately
   b. Physician may choose to remove catheter or to replace it over a guidewire
   c. Blood cultures usually drawn from a peripheral vein as well as the central line

d. Patient usually given antibiotic therapy and may be given anticoagulant therapy

e. An implanted vascular access device is not removed or used until the origin of the infection is determined

f. Treat patient for sepsis if he develops sudden chills with fever, general malaise, headache, nausea, vomiting, hypotension, and cyanosis

4. Preventive measures

a. Maintain aseptic techniques during insertion of the central venous catheter

b. Wash hands before donning gloves for catheter insertion, dressing changes, and manipulation of the catheter

c. Use sterile gloves and mask when performing dressing changes

d. Assess equipment for package integrity and sterility before use

e. Change dressing at established intervals in compliance with standards

1) Gauze dressings

• Occlusive, with all edges secured with an adhesive material

• Change every 48 hours, and immediately if integrity of dressing is compromised

2) Transparent semipermeable membrane: change at least every 3 to 7 days, and immediately if integrity of dressing is compromised

Q. Indwelling Central Venous Catheter Complications: Skin Erosion

1. Description

a. Skin tear over the portal septum of an implanted vascular access device or an implanted catheter

b. Usually seen in patients with poor nutritional status, who are extremely thin, or have had extreme weight loss

c. May be seen as a result of trauma to the area over the portal septum or along the catheter line, such as a patient fall with direct injury or tearing of skin over the area

2. Signs and symptoms

a. Visible skin abrasions or tears over a port or catheter

b. May be with or without redness and/or edema

3. Interventions

a. Notify physician

b. Catheter is usually removed

c. Apply sterile dressing to damaged skin and treat area to prevent infection

4. Preventive measures

a. Maintain good nutritional status

b. Avoid activities that place the implanted portal septum or tunneled catheter at high risk for injury

c. Avoid pressure to area surrounding catheter or implanted port

d. Rotate access site with a needle each time implanted port is accessed

PART SEVEN TERMINATION OF INTRAVENOUS THERAPY

I. TERMINATION OF INTRAVENOUS THERAPY

A. Assessment

1. Determination
   a. Patient need
   b. Patient response to therapy
   c. Achievement of expected outcome
   d. Patient or legally authorized representative refuses to continue therapy or requests to discontinue therapy
2. Physician's order
   a. Order must be clearly written and signed
   b. Verbal orders taken from a physician in a hospital setting are written in the medical record by the licensed nurse and signed by the physician within 24 hours
   c. Verbal orders taken from a physician regarding a patient in a homecare setting are sent to the physician within 24 hours, and follow-up is initiated if the order is not signed by the physician within 4 to 5 days
   d. Any intervention resulting in the discontinuation of therapy is communicated to the physician and an order is written to discontinue the therapy

B. Cannula Removal

1. Peripheral-short
   a. Aseptic technique should be used to prevent bacteria from entering the site
   b. Cannulae should be removed in accordance with the *Intravenous Nursing Standards of Practice*
   c. Cannula removal requires the application of pressure and a dry, sterile dressing to the site
   d. Cannula integrity should be assessed on removal
   e. Cannula defects should be reported to the manufacturer and regulatory agencies
2. Peripheral-midline
   a. Optimal dwell time is unknown
   b. Maximum dwell time is 2 to 4 weeks
   c. Longer dwell times should be based on the professional judgment of the nurse after consideration of certain factors
      1) Length of therapy remaining
      2) Patient's peripheral venous status
      3) Patient's condition
      4) Vein condition in which cannula resides
      5) Skin integrity
   d. Catheter should be removed immediately on suspected contamination, complication, or when therapy has been discontinued

   e. Caution should be used in catheter removal, particularly when the catheter has remained in place for an extended time period
   f. Consideration should be given to abduction of the arm for catheter removal
   g. Physician should be notified if resistance is encountered when attempting to remove the catheter
   h. On catheter removal, pressure should be applied over the site and a sterile gauze dressing with antiseptic ointment should be applied
   i. Catheter integrity should be assessed on removal and defects should be reported to the manufacturer and regulatory agencies
3. Arterial
   a. Aseptic technique should be used to prevent bacteria from entering the site
   b. Catheters should be removed in accordance with the *Intravenous Nursing Standards of Practice*
   c. Physician's order should be verified for removal of an arterial catheter, unless circumstances as previously stated demand catheter removal
   d. On catheter removal, digital pressure should be applied to the site until hemostasis occurs, and a sterile, dry pressure dressing should be applied
   e. The circulatory status distal to the area of cannulation should be assessed and documented after catheter removal
   f. Catheter integrity should be assessed on removal and defects should be reported to the manufacturer and regulatory agencies
4. Peripherally inserted central catheter
   a. Optimal dwell time is unknown
   b. Catheter should be assessed frequently for complications
   c. Catheter should be removed immediately on suspected contamination or complication and when no longer appropriate for the prescribed therapy
   d. Caution should be used in catheter removal, particularly when the catheter has remained in place for an extended time period
   e. Precautions should be taken against an air embolism during catheter removal
   f. Consideration should be given to abduction of the arm for catheter removal
   g. Physician should be notified if resistance is encountered when attempting to remove the catheter
   h. On catheter removal, pressure should be applied over the site, and a sterile gauze dressing with antiseptic ointment should be applied
   i. Dressing should be changed and site assessed every 24 hours until the site is epithelialized
   j. Catheter integrity should be assessed on removal and defects should be reported to the manufacturer and regulatory agencies
5. Nontunneled/nonimplanted central
   a. Optimal dwell time is unknown
   b. Cannula and site should be assessed frequently for complications
   c. Cannula should be removed immediately on suspected contamination or

complication in compliance with the *Intravenous Nursing Standards of Practice*

   d. Aseptic technique should be used to prevent bacteria from entering the site and circulation

   e. Organizational policy should be established based on state statutes and/or the state Nurse Practice Act to dictate the removal of a central venous catheter

     1) Removal of certain central venous catheters may constitute a medical act

     2) Policy must be clear about who can remove each type of central venous catheter

     3) Usually subclavian, jugular, and peripherally inserted central venous catheters are removed by the registered nurse according to agency policies and procedures

     4) Physician should be asked to remove catheter when nurse meets resistance

   f. On catheter removal, pressure should be applied over the site, and a sterile gauze dressing with antiseptic ointment should be applied

   g. Catheter integrity should be assessed on removal and defects should be reported to the manufacturer and regulatory agencies

6. Tunneled catheter

   a. Optimal dwell time is unknown

   b. Catheter, along cannula path, and site should be assessed frequently for complications

   c. Catheter should be removed by a physician because catheter removal may require the dissection of a Dacron cuff from the subcutaneous tissue

   d. Catheter tip should be cultured if a catheter-related infection is suspected

   e. Catheter site should be monitored for healing after catheter removal

7. Implanted port

   a. Optimal dwell time is unknown

   b. Cannula path under skin (if palpable) and site over port should be assessed frequently for complication

   c. Port and attached catheter should be removed by a physician

   d. Catheter site should be monitored for healing after catheter removal

C. Documentation

1. Date and time
2. Observations

   a. Subjective

     1) Patient's perceptions of any feelings or symptoms, such as pain at insertion site or tingling sensation as catheter is removed

     2) Patient's perceptions of what he or she believes regarding therapy, such as therapy did or did not help

   b. Objective

     1) Visible observations, such as erythema, edema, and blanching

     2) Site and surrounding area observed for untoward reactions with each complication and the severity documented

    3. Cannula integrity

    4. Control of bleeding

    5. Condition of the surrounding tissue

    6. Complications, interventions, and culturing if necessary

    7. Type of sterile dressing applied

    8. Name and title of person removing cannula

D. Postcannula Removal (complications may occur and necessitate interventions with documentation)

    1. Observe and monitor for potential complications

        a. Peripheral

            1) Site and surrounding area

            2) Involved extremity

        b. Arterial

            1) Site and surrounding area

            2) Circulation of involved extremity

            3) Delayed systemic reactions in patient

        c. Central

            1) Site and surrounding area

            2) Systemic complications

    2. Interventions

        a. Dressing changes

        b. Application of antimicrobials

        c. Interventions for complications

REFERENCES

Adelman RD, Solhung ML. Pathophysiology of body fluids and fluid therapy. In *Nelson Textbook of Pediatrics*, 15th ed., edited by Behrman RE, Kliegman RM, and Arvin AM. Philadelphia, PA: Saunders, 1996:185–222.

American Association of Blood Banks. *Standard for Blood Banks and Transfusion Services*, 17th ed., edited by Klein HG. Bethesda, MD: AABB, 1996

American Association of Blood Banks. *Technical Manual*, 12th ed., edited by Vengelen-Tyler V. Bethesda, MD: AABB, 1996:449–459.

American Society of Hospital Pharmacists. ASHP report: ASHP therapeutic position statement on the institutional use of 0.9% sodium chloride injection to maintain patency of peripheral indwelling intermittent infusion devices. *American Journal of Hospital Pharmacy* 1994;51:1572–1574.

Andris DA, Krzywda EA. Catheter pinch-off syndrome: recognition and management. *Journal of Intravenous Nursing* 1997;20(5):233–237.

Bagnall-Reeb H. Diagnosis of central venous access device occlusion. *Journal of Intravenous Nursing* 1998;21(5S):S115–S121.

Balstreri L, DeCicco M, Matoure M, et al. Central venous catheter-related thrombosis in clinically asymptomatic oncology patients: A phlebographic study. *European Journal of Radiology* 1995;20:108–111.

Bern MM, Lokich JJ, Wallach SR, et al. Very low doses of warfarin can prevent thrombosis in central venous catheters: A randomized prospective trial. *American College of Physicians* 1990;112:423–428.

Berry RK. Patient education. In *Intravenous Therapy: Clinical Principles and Practice,* edited by Terry J, Baranowski L, Lonsway RA, and Hedrick C. Philadelphia, PA: Saunders, 1995:447–454.

Black R. Vein extravasation: A severe complication of IV therapy. *Parenterals* 1998;6(4):5–8, 12.

Crow S. Prevention of intravascular infections ways and means. *Journal of Intravenous Nursing* 1996;19(4):175–181.

Hadaway LC. Anatomy and physiology related to intravenous therapy. In *Intravenous Therapy: Clinical Principles and Practice,* edited by Terry J, Baranowski L, Lonsway RA, Hedrick C. Philadelphia, PA: WB Saunders, 1995:81–110.

Hadaway LC. Major thrombotic and nonthrombotic complications. *Journal of Intravenous Nursing* 1998;21(5S):S143–S160.

Hastings-Tolsma M, Yucha CB. IV infiltration: No clear signs, no clear treatment? *RN* 1994;57(12):34–39.

Health Care Advisory Board. *Fact Brief: IV Teams.* Washington, DC: HCAB, 001–219–839, December 1998.

Horner KA. Technology assessment of two needleless systems. *Journal of Intravenous Nursing* 1998;21(4):203–208.

Hunter ES, Bell E, Straub MB, Coyle G. Relationship of local IV complications and the method of intermittent IV access. *Journal of Intravenous Nursing* 1995;18(4):202–206.

Ingle JF. Rare complications of vascular access devices. *Seminars in Oncology Nursing* 1995;11(3):1346–1348.

Intravenous Nurses Society. Intravenous Nursing Standards of Practice (revised 1998). *Journal of Intravenous Nursing* 1998;21(1):suppl.

Intravenous Nurses Society. Position paper: Midline and midclavicular catheters. *Journal of Intravenous Nursing* 1997;20(4):175–176.

Intravenous Nurses Society. Position paper: Peripherally inserted central catheters. *Journal of Intravenous Nursing* 1997;20(4):176–178.

Jensen BL. Types of intravenous therapy equipment. In *Intravenous Therapy: Clinical Principles and Practice,* edited by Terry J, Baranowski L, Lonsway RA, and Hedrick C. Philadelphia, PA: Saunders, 1995:303–338.

Joint Commission on Accreditation of Health Care Organizations. CAMH refreshed core, *Comprehensive Accreditation Manual for Hospitals.* Oakbrook Terrace, IL: JCAHO, 1999;Tx. 7.5.3, 7.5.4, 7.5.5.

Joint Commission on Accreditation of Health Care Organizations. *Comprehensive Accreditation Manual for Home Care.* Oakbrook Terrace, IL: JCAHO, 1996.

Jones GR. A practical guide to evaluation and treatment of infections in patients with central venous catheters. *Journal of Intravenous Nursing* 1998:21(5S):S134–142.

Kaplan LK. Filtration: An overview. *Infusion* 1996;3(1):29–32.

Kearns PJ, Coleman S, Wehner JH. Complications of long-arm catheters: A randomized trial of central versus peripheral tip location. *Journal of Parenteral and Enteral Nutrition* 1996;20(1):20–24.

Klotz HP, Schopke W, Kohler A, et al. Catheter fracture: A rate complication of totally implanted subclavian venous access devices. *Journal of Surgical Oncology* 1996;62:222–225.

Klotz RS. The effects of intravenous solutions on fluid and electrolyte balance. *Journal of Intravenous Nursing* 1998;21(1):20–26.

Kruse JA, Shah NJ. Detection and prevention of central venous catheter-related infections. *Nutrition Clinical Practice* 1993;8:163–170.

Kupensky DT. Applying current research to influence clinical practice: Utilization of midline catheters. *Journal of Intravenous Nursing* 1998;219(5):271–274.

Kupensky DT. Use of hydrochloric acid to restore patency in an occluded implanted port. *Journal of Intravenous Nursing* 1995;18(4):198–201.

Larson EL. APIC guideline for hand washing and hand antisepsis in health care settings. *American Journal of Infection Control* 1995;23:251–269.

Lau C. Transparent and gauze dressings and their effect on infection rates of central venous catheters: A review of past and current literature. *Journal of Intravenous Nursing* 1996;19(5):240–245.

Lonsway RA, Acevedo M. Patient assessment. In *Intravenous Therapy: Clinical Principles and Practice,* edited by Terry J, Baranowski L, Lonsway RA, and Hedrick C. Philadelphia, PA: Saunders, 1995:359–364.

Lonsway RA, Terry J. Fluids and electrolytes. In *Intravenous Therapy: Clinical Principles and Practice,* edited by Terry J, Baranowski L, Lonsway RA, and Hedrick C. Philadelphia, PA: Saunders, 1995:118–120.

Maki DG. Complications associated with IV therapy. *Journal of Vascular Access Devices* 1994;1(1):8–9.

Maki DG, Mermel LA. Transparent polyurethane dressings do not increase the risk of CVC-related BSI: A meta-analysis of prospective randomized trials. Abstract presented at the annual meeting of the Society for Healthcare Epidemiology of America, St. Louis, MO, April 1997.

Maki DG, Stolz SS, Wheeler S, Mermel DO. A prospective, randomized trial of gauze and two polyurethane dressings for site care of pulmonary artery catheters: Implications for catheter management. *Critical Care Medicine* 1994;22(11):1729–1737.

Miller JM, Goetz AM, Squier C, Muder RR. Reduction in nosocomial intravenous device-related bacteremias after institution of an intravenous therapy team. *Journal of Intravenous Nursing* 1996;19(2):103–106.

Monsuez J-J, Douard M-C, Martin-Bouyer Y. Catheter fragments embolization. *Angiology* 1997;48(2):117–120.

O'Farrell L, Griffith JW, Lang CM. Histologic development of the sheath that forms around long-term implanted central venous catheters. *Journal of Parenteral Enteral and Nutrition* 1996;20 (2):156–158.

Orr ME, Ryder MA. Vascular access devices: Perspectives on designs, complications and management. *Nutrition Clinical Practice* 1993;8:145–152.

Parisian S. The potential for adverse reactions due to the presence of additives and preservatives in intravenous solutions and medications. *Journal of Vascular Access Devices* 1996;1(1):5–14.

Pearson ML. Guideline for prevention of intravascular device-related infections. *Infection Control and Hospital Epidemiology* 1996;17(7):438–473.

Perdue M. Intravenous complications. In *Intravenous Therapy: Clinical Principles and Practice,* edited by Terry J, Baranowski L, Lonsway RA, and Hedrick C. Philadelphia, PA: Saunders, 1995:419–445.

Perucca R. Changing and discontinuing intravenous therapy. In *Intravenous Therapy: Clinical Principles and Practice,* edited by Terry J, Baranowski L, Lonsway RA, and Hedrick C. Philadelphia, PA: Saunders, 1995:400–405.

Perucca R. Intravenous monitoring and catheter care. In *Intravenous Therapy: Clinical Principles and Practice,* edited by Terry J, Baranowski L, Lonsway RA, and Hedrick C. Philadelphia, PA: Saunders, 1995:392–399.

Perucca R. Obtaining vascular access. In *Intravenous Therapy: Clinical Principles and Practice,* edited by Terry J, Baranowski L, Lonsway RA, and Hedrick C. Philadelphia, PA: Saunders, 1995:379–391.

Perucca R, Hedrick C, Terry J, Johnson J. Infection control. In *Intravenous Therapy: Clinical Principles and Practice,* edited by Terry J, Baranowski L, Lonsway RA, and Hedrick C. Philadelphia, PA: Saunders, 1995:151–164.

Phillips LD. *Manual of IV Therapeutics,* 2nd ed. Philadelphia, PA: FA Davis, 1997:76–79, 123–125, 186–217, 232–256, 280, 320–323, 366, 394–396, 466–468.

Reed T, Phillips S. Management of central venous catheter occlusion and repairs. *Journal of Intravenous Nursing* 1996;19(60):289–294.

Rohrer MJ, Anderson FA. Anticoagulant therapy for deep vein thrombosis: Its proper application. *Seminars in Vascular Surgery* 1996;9:13–20.

Roye GD, Breazeale EE, Byrnes JPM, et al. Management of catheter emboli. *Southern Medical Journal* 1996;89(7):714–718.

Sansivero GE. Venous anatomy and physiology. *Journal of Intravenous Nursing* 1998; 21(5S):S107–S114.

Sherertz RJ, Heard SO, Raad II. Diagnosis of triple-lumen catheter infection: Comparison of roll plate, sonication, and flushing methodologies. *Journal of Clinical Microbiology* 1997;35:641–646.

Terry J, Hedrick C. Parenteral fluids. In *Intravenous Therapy: Clinical Principles and Practice,* edited by Terry J, Baranowski L, Lonsway RA, and Hedrick C. Philadelphia, PA: Saunders, 1995:151–164.

Treston-Aurand J, Olmsted RN, Allen-Bridson K, Craig CP. Impact of dressing materials on central venous catheter infection rates. *Journal of Intravenous Nursing* 1997;20(4):201–206.

US Department of Health and Human Services, Public Health Service, Centers for Disease Control and Prevention. Guideline for prevention of intravascular device-related infections. *American Journal of Infection Control* 1996;24:262–293.

US Department of Labor. Occupational Safety and Health Administration. *Occupational Safe Exposure to Bloodborne Pathogens: Final Rule.* Washington, DC: OSHA Docket No. H–370, December 6, 1991.

US Department of Veterans Affairs. Veterans Health Services and Research Administration. *Veterans Health Administration IV (Intravenous) Therapy Teams.* Washington, DC: VHA, Directive 10–92–025, Feb. 20, 1992.

Weinstein SM. *Plumer's Principles & Practices of Intravenous Therapy,* 5th ed. Philadelphia, PA: Lippincott, 1993:45–62, 76–94, 186–218, 366–368.

Weir JA. Blood component therapy. In *Intravenous Therapy: Clinical Principles and Practice,* edited by Terry J, Baranowski L, Lonsway RA, and Hedrick C. Philadelphia, PA: Saunders, 1995:171–175.

Williams HF. Integrating the Occupational Safety & Health Administration mandates on bloodborne pathogens in the practice setting. *Journal of Intravenous Nursing* 1995;18(6S):S9–S16.

Williams PL, Warwick R, Dyson M, et al. *Gray's Anatomy,* 37th ed. New York: Churchill Livingston, 1989:684–688, 691–692, 709–712, 720–723, 806, 919–968.

CHAPTER 2

Fluid and Electrolyte Balance

Judy Hankins, BSN, CRNI

I. BODY COMPOSITION AND REGULATION OF BODY FLUIDS

A. Composed of Fluids, Lymph, Cell Solids, Fat, and Minerals

B. Varies Depending on Age, Gender, and Size

C. Fluids

1. Accounts for approximately 60% of the body weight for an adult and 80% for infants
2. Adult body weight is attained by puberty
   a. Increased fat stores are found in females; females have less fluid content than males
   b. Increased body fat content generally comes with aging, accompanied by decrease in fluid volumes
3. Fluids normally are lost through various routes
   a. Kidneys as urine
   b. Skin as sweat
   c. Lungs as water vapor
   d. Gastrointestinal tract as vomitus and diarrhea[1]
4. Fluid compartments
   a. Two major fluid compartments: intracellular and extracellular
      1) Both are relatively equal in infants[2]
      2) Rapid changes occur in the first 6 months of life
      3) By age 3 years, intracellular fluid (ICF) decreases to approximately 36%
      4) By puberty, the percentage approximates that of an adult
   b. Intracellular fluid
      1) Fluid within the cells
      2) Largest portion of adult body weight (40%); equivalent to approximately 25 liters

c. Extracellular fluid (ECF)
1) Fluids located outside the cells with a volume of approximately 12 liters[3]
2) Lymph, gastrointestinal secretions, cerebrospinal fluid, sweat, ocular fluids, and pleural, synovial, and pericardial fluids are also included
3) Further divided into the interstitial and intravascular fluids
4) Interstitial fluid
   • Located between cells
   • Comprises approximately 15% of total body weight
5) Intravascular fluid
   • Located in arteries, veins, and capillaries
   • Volume of approximately 5 to 6 liters in the average adult
   • Components include approximately 3 liters of plasma
   • Approximately 2 to 3 liters of red blood cells are suspended in the plasma
5. Electrolytes
   a. Substances that dissociate in solution and have the ability to conduct an electrical charge
   1) Negatively charged particles are called anions
   2) Positively charged particles are called cations
   b. Anions and cations are located in ICF and ECF
   1) Cations in ICF
      • Potassium (major cation)
      • Magnesium
      • Limited amount of sodium
   2) Anions in ICF
      • Phosphate (major anion)
      • Chloride
      • Bicarbonate
   3) Cations in ECF
      • Sodium (major cation)
      • Calcium
      • Magnesium
      • Potassium
   4) Anions in ECF
      • Chloride (major anion)
      • Phosphate
      • Bicarbonate
      • Sulfate
      • Proteinate
      • Organic acids
6. Nonelectrolyte solutes
   a. No dissociation into ions
   b. Measured as weight per solution
   c. Examples include glucose, creatinine, urea, and bilirubin[5]

D. Homeostatic Mechanisms

1. Overview
   a. Internal chemical balance is necessary for normal bodily function
   b. Several organs are responsible for ensuring balance (homeostasis)
2. Renal system
   a. Kidneys act as major regulator of the body's water balance
   b. Body's water balance controlled by urine output
   c. Electrolytes are regulated through retention or excretion of urine
   d. Acid-base balance is maintained through excretion of hydrogen ions and generation of bicarbonate ions[6]
   e. Function in the excretion of metabolic wastes and toxic chemicals
3. Cardiac system
   a. Heart and blood vessels are responsible for circulating the blood through the kidneys, enabling urine production
   b. Fluid regulation is assisted by the cardiovascular system through fluid volume, pressure sensors, and atrial natriuretic factor[7]
4. Respiratory system
   a. Lungs remove water through exhalation
   b. Assists in the acid-base balance maintenance through regulation of hydrogen ions
5. Endocrine system
   a. Regulate those chemical reactions related to metabolism, growth, and reproduction
   b. Endocrine glands that control these reactions include the pituitary, adrenal, parathyroid, and thyroid
   c. Pituitary gland
      1) Signals received by hypothalamus from nervous system and electrolytes are transmitted to the pituitary
      2) Antidiuretic hormone (ADH) is secreted by the hypothalamus and stored in the posterior pituitary, and is important for regulating renal water excretion and conservation
   d. Andrenal gland
      1) Comprised of two components: adrenal cortex and adrenal medulla
      2) Of the two components, adrenal cortex (outside layer of adrenal gland) is more influential on fluid and electrolyte balance
      3) Aldosterone, a mineralocorticoid, is secreted by the adrenal cortex
         • Causes potassium excretion
         • Causes fluid volume restoration through sodium retention
      4) Cortisol also influences potassium excretion and sodium and fluid retention
   e. Parathyroid gland
      1) Production of parathyroid hormone affecting the regulation of calcium and phosphate

2) Increased parathyroid levels result in increased calcium level and decreased phosphate level

3) Opposite effect with decreased hormone level

f. Thyroid gland

1) Secretes calcitonin secretion to regulate calcium levels

2) Increased calcitonin levels lead to decreased calcium levels

II. PATIENT ASSESSMENT

A. Helps Determine Fluid and Electrolyte Status

B. Necessary for Treatment Plan Development

C. History Can Reveal Valuable Information about the Patient's Health Status and Potential for Fluid and Electrolyte Imbalances

1. Disease/injury status
   a. Renal, cardiac, respiratory, and endocrine system diseases
   b. Chronic alcoholism
   c. Carcinoma
   d. Massive trauma, including burns and crushing injuries
2. Medications
   a. Diuretics
      1) Fluid and electrolyte depletion
      2) Possible electrolyte excess (specific electrolyte dependent on type of diuretic)
   b. Laxatives possibly lead to potassium deficits
   c. Corticosteroids
      1) Possible fluid and electrolyte retention
      2) Potassium deficit
      3) Respiratory and metabolic alkalosis
   d. Inappropriate use of intravenous solutions
      1) Excessive use of sodium-containing solutions can result in fluid volume excess and hypernatremia
      2) Administration of electrolyte-free intravenous solutions can lead to electrolyte deficits
      3) Use of electrolyte-containing fluids could lead to excesses depending on the content
3. Fluid status
   a. Output exceeding intake may create fluid volume deficits or electrolyte imbalances
   b. Abnormal fluid loss through vomitus, gastrointestinal suctioning, fistulas, profuse perspiration, or diarrhea may result in imbalances
   c. Patient's activity and location of activity just prior to assessment can reveal if imbalance is related to activity level or excessive environmental temperature
4. Age

a. Takes longer and is more difficult for the elderly to regain homeostasis
b. Increased risk of fluid volume deficit with aging
  1) Reduction in total body fluid
  2) Diminished renal function
  3) Increased difficulty for respiratory system to maintain a normal pH
  4) Decreased skin turgor makes it more difficult to determine fluid status
  5) Poor intake or excessive fluid losses may occur due to confusion, decreased thirst threshold, or inability to obtain fluids, and diuretic/laxative use (most common problem is hypernatremia)
  6) Osteoporosis related to calcium deficits

D. Laboratory Data

1. Serum osmolality
  a. Measures the number of particles contained in a solution
  b. Primarily affected by the serum sodium content
  c. Concentration increases with dehydration and hyperglycemia
  d. Concentration decreases with fluid volume excess
2. Hematocrit
  a. Measures the percentage of red blood cells as compared with the plasma in whole blood
  b. Normal range is 44 to 52% for males and 39 to 47% for females
  c. Decreases with fluid volume excess as a result of the increased fluid diluting red blood cells
  d. Increases in dehydration as a result of less fluid available to dilute the cells
3. Blood urea nitrogen (BUN)
  a. Measures the amount of urea, the end product of protein metabolism, found in the serum
    1) Formed in the liver
    2) Picked up by the circulating blood
    3) Excreted through the renal system
  b. Normal adult level: 10 to 20 mg/dL
  c. Low BUN may result from overhydration, intravenous therapy, and low protein intake[9]
  d. Increased levels result from dehydration, excessive protein intake, diabetes mellitus, gastrointestinal bleeding, and renal disease
4. Serum creatinine
  a. Measurement of the serum level of creatinine, a byproduct of muscle catabolism, is directly proportional to the muscle mass
  b. Circulates in the blood, is filtered by glomeruli, and is not reabsorbed by the renal tubules

c. Generally not affected by diet or fluid levels and is a more sensitive indicator of renal disease

5. Serum electrolytes
   a. Measures the electrolytes found in the body
      1) Sodium
      2) Potassium
      3) Calcium
      4) Magnesium
      5) Phosphorus
      6) Chloride
      7) Bicarbonate
   b. Affected by fluid and electrolyte intake and excretion (see "Fluid Imbalances" and "Electrolyte Imbalances")

6. Arterial blood gases (ABGs)
   a. Measurement of pH, $PaCO_2$, PaO_2, bicarbonate, and base excess levels
   b. Used to evaluate acid-base balance (see "Acid-Base Balance and Imbalance" for further discussion)

7. Urinary specific gravity
   a. Measures the quantity and nature of particles in the urine
   b. Normal value is 1.003 to 1.030
   c. Affected by hydration status, renal status, and the number and size of particles in urine; large molecules such as glucose, protein, and radiologic contrast media will elevate results out of proportion to actual results

8. Urine osmolality
   a. Measures the number of particles, ions, and molecules in urine
   b. Not overly influenced by the size of the molecules
   c. Urine osmolality in conjunction with serum osmolality generally is considered a more accurate indication of renal concentrating ability than is the specific gravity measurement[11]

E. Clinical Assessment Parameters

1. Overall responsibilities
   a. Clinical assessment should be performed on patient admission and monitored on a continuing basis throughout the course of treatment
   b. Shared responsibility with emphasis for nursing staff because of increased patient contact
   c. Regular documentation
   d. Report any unusual or abnormal findings to the physician

2. Comparison of fluid intake and output
   a. Awareness of intake and output is needed for all patients, especially those with possible fluid and electrolyte imbalances
   b. Intake measurement includes all oral fluids, enteral feedings, other tube feedings, and parenteral solutions

    c. Individual volumes and the time of day are important for accurate comparison between intake and output and with body weight and should be totalled for a 24-hour period

    d. Output measurement includes urine, diarrhea, fistula drainage, vomitus, and any drainage obtained through suctioning

    e. Other fluid losses are important but not as easily measured

       1) Perspiration, respirations (particularly hyperventilation, respirator use, etc.), and drainage from lesions

       2) Document and quantify as much as possible, particularly in situations in which strict intake and output required

       3) Time of day also important

    f. Comparison of intake and output totals is important

       1) When total intake greater than output, fluid volume overload possible

       2) When output exceeds intake, fluid volume deficit possible

       3) Electrolyte imbalances possible from fluid volume deficits or excesses

       4) Apprise physician of abnormal findings

3. Urine

    a. Urine volume and concentration are indicators of homeostasis

       1) Urine volume is important component of total output for a patient

       2) Low urine volume may indicate fluid volume deficit

       3) High urine volume may suggest fluid volume excess

    b. Urine concentration also may indicate fluid imbalances

       1) Urine more concentrated with fluid volume deficit

       2) Urine less concentrated with fluid volume excess

       3) Urine concentration and volume are indicative of functioning renal and endocrine (ADH and aldosterone levels) systems

       4) Document findings and report abnormalities to physician

4. Skin and tongue turgor

    a. Tissue turgor is assessed by pinching the skin and observing the results on release of the skin

       1) With normal fluid balance, skin quickly returns to its normal position

       2) With fluid volume deficit, skin remains slightly elevated for several seconds

    b. Assessment sites for checking skin turgor include over the forearm, dorsum of the hand, forehead, and sternum, with the latter two areas generally considered the best sites

    c. Possible exceptions include checking skin turgor in the infant and elderly patient

       1) Depressed skin turgor, particularly in infants, may be a false indicator in the presence of malnutrition

       2) Normal skin turgor may be deceptive in indicating fluid volume deficit for obese infants[12]

          3) In older adults, due to a decrease in the skin's elasticity, assessment of skin turgor may not be a good indicator of fluid balance

          4) The best test sites for older adults are the sternum and forehead[13]

    d. Observation of the tongue reveals one longitudinal furrow under normal conditions

          1) Increase in number of furrows is indicative of reduced tissue volume related to fluid volume deficit

          2) With hypernatremia, the tongue may appear red and swollen

5. Thirst

    a. The presence or absence of thirst may be a sign of fluid imbalance

    b. This mechanism ensures an adequate fluid volume as long as thirst is present, fluid is available, and losses are not abnormally high

    c. Thirst is normally present but may be altered by certain conditions

          1) Nausea

          2) Vomiting

          3) Altered states of consciousness

          4) Inability to respond, including emotional factors

          5) Increasing age (older adult)

6. Tearing and salivation

    a. Tearing and salivation, normally observed, may not be present when there is a deficit in fluid volume

    b. A tearless cry or the lack of salivation in an infant over 3 months old is a good indicator of fluid volume deficit (becomes obvious with a 5% loss)[14]

7. Body weight

    a. Body weight is used as an indicator of fluid status

    b. 1 kilogram of body weight gained or lost is equal to approximately 1 liter of fluid

    c. Weight loss may be the result of several factors

          1) Can occur from loss of tissue from malnutrition secondary to lack of eating or receiving supplements (parenteral or enteral nutrition)

          2) Is more often indicative of fluid loss

             • Rapid fluid loss of 2% of the total body weight indicative of mild fluid volume deficit

             • A loss of 5% indicative of moderate deficit

             • A loss of 8% indicative of severe deficit

          3) Severe fluid volume deficit not always signaled by a loss of body weight, particularly when fluid is pulled from vascular system and trapped in a cavity, bowel, etc., as in third-spacing

    d. Rapid weight gain often indicates an increased fluid volume

          1) Gain can occur in any fluid compartment

- Overload in vascular space as a result of excessive administration of intravenous fluids or an excess of sodium
  - Body's inability to excrete fluid (renal disease, ascites, etc.)
2) Percentage of weight gain indicates severity of the excess: rapid weight gain of 2% indicates mild fluid volume excess; 5% indicates moderate excess; 8% indicates severe excess[15]
  e. Daily weight recordings are used for comparisons to detect losses or gains
    1) Weight taken at same time every day
    2) Best time is in the morning after voiding and before eating
    3) For accuracy, same type of scales should be used and same type of clothing should be worn each day
    4) Dry clothing worn to prevent additional nonbody weight
    5) Findings should be recorded in a manner for easy day-to-day comparison of losses or gains
8. Edema
  a. Edema is excessive fluid in the interstitial space
    1) Localized edema may occur as a result of inflammation
    2) Generalized edema may result from excessive sodium and water retention or from altered capillary hemodynamics
  b. Generally, edema is more visible in dependent areas such as the feet and ankles
  c. Edema in the back and buttocks is common in patients confined to bed
  d. Edema is often classified according to the severity of the swelling
    1) Barely detectible edema rated as +1
    2) Severe edema rated as +4
    3) Degree of pitting best assessed over a bony prominence
9. Appearance and temperature of the skin
  a. Appearance and temperature of the skin may be affected by fluid and electrolyte imbalances
  b. Pale skin may result from peripheral vasoconstriction secondary to fluid volume deficit
  c. Warm, flushed skin may occur from vasodilation, as found with metabolic acidosis[16]
  d. Skin temperature may indicate imbalances
    1) With hypovolemia, skin may be cool to the touch
    2) With hypernatremic dehydration, skin temperature may be elevated
10. Vital signs
  a. One of the first and often easiest means of assessment and should be documented for easy comparison
  b. Temperature
    1) Elevated temperature may result in loss of fluids and electrolytes from excessive sweating
    2) Temperature may indicate an imbalance

• May increase with fluid volume deficits
• May decrease with hypovolemia
c. Pulse
1) Increased heart rate in an attempt to maintain cardiac output with a fluid volume deficit; pulse usually is weak with fluid volume deficit and full and bounding with fluid volume excess
2) Potassium and magnesium deficits and sodium excess may cause increased heart rate
3) Decreased heart rate may result from severe hyperkalemia or hypermagnesemia
4) Irregularities in heart rate with potassium imbalances or magnesium deficit
5) Electrocardiogram (ECG) changes possible with potassium, calcium, and magnesium excesses or deficits as related to regularity
d. Respirations
1) Increased respiratory rate may lead to increased fluid loss
2) Fluid volume deficit possible from increased production of respiratory secretions
3) Shortness of breath and moist rales seen with fluid volume excess
4) Mechanical ventilation associated with fluid gain
5) Deep, rapid respirations indicative of respiratory alkalosis or compensation for metabolic acidosis
6) Slow, shallow respirations indicative of respiratory acidosis or compensation for metabolic alkalosis
e. Blood pressure
1) Increased blood pressure with fluid volume excess
2) Decreased blood pressure with fluid volume deficit
3) Decreased blood pressure with magnesium excess from decreased vascular resistance
4) Changes in blood pressure with sodium imbalances secondary to fluid volume levels
5) Postural hypotension possible with hypokalemia
6) Possible decreased blood pressure related to hypophosphatemia
11. Appearance of the oral cavity
a. Normally, the oral mucous membranes are moist
b. Possibly altered in individuals who breathe mainly through the mouth
c. Sticky, dry mucous membranes may be indicative of fluid volume deficit or hypernatremia
12. Central venous pressure
a. Measurement of mean right atrial pressure
b. Readings should be taken with the patient in the same position each time

    c. Low readings may be related to a decrease in fluid volume
    d. High readings may be related to an increased blood volume
13. Neurological indicators
    a. Changes may occur in sensorium, including levels of awareness, orientation, and consciousness[17] from acid-base and electrolyte imbalances
       1) Degree of changes directly related to severity of imbalance
       2) Restlessness and confusion may result from fluid volume deficit
    b. Disturbances in neuromuscular excitability may occur as a result of electrolyte imbalances
       1) Increased excitability seen with calcium and magnesium deficits
       2) Depressed neuromuscular activity seen with excesses of calcium and magnesium
    c. Neuromotor symptoms result from metabolic alkalosis, which decreases calcium ionization
       1) Tingling of fingers and toes
       2) Hypertonic muscles
       3) Dizziness
    d. Chvostek's and Trousseau's signs are useful in determining calcium and magnesium imbalances
       1) Chvostek's sign elicited by tapping facial nerve slightly anterior to earlobe
       2) Positive Chvostek's sign indicated by unilateral contraction of facial and eyelid muscles
       3) Trousseau's sign created by inflating blood pressure cuff placed on upper arm to a level above systolic pressure
       4) Positive Trousseau's sign indicated by hand spasm, resulting from decreased blood supply
    e. Other neuromotor symptoms are related to potassium imbalances; they vary depending on level excesses or deficits (see "Fluid and Electrolyte Imbalances: Potassium")
14. Other indicators
    a. Changes in the circulating volume of fluid are detected by observation of the neck and hand veins
    b. In a dependent position and in the presence of a fluid volume deficit, neck veins are flat and filling of hand veins is delayed
    c. With increased plasma volume, emptying of hand veins is delayed and veins appear engorged

III. FLUID IMBALANCES

A. Fluid Volume Excess (hypervolemia)

  1. Description
     a. An increase in the fluid volume of the extracellular compartment
     b. Can occur in the intravascular or interstitial compartments, or both

c. Generally retains the same proportion of water and electrolytes

2. Etiology

    a. Intake of sodium and water

        1) Excessive intake of intravenous solutions

          • Rapid administration of solutions

          • Continuous or excessive use of sodium-containing solutions leading to water retention

        2) Ingestion of sodium-containing foods in patients with renal or cardiac disease resulting in increased thirst and fluid intake

        3) Oral or intravenous medications containing sodium may lead to fluid retention

    b. Conservation of water and sodium

        1) Abnormal antidiuretic hormone (ADH) production or increased aldosterone, as occurs postoperatively

        2) Circulating intravascular volume often decreased with congestive heart failure, renal diseases, and cirrhosis of the liver

          • Subsequent renin and aldosterone production lead to increased water and sodium conservation

        3) Corticosteroid therapy will increase water and sodium retention

    c. Fluid shifts

        1) Shift of fluid from interstitial to vascular space may increase fluid volume excess

        2) Possible during treatment of burns or with use of hypertonic intravenous solutions or medications

    d. Inability to excrete fluids

        1) Secondary to renal diseases resulting in decreased renal function leading to decreased output

        2) Continuous fluid ingestion then leads to an intake that exceeds output

3. Signs and symptoms (dependent on severity and location of excess)

    a. Elevated blood pressure

    b. Increased pulse rate, bounding

    c. Possible extra heart sound

    d. Increased central venous pressure

    e. Distended neck veins

    f. Engorged peripheral veins with slowed hand vein emptying

    g. Pulmonary edema

        1) Shortness of breath

        2) Moist rales

        3) Increased respirations

    h. Body weight increases as fluid increases in the extracellular compartment (exception: if fluid excess is caused by fluid shift between compartments)

    i. Peripheral edema, possibly pitting edema in dependent areas such as the feet and ankles

1) Determined by applying pressure for several seconds
2) If edema present, the indention from finger pressure remains
3) Severity measured by size of indention and length of time required to disappear

    j. Ascites
1) Subsequent shortness of breath as a result of increased pressure on diaphragm
2) Drop in cardiac output as a result of poor right ventricle filling

    k. Diagnostic testing
1) Hematocrit: decreased as a result of hemodilution
2) ABGs: decreased oxygen content, decreased $PaCO_2$, and increased pH
3) Chest x-ray: pulmonary vascular congestion
4) Serum sodium and osmolality: possibly decreased as a result of excessive fluid retention, particularly if renal disease is present
5) BUN and creatinine levels: increased with renal or cardiac failure

    l. Urine-specific gravity: decreased as kidneys try to excrete excessive fluid

4. Treatment
    a. Elimination of precipitating factors and return of ECF to a normal level
    b. Sodium and water restriction
    c. Diuretic therapy
    d. Bed rest

5. Nursing interventions
    a. Continue to assess clinical parameters such as vital signs, body weight, and edema
    b. Frequently monitor intake and output
    c. If diuretic therapy is used, document response
    d. Observe for any signs of overcorrection resulting in a fluid volume deficit
    e. Monitor for related conditions such as pulmonary edema and ascites
    f. Document all pertinent observations and report abnormal findings to the physician

B. Fluid Volume Deficit (hypovolemia)

1. Description
    a. Decreased fluid volume in the extracellular compartment
    b. With fluid loss, electrolytes are lost, further complicating the body's ability to retain water
    c. Inadequate fluid intake is a factor
    d. Possible related problems include acid-base, fluid, and/or electrolyte imbalances

2. Etiology
   a. Abnormal fluid loss
      1) Gastrointestinal tract is most common route
         • Vomiting
         • Suctioning
         • Diarrhea
         • Fistulas
         • Laxative abuse
      2) Fluid lost by way of the skin
         • Insensible fluid loss used as mechanism to regulate temperature within body
         • Elevated temperatures as a result of illness or strenuous activity causing body to dissipate heat, resulting in increased fluid loss
         • Any breaks in the skin, such as burns and wounds, allowing fluid to escape body
      3) Hemorrhage rapidly decreasing fluid volume in the intravascular space
         • Surgery
         • Trauma
         • Bleeding disorders
         • Accidental disconnection of intravenous tubing from venipuncture device or from central line catheters
      4) Renal disease or use of diuretics
      5) Fluid shifting from one area to another, where it cannot be readily used by the body (third spacing)
         • Ascites
         • Internal bleeding
         • Burns
         • Fluid trapped in bowel or body cavities, such as the pleural, pericardial, or peritoneal spaces
   b. Decreased intake
      1) Failure to prescribe or deliver adequate amounts of intravenous solutions
      2) Lack of available fluids, such as with infants or older adults who are physically unable to get to a fluid source
      3) Alteration of the thirst mechanism
      4) Older adults have a decreased sense of thirst and may not seek adequate replacement
      5) Difficulty communicating the need for fluid
         • Infants
         • Comatose patients
3. Signs and symptoms (directly related to severity of the deficiency)
   a. Weight loss (particularly with rapid fluid loss) except with third-spacing
   b. Decreased central venous pressure

    c. Flattened jugular veins (in the supine position)

    d. Slowed hand vein filling

    e. Decreased blood pressure as a result of decreased circulating volume

    f. Postural hypotension

    g. Neurological indicators such as muscle weakness, dizziness, lethargy, and confusion from decreased tissue perfusion

    h. Weak, rapid pulse in an attempt to maintain an adequate circulating volume within the vascular system

    i. Decreased urine output as the body tries to conserve fluid (in hypovolemic states, the urinary output typically is less than 30 ml/hr)

    j. Decreased skin turgor

    k. Soft, small tongue with several longitudinal furrows instead of the normal one furrow

    l. Pinched facial expression

    m. Soft, sunken eyes

    n. With severe losses, patient may go into shock

        1) Cool, clammy extremities

        2) Diaphoresis

        3) Sharp drop in urine output

        4) Coma

    o. Laboratory data

        1) Serum BUN: decreased

        2) Hematocrit: decreased (unless deficit is caused by bleeding)

        3) Serum electrolytes, serum osmolality, and acid-base balance: dependent on cause of deficit and the type of fluid lost

        4) Urine-specific gravity: increased

        5) Urine osmolality: increased

4. Treatment

    a. Correction of the cause of the deficit

    b. Restoration of the ECF level

    c. Initially, fluid replacement with an isotonic electrolyte solution such as lactated Ringer's

        1) Prompt vascular access should be initiated in accordance with the *Intravenous Nursing Standards of Practice*

        2) Gauge of venipuncture device is sufficient to carry adequate volumes of solution for replacement

    d. Replacement rate is dependent on the severity of the deficit

    e. Once volume replacement is achieved, replacement solutions are chosen to provide free water to assist the kidneys in excreting wastes

    f. Possible fluid challenge test necessary if oliguria is present to determine the cause

        1) Intravenous solutions administered according to a specific plan

        2) Patient monitored closely

- Increased urinary output indicating that oliguria was related to the hypovolemia
- No change in the output possibly indicating the cause to be renal failure or decreased cardiac function

5. Nursing interventions
   a. Assess vital signs, urinary output, hemodynamic pressures, laboratory findings, and body weight
   b. Monitor the rate of intravenous solution administration
   c. With rehydration, look for a drop in hematocrit that may necessitate blood administration

IV. ELECTROLYTE IMBALANCES

A. Sodium

1. Overview
   a. The major electrolyte (cation) in the ECF
   b. Important functions in the body
      1) Controls water distribution
      2) Maintains volume of ECF
      3) Promotes irritability of nerve and muscle tissue
      4) Transmits nerve impulses
      5) Maintains acid-base balance
   c. Normal serum sodium value: 135 to 145 mEq/L
2. Hyponatremia
   a. Definition
      1) Sodium deficit
      2) Level below 135 mEq/L
   b. Etiology
      1) Excessive intake of water
         - Administration of excessive water or dextrose-containing intravenous solutions resulting in water excess (edema) and dilution of sodium concentration
         - Excessive fluid intake as a result of a chronic psychiatric disorder, psychogenic polydipsia resulting in dilutional hyponatremia
         - Syndrome of Inappropriate Antidiuretic Hormone (SIADH): inappropriate secretion of ADH resulting in excessive water retention
      2) Excessive sodium loss
         - Use of diuretics
         - Adrenal insufficiency resulting in stimulation of the ADH and increased water retention leading to hyponatremia
         - Excessive sweating, such as occurs in children with cystic fibrosis, increasing loss of sodium
   c. Signs and symptoms (dependent on cause and rate of onset)

1) A decrease in plasma osmolality may result in fluid being pulled into cells; signs and symptoms relative to affected cells
- Overhydration of brain cells results in nausea, vomiting, weakness, muscular twitching, confusion, and coma

2) Deficit due to water gain results in same symptoms of hypervolemia
- Weight gain
- Edema

3) Deficit caused by fluid loss results in signs and symptoms of hypovolemia
- Hypotension
- Dizziness

4) Laboratory data
- Serum sodium level: below 135 mEq/L
- Serum osmolality: decreased
- Urine sodium and specific gravity: increased (with SIADH); decreased (with excessive sodium losses)

d. Treatment
1) Dependent on etiology
2) Deficit as a result of loss of fluids
- Sodium and fluid replacement orally or with intravenous solutions
- Hypertonic sodium chloride intravenous solutions for extremely low sodium levels

3) Deficit related to fluid gain
- Diuretics to excrete excess fluid
- Hypertonic sodium chloride solutions along with loop diuretics for severe hyponatremia

4) Deficit as a result of SIADH
- Removal of cause
- Diuretics
- Fluid restriction
- Medication to inhibit action of ADH (chronic SIADH)

e. Nursing interventions
1) Assess patient for clinical signs and symptoms
2) Monitor laboratory values
3) Administer medications and intravenous solutions as ordered
4) Document observations and interventions, especially when giving hypertonic sodium chloride
5) Notify physician of abnormal findings

3. Hypernatremia
a. Definition
1) Sodium excess
2) Serum level about 145 mEq/L

b. Etiology
1) Excessive sodium

- Intravenous administration of sodium-containing solutions or medications
- Decreased excretion of sodium, such as with primary aldosteronism

2) Increased water loss
- Burns
- Diaphoresis
- Increased insensible fluid loss from the lungs
- Impaired thirst or inability to get water (normally with hypernatremia, thirst response is initiated and thirst satisfied by fluid intake, which replaces volume deficit)
- Osmotic diuresis, such as from administration of mannitol or elevated glucose level
- Diabetes insipidus (a lack of functioning ADH)

c. Signs and symptoms (many related to intracellular volume; more apparent increases)

1) Moderate imbalance first evident by restlessness, fatigue, and weakness; more prominent signs develop as cells become more dehydrated

2) Neurological signs
- Agitation
- Delirium
- Seizures
- Coma

3) Thirst

4) Dry and sticky mucous membranes

5) Decreased saliva and tears

6) Rough, red, dry tongue possibly becoming swollen, creating speech difficulties

7) Elevated temperature

8) Flushed skin

9) Diagnostic data
- Serum sodium level: elevated
- Serum osmolality: elevated
- Central venous pressure: low due to fluid loss
- Urine-specific gravity: increases as the kidneys attempt to conserve water
- ADH levels or vasopressin test: if diabetes insipidus suspected

d. Treatment

1) Restoration of sodium to a normal level

2) Dependent on etiology

3) Related to sodium excess: sodium restriction

4) Related to water loss
- Replacement with oral fluids or intravenous solutions with hypotonic electrolyte solutions or 5% dextrose in water
- Replacement done with caution to prevent rapid correction

due to possible shift of water into brain cells resulting in cerebral edema
- Diuretics (to help prevent cerebral edema)

e. Nursing interventions
1) Assess patient for clinical signs and symptoms
2) Establish patent intravenous line
3) Monitor venipuncture site and flow rate
4) When intravenous therapy is used, closely monitor for signs of cerebral edema and immediately report any signs to the physician
5) Document observations and interventions
6) Notify physician of abnormal findings
7) Institute precautions as needed for patient orientation and safety secondary to confusion, delirium, and seizures

B. Potassium

1. Overview
a. The main cation in the intracellular compartment; small amount of potassium in the ECF
b. Balance of intracellular and extracellular potassium is maintained through the action of the sodium-potassium pump
c. Kidneys act as the main regulators
1) Kidneys respond to increased serum levels of potassium by promoting greater potassium excretion in urine
2) Increased levels stimulate aldosterone production, leading to increased sodium and water retention and potassium excretion
d. Maintenance of adequate levels is dependent on regular replenishment
e. Important functions in the body
1) Controls osmotic pressure within the cells
2) Influences action of the kidneys
3) Assists in regulating acid-base balance
4) Helps to maintain neuromuscular activity, particularly the cardiac system
f. Normal serum potassium level: 3.5 to 5.0 mEq/L
2. Hypokalemia
a. Definition
1) Potassium deficit
2) Serum level below 3.5 mEq/L
b. Etiology
1) Potassium loss (major cause)
- Main cause is the use of diuretics, particularly loop diuretics (furosemide and ethacrynic acid) and thiazides
- Increased aldosterone levels
- Abnormal losses through gastrointestinal fluids such as gastric suctioning, vomitus, diarrhea, and fistulas

- Severe trauma
- Osmotic diuresis
- Increased sweating

2) Inadequate intake
- Inadequate replacement in parenteral or total parenteral nutrition solutions
- Potassium-poor diet (rare)

3) Stress
- Physical or emotional stress leads to increased release of aldosterone and epinephrine, which increase urinary potassium loss and shift potassium into the cells

4) Potassium movement into cells from extracellular space
- Alkalosis
- Tissue repair from trauma or burns
- Increased glucose (TPN solutions)
- Insulin

c. Signs and symptoms (level generally below 3 mEq/L before indicators are present)[18]

1) Slowed muscle and nerve impulse transmission
- Fatigue
- Leg cramps
- Paresthesias
- Muscle weakness
- Drowsiness
- Diminished deep tendon reflexes
- Nausea
- Vomiting
- Decreased bowel motility

2) Altered cardiac function
- Irregular pulse
- Dysrhythmias
- Increased sensitivity to digitalis

3) Diagnostic data
- Serum potassium level: below 3.5 mEq/L
- ABGs: metabolic alkalosis
- Urine potassium level: some loss (because the kidneys have difficulty conserving potassium)
- ECG: ST segment depression, flattened T waves, and a U wave possibly superimposed on the T giving the impression of a prolonged QT interval[19]

d. Treatment
1) Mild depletions treated with diet or supplements
2) Extremely low levels are usually treated with intravenous potassium
- Potassium acetate
- Potassium phosphate

- Potassium chloride (most frequently used)
3) Administration of a nonpotassium-containing solution may be necessary first to ensure adequate hydration and renal function
4) Potassium chloride must be diluted before administration
   - Must not be given IV push
   - Concentration generally does not exceed 40 mEq/L
   - Flow rate should not exceed 20 mEq/hr except in cases of severe depletion in which maximum concentration should not exceed 80 mEq/L[20]
   - Caution necessary when administering high concentrations at a rapid rate because of potential for cardiac side effects
e. Nursing interventions
   1) Assess patient for clinical signs and symptoms
   2) Initiate an intravenous line
   3) Administer properly diluted potassium admixtures
   4) Observe the patient and the venipuncture site for possible vascular intolerance
   5) Be alert for complaints of pain related to intravenous administration
      - Decrease flow rate
      - Further dilute admixture
      - Initiate secondary intravenous line
   6) Monitor ECG readings on an ongoing basis
   7) Monitor serum potassium levels on an ongoing basis
   8) Document observations and interventions
   9) Notify physician of abnormal findings
3. Hyperkalemia
   a. Definition
      1) Potassium excess
      2) Serum level above 5.0 mEq/L
      3) Frequently associated with renal disease
   b. Etiology
      1) Increased intake
         - Intravenous administration of inappropriate amounts of potassium
         - Inadequately diluted potassium-containing solutions
         - Renal disease; even small amounts of potassium may be problematic
         - Aged blood; potassium released with breakdown of blood cells and may become excessive
      2) Decreased excretion
         - Renal disease—acute or chronic failure
         - Use of potassium-sparing diuretics may result in fluid volume elimination greater than potassium excretion; similar problems possible with any ECF depletion
         - Decreased secretion of aldosterone

      3) Potassium shift from the cells to extracellular fluid
- Metabolic acidosis causes positively charged hydrogen ions to enter the cells and forces potassium cations out of the cells
- Hyperglycemia where potassium is pulled from the cells as water moves out of the cells in attempt to dilute concentrated glucose content
- Breakdown of cells allows excessive potassium to enter extracellular compartments as a result of burns, trauma, and sepsis

      4) Improper technique in obtaining blood samples indicating false high levels of potassium (considered if levels are excessive without any clinical signs)
- Tourniquet left on too long
- Hemolysis of the blood cells
- Delayed separation of serum and cells
- Blood samples drawn in close proximity of an infusing potassium-containing intravenous solution

  c. Signs and symptoms

      1) Clinical picture is usually related to altered cardiac or neuromuscular activity

      2) Impulses necessary for sending messages to the nerves and muscles are altered, creating an increase in neuromuscular excitability
- Paresthesias (face, tongue, hands, and feet)
- Gastrointestinal hyperactivity (diarrhea, nausea, abdominal cramping)
- Irritability

      3) As the level increases, the cardiac and neuromuscular cells of the lower extremities are unable to handle the rapid signals
- Weakness progressing to body and arms
- Heart rate affected eventually leading to atrial and/or ventricular fibrillation and heart block

      4) Diagnostic data
- Serum potassium level: above 5.5 mEq/L
- ABGs: metabolic acidosis
- ECG: high-tented T waves, absences of P waves, and prolonged QRS complexes, indicating impending cardiac arrest

  d. Treatment

      1) Eliminate the cause

      2) Mild excesses treated with cation exchange resins

      3) Use of intravenous hypertonic glucose and insulin for temporary treatment of moderate to severe excesses
- Potassium shifts back into the cells
- Once started, this form of treatment continued until normal levels attained

      4) Sodium bicarbonate

- Temporary treatment that shifts potassium into the cells
- Reduction lasting for only 1 to 2 hours[21]
5) Calcium gluconate
- Used in severe cases when cardiac abnormalities present
- Effects of potassium on the myocardiurn antagonized
- Only a temporary effect, lasting approximately 1 hour
6) Dialysis including hemo- or peritoneal dialysis to remove excess potassium in severe hyperkalemia
e. Nursing interventions
1) Assess patient for clinical signs and symptoms
2) Monitor intake and output and serum potassium level
3) Evaluate ECG for changes
4) Initiate intravenous access for administration of insulin, dextrose, or sodium bicarbonate
5) Monitor patient for signs and symptoms of potassium shift, rebound hypoglycemia, or sodium excess during administration
6) Use calcium gluconate cautiously with patients receiving digitalis
- Monitor ECG
- Observe for signs of digitalis toxicity
- Stop medication immediately if bradycardia occurs
7) Document observations and interventions
8) Notify physician of abnormal findings

C. Calcium

1. Overview
   a. Cation with important body functions
   1) Formation of teeth and bones
   2) Muscle contraction
   3) Normal clotting
   4) Neural function
   b. Available as ionized, bound, and complex
   1) Approximately 50% of total volume is in ionized form
   2) Slightly less occurs in bound form
   3) Small percentage is in complex form
   c. Approximately 1 to 2% of the total calcium is found in the ECF
   d. Regulated by the parathyroid hormone and calcitonin
   e. Eliminated through the gastrointestinal tract, urinary tract, and sweat; also deposited in the bone
   f. Reciprocal relationship with phosphorus
   g. Normal serum calcium level: 8.9 to 10.3 mg/dL (ionized portion is approximately half the total value)[22]
2. Hypocalcemia
   a. Definition
   1) Calcium deficit
   2) Serum level below 4.6 mEq/L
   b. Etiology

1) Reduced intestinal absorption
   - Vitamin D deficiency
   - Decreased intake
   - Small bowel disease
   - Continuous infusion of calcium-free intravenous solutions
2) Increased calcium losses
   - Diuretics
   - Renal disease
   - Fistulas
   - Burns
   - Infections
3) Altered regulation: hypoparathyroidism secondary to surgery or injury to the parathyroid glands
4) Phosphorus or magnesium imbalances
   - Increased phosphorus levels lead to decreased calcium levels due to reciprocal relationship of calcium and phosphorus
   - Increased bone uptake of calcium results in decreased magnesium levels in bone
5) Other causes
   - Acute pancreatitis
   - Alkalosis
   - Decreased serum albumin

c. Signs and symptoms (primarily related to neuromuscular activity)
1) Numbness and tingling of the fingers, toes, and circumoral region
2) Tetany
3) Convulsions
4) Hyperactive deep tendon reflexes
5) Muscle cramps
6) Positive Trousseau's and Chvostek's signs
7) Mental changes
   - Depression
   - Confusion
8) Respiratory effects (seen with more severe deficits)
   - Dyspnea
   - Stridor
   - Spasm of the laryngeal muscles
9) Diagnostic data
   - Serum calcium level: below 4.6 mEq/L
   - Serum phosphorus level: may be elevated
   - Serum magnesium: decreased
   - ECG: prolonged QT interval and ST segment

d. Treatment
1) Emergency treatment is required as acute hypocalcemia is a potentially life-threatening situation
2) Correct cause as quickly as possible

3) Administration of oral or intravenous calcium
- Calcium chloride (more concentrated form)
- Calcium gluconate (drug of choice)

4) Caution is used in intravenous calcium administration as extravasation may result in cellulitis, necrosis, and sloughing of tissue

e. Nursing interventions
1) Assess patient for clinical signs and symptoms
2) Initiate intravenous line for rapid calcium administration
3) Monitor laboratory values and ECG
4) Protect the patient if tetany is present
5) Institute precautions related to respiratory problems
6) Document observations and interventions
7) Notify physician of abnormal findings

3. Hypercalcemia
a. Definition
1) Calcium excess
2) Serum level above 5.1 mEq/L
3) Increases may occur in the total serum calcium or free ionized calcium[23]

b. Etiology
1) Calcium loss from bone
- Hyperparathyroidism
- Malignancy (as a result of the release of parathyroid hormone, bone metastasis, or medications)
- Prolonged immobilization or multiple fractures resulting in calcium release from the bones
2) Increased intake
- Excessive administration of intravenous calcium
- Use of calcium-containing antacids
3) Decreased excretion of calcium
- Renal disease
- Hyperparathyroidism
- Medications such as thiazides
4) Excess ionized calcium level from acidosis

c. Signs and symptoms (vary according to serum level)
1) Initial symptoms may be misleading because of an association with a variety of disorders
- Anorexia
- Fatigue
- Lethargy
- Muscle weakness
- Nausea
- Vomiting
- Dehydration
- Constipation

2) Decreased ability of the kidneys to concentrate urine
   • Polyuria
   • Polydipsia
3) Other signs and symptoms
   • Bone pain
   • Generalized osteoporosis
   • Personality changes ranging from neurotic behavior to psychosis
4) Diagnostic data
   • Serum calcium level: increased
   • ECG: shortened ST segment and QT interval, a widened and rounded T wave, and a slightly widened QRS and PR interval
d. Treatment
   1) Elimination of cause
   2) Reduction of calcium level
   3) Intravenous administration of 0.45% or 0.9% sodium chloride
      • In absence of renal disease to dilute the body fluids
      • Helpful in eliminating calcium for severe hypercalcemia
   4) Furosemide (Lasix) loop diuretic may be used to increase urinary excretion of calcium
   5) Calcitonin for temporary correction
   6) Chemotherapy or radiation therapy to reduce the tumor if the excess is related to malignancy
   7) Corticosteroids to reduce bone turnover and reabsorption by the renal system
   8) Plicamycin (Mithracin) may be used to inhibit bone reabsorption
e. Nursing interventions
   1) Assess patient for clinical signs and symptoms
   2) Monitor patient for indicators of calcium excess
      • Serum level
      • ECG
      • Renal function
   3) Administer medications as ordered while observing for side effects
   4) Document observations and interventions
   5) Notify physician of abnormal findings

D. Magnesium

1. Overview
   a. Cation located primarily in the cells of bones and muscles
   b. Small percentage is found in the ECF compartment
   c. Excreted mainly by the kidneys
   d. Close to one-third of the magnesium is bound to protein
      1) Most of remaining electrolyte occurring as free or ionized
      2) Serum levels not an accurate reflection of total amount of magnesium in body
   e. Important functions in the body
      1) Activates enzymes

2) Affects protein and carbohydrate metabolism

3) Directly acts on the myoneural junction affecting neuromuscular irritability and contractility

4) Acts on skeletal muscle by depressing acetylcholine release at the synaptic junction

5) Affects cardiovascular system by contributing to vasodilation leading to changes in blood pressure and cardiac output[24]

  f. Levels and actions of magnesium are interdependent with those of calcium and potassium

  g. Normal serum magnesium level: 1.3 to 2.1 mEq/L

2. Hypomagnesemia

  a. Definition

    1) Magnesium deficit

    2) Serum level below 1.3 mEq/L

  b. Etiology

    1) Decreased intake

- Dietary insufficiency
- Refeeding after starvation
- Continuous use of magnesium-free parenteral solutions

    2) Improper gastrointestinal absorption

- Malabsorption syndrome
- Small bowel resection
- Colitis

    3) Increased elimination

- Prolonged diarrhea
- Vomiting
- Nasogastric suctioning
- Intestinal fistulas
- Some medications including laxatives, diuretics, Cisplatin (Platinol), Amphotericin B (Fungizone), and aminoglycosides may enhance excretion through the renal system

    4) Chronic alcoholism

- Primary cause
- Result of poor dietary intake, intestinal malabsorption, diarrhea, and increased urinary output

  c. Signs and symptoms

    1) Neuromuscular indicators

- Positive Trousseau's and Chvostek's signs
- Increased reflexes
- Tremors
- Convulsions
- Tetany
- Paresthesias
- Painfully cold sensations in hands and feet

    2) Mental indicators

- Depression
- Personality disorders

- Confusion
- Delirium
3) Cardiovascular indicators
  - Dysrhythmias such as ventricular tachycardia and ventricular fibrillation
  - Increased risk for digitalis toxicity
4) Diagnostic data
  - Serum magnesium level: below 1.3 mEq/L
  - Urine magnesium level: increased
  - Serum calcium: often low
  - ECG: prolonged PR interval and a widening QRS complex depending on the severity of the deficit; possible ST segment depression and broad, flat T waves
d. Treatment
  1) Prevention is the key to management
  2) Oral, intramuscular, or intravenous supplements once the deficit occurs
     - Oral supplements to treat mild to moderate deficits and continuing losses
     - Intravenous magnesium (magnesium sulfate as drug of choice) for treating severe deficits
e. Nursing interventions
  1) Assess patient for clinical signs and symptoms
  2) Consider the degree of loss and renal status when giving magnesium as it is eliminated by the kidneys
  3) Ensure urinary output of at least 100 ml every 4 hours[25]
  4) Periodically check knee-jerk reflexes
     - Keep in mind that deep tendon reflexes disappear just before depressed respirations
     - Notify physician if reflex is absent
  5) Assess vital signs frequently to detect any decreases in blood pressure or labored respirations when large doses of magnesium are given
  6) Monitor serum levels
  7) Prepare to counteract respiratory arrest before administering magnesium in case the magnesium level becomes excessive
  8) Institute seizure precautions
  9) Stop the intravenous infusion immediately should any side effects appear
  10) Have calcium gluconate readily available to reverse signs of magnesium overload
  11) Document observations and interventions
  12) Notify physician of abnormal findings
3. Hypermagnesemia
  a. Definition
    1) Magnesium excess
    2) Serum level above 2.1 mEq/L

b. Etiology
   1) Decreased elimination
      • Renal disease is the major cause; often associated with additional magnesium intake
      • Endocrine disturbances including hypothyroidism, hyperparathyroidism, and Addison's disease
   2) Increased intake
      • Medications including laxatives and antacids
      • Continued or excessive intravenous administration, such as with treatment for eclampsia
c. Signs and symptoms (usually not present until levels become excessively elevated)
   1) Interference with neuromuscular transmission
      • Increased muscle weakness
      • Paralysis
      • Decreased deep tendon reflexes
      • Respiratory muscle depression with eventual paralysis (at higher levels)
   2) Gastrointestinal indicators
      • Nausea
      • Vomiting
   3) Cardiovascular indicators (become increasingly severe with rising levels)
      • Flushing and sensation of skin warmth as a result of vasodilation (at low serum levels)
      • Pulse rate may decrease (bradycardia) eventually leading to heart block (with increasing levels)
   4) Diagnostic data
      • Serum magnesium level: increased
      • ECG: prolonged PR, QT, and QRS intervals; heart block and cardiac arrest with severely increased levels
d. Treatment (dependent on severity of imbalance)
   1) Prevention is the key
   2) Elimination of the cause is important
   3) 0.45% sodium chloride solution given intravenously along with diuretics to help facilitate elimination of the excess magnesium for moderate cases not complicated by renal disease
   4) Calcium gluconate given intravenously as a temporary measure to antagonize the action of the magnesium for more severe excesses
   5) With renal impairment, dialysis may be the only method to eliminate the excessive magnesium ions
e. Nursing interventions
   1) Assess patient for clinical signs and symptoms
   2) Monitor serum magnesium levels
   3) Have equipment readily accessible to assist respirations
   4) Initiate an intravenous line (for severe cases) according to established standards

5) Monitor the site and flow rate on a continuing basis
6) Document observations and interventions
7) Notify physician of abnormal findings
8) Provide patient teaching, including cautions about the use of over-the-counter magnesium-containing medications

E. Phosphate

1. Overview
    a. Located in the intracellular and extracellular compartments; only a small amount is located intracellularly
    b. Major anion in the ICF, primarily found in the bones and teeth
    c. Ability to shift between compartments; usually present in the body in the form of phosphate (the two terms, phosphorus and phosphate, are frequently used interchangeably)
    d. Metabolism and homeostasis of phosphates are related to calcium metabolism
        1) Concentrations of both controlled by parathyroid gland
        2) Vitamin D necessary for their absorption from the gastrointestinal tract
        3) Calcium and phosphate have an inverse proportional relationship
    e. Important functions in the body
        1) Metabolism of carbohydrates, fats, and protein
        2) Transfer of energy
        3) Maintenance of acid-base balance (primary urinary buffer)
        4) Promotion of muscle and nerve activity
    f. Normal serum phosphate level: 2.5 to 4.5 mg/dL
2. Hypophosphatemia
    a. Definition
        1) Phosphate deficit
        2) Serum level below 2.5 mg/dL
    b. Etiology
        1) Transient intracellular shifts (phosphate movement into cells)
            • Administration of high concentrations of glucose
            • Increased intracellular pH (as occurs in respiratory alkalosis)
        2) Increased losses
            • Diuretics (thiazides)
            • Hypokalemia
            • Hyperparathyroidism
            • Hypomagnesemia
        3) Reduced intestinal absorption
            • Antacid use
            • Vomiting
            • Diarrhea
            • Malabsorption syndromes
            • Alcoholism
    c. Signs and symptoms (related to how rapidly the deficit occurs)

1) Chronic deficits demonstrate subtle indicators
   - Bone pain
   - Memory loss
   - Muscle weakness
2) Acute losses result in more severe signs and symptoms
   - Paresthesias
   - Muscle pain
   - Seizures
   - Numbness
   - Coma
3) Cardiovascular indicators
   - Dysrhythmias
   - Heart failure
   - Shock
4) Respiratory muscle weakness may lead to respiratory failure
5) Altered red blood cell makeup and ability of red and white blood cells to function
6) Laboratory data
   - Serum phosphate level: low
   - Serum magnesium and potassium levels: low
   - Parathyroid hormone level: elevated if deficit is caused by hyperparathyroidism

d. Treatment
   1) Prevention through education regarding proper use of antacids
   2) Oral supplements for mild to moderate losses
   3) Intravenous administration of the electrolyte necessary for more severe deficits
      - Sodium phosphate
      - Potassium phosphate

e. Nursing interventions
   1) Assess patient for clinical signs and symptoms
   2) Monitor laboratory tests
   3) Take appropriate actions, such as seizure precautions
   4) Initiate an intravenous line to administer intravenous supplements for severe deficits
   5) Use caution in monitoring the line when potassium phosphate is used; infiltrations may lead to necrosis and sloughing of affected tissue
   6) Observe for possible hypocalcemia as the phosphate deficit is corrected
   7) Document observations and interventions
   8) Notify physician of abnormal findings

3. Hyperphosphatemia
   a. Definition
      1) Phosphate excess
      2) Serum level above 4.5 mg/dL
   b. Etiology

1) Renal disease (a major cause; acute and chronic renal failure) decreases the kidney's ability to excrete phosphate
2) Increased intake
   • Oral intake
   • Gastrointestinal absorption related to vitamin D excess
   • Phosphorus-containing enemas and laxatives
3) Compartmental shifting
   • Respiratory acidosis and decreased cell utilization
   • Cellular breakdown such as with cytoxic medications

c. Signs and symptoms
1) Signs and symptoms are relatively nonexistent
2) Those present are a result of the reciprocal action of phosphate and calcium
3) Indicators are usually related to a calcium deficit
   • Neuromuscular symptoms including tetany and hyperactive reflexes
   • Soft tissue calcification with calcium phosphate deposits in the lungs, kidneys, heart, and corneas; deposits may interrupt normal function of the affected organ or area with site-specific signs and symptoms
4) Laboratory data
   • Serum phosphorus level: elevated; greater than 4.4 mg/dL
   • Serum calcium level: decreased
   • Serum creatinine level: elevated if the cause is thought to be connected to renal disease

d. Treatment
1) Prevention is the key
2) Restriction of dietary intake
3) Phosphate-binding gels or antacids to help increase intestinal elimination of excessive phosphate
4) Hemodialysis possible in severe cases, particularly with renal involvement
5) Cause related to neoplastic disease
   • Maintenance of fluid balance
   • Treat electrolyte imbalances (hyperkalemia, hypocalcemia, hyperuricemia, and hyperphosphatemia)
   • Hemodialysis (renal failure)[26]

e. Nursing interventions
1) Assess patient for clinical signs and symptoms
2) Monitor serum phosphate levels
3) Document observations and interventions
4) Notify physician of abnormal findings

F. Chloride

1. Overview
   a. Primary anion in the ECF

b. Important functions in the body
   1) Maintenance of tonicity
   2) Regulation of acid-base balance
   3) Reabsorption of sodium
c. Direct relationship with sodium and potassium
   1) With increased levels of sodium or potassium, chloride level also increases
   2) Inverse relationship with bicarbonate
d. Filtered out of the ECF by the kidney glomeruli
e. Amount needed to maintain balance is reabsorbed by the renal tubules
f. Normal serum chloride level: 97 to 100 mEq/L

2. Hypochloremia
   a. Definition
      1) Chloride deficit
      2) Serum level below 97 mEq/L
   b. Etiology
      1) Generally associated with sodium and potassium deficits
      2) A loss of gastric juices or prolonged vomiting may result in hypochloremic alkalosis
      3) Possible decreased renal chloride reabsorption
   c. Signs and symptoms
      1) Usually related to the attached cation (sodium or potassium)
      2) Laboratory data
         • Serum chloride level: decreased
         • Serum sodium and potassium levels: decreased
         • ABGs: alkalosis possible
   d. Treatment
      1) Eliminate the cause
      2) Electrolyte replacement
      3) Replacement for severe deficits is dependent on the status of the other electrolytes as chloride generally travels in pairs
      4) Intravenous sodium chloride or potassium chloride solutions may be indicated
   e. Nursing interventions
      1) Assess patient for clinical signs and symptoms
      2) Monitor serum chloride levels
      3) Initiate intravenous line as needed for severe deficits
      4) Document observations and interventions
      5) Notify physician of abnormal findings

3. Hyperchloremia
   a. Definition
      1) Chloride excess
      2) Serum levels above 110 mEq/L
   b. Etiology
      1) Increased intake from continuous or excessive intravenous

administration of potassium- or sodium-containing solutions (particularly hypertonic sodium chloride solutions)

2) During metabolic acidosis as a result of an excessive loss of bicarbonate or dehydration[27]

c. Signs and symptoms

1) Similar to those associated with the excessive cation

2) Laboratory data

- Serum chloride level: increased
- ABGs: acidosis
- Renal function tests: reflective of renal disease
- Serum sodium or potassium levels: may be elevated (as chloride usually associated with these electrolytes)

d. Treatment

1) Eliminate the cause

2) Monitor signs and symptoms

3) Decrease the cation level with subsequent decrease in loss of chloride (if the excess is related to an increased cation level)

e. Nursing interventions

1) Assess patient for clinical signs and symptoms

2) Monitor serum chloride level

3) Initiate intravenous line for administration of medications as indicated

4) Document observations and interventions

5) Notify physician of abnormal findings

V. REPLACEMENT FLUIDS

A. Overview

1. The body maintains a balance of fluids and electrolytes through various processes

a. Diffusion

b. Osmosis

c. Active transport

d. Filtration

2. Maintenance of an adequate volume is important as most of the body is composed of fluids

3. When there is an abnormal loss of body fluid, this volume may be replaced by the use of intravenous solutions

B. Tonicity

1. Basic concepts

a. Fluids and electrolytes within the body continually move from one compartment to another to maintain homeostasis

1) Some of the molecules move easily from one compartment to another while larger ones are not as mobile

           2) Those molecules not shifting as easily impact the movement of water between the intracellular and extracellular compartments

      b. The mobility of fluids and electrolytes is affected by the permeability of the membrane and the size and composition of the molecule

      c. Tonicity denotes this dynamic process, representing the number of particles in a solution that has an osmotic effect on the movement of water

2. Hypotonic solutions

      a. Those with fewer particles having an osmolality of less than 240 mOsm/kg

      b. Has a concentration less than that of body fluids

      c. When used, water moves from the intravascular space into the intracellular compartment

           1) For example, when blood cells are placed in hypotonic solution, fluid is drawn into the blood cells

           2) Depending on degree of hypotonicity, the volume of fluid being pulled into the blood cells may cause them to swell and burst

      d. An example is 0.45% sodium chloride

      e. During administration of hypotonic solutions, patients require close monitoring

      f. Sterile water is never used without additives because of its hypotonicity

3. Isotonic solutions

      a. Have the same tonicity as plasma, with an osmolality ranging from 240 to 340 mOsm/kg

      b. The osmotic pressure is the same within the intracellular and extracellular compartments

      c. Water will not have the tendency to shift from one compartment to the other

      d. Examples include 0.9% sodium chloride, 5% dextrose in water, and lactated Ringer's solution

           1) Expand the ECF

           2) Will not initiate movement of fluid from or into the blood cells

4. Hypertonic solutions

      a. Have an osmolality greater than 340 mOsm/kg

      b. Have a greater number of particles and exert more osmotic pressure than do normal body fluids

      c. When used, fluid is pulled into the vascular system

           1) For example, when blood cells are placed in hypertonic solutions, fluid is drawn out of the blood cells

           2) This causes the cells to shrink

      d. Examples include 3% and 5% sodium chloride solutions and 50% dextrose in water

e. Patients require close monitoring while receiving hypertonic solutions to prevent fluid overload

C. Selection Parameters

1. Basic concepts
   a. When replacing abnormal fluid and electrolyte losses, selection of the replacement fluid takes individual needs into account
   b. These needs include type and amount of fluid and electrolyte losses, activity, and clinical status
2. Osmolality
   a. A hypertonic solution may be the best choice to decrease ICF volume or for volume expansion
   b. An isotonic solution may be needed to expand intravascular volume rapidly
   c. A hypotonic solution may be necessary to treat excess electrolyte imbalances
3. Electrolytes
   a. Electrolyte balance is necessary to maintain homeostasis
   b. Intravenous administration of electrolyte supplements may be required to replace abnormal losses
   c. The need for replacement is determined by monitoring laboratory findings and clinical signs and symptoms
   d. Electrolyte excess can create equal or even greater complications than electrolyte deficits
      1) Hypotonic solutions used to dilute concentration
      2) Electrolyte solution used that will have an antagonistic effect (i.e., calcium gluconate to treat hyperkalemia)
4. Activity: increased activity accelerates the use of calories and the loss of fluids and electrolytes
5. Clinical status
   a. Continually monitoring the clinical status is necessary to determine the need to initiate or readjust intravenous fluid delivery
      1) Body weight
      2) Intake-output status
      3) Vital signs
      4) Skin turgor
      5) Diagnostic findings
      6) Central venous pressure
   b. Disease states/conditions, such as renal and endocrine diseases, influence the fluid status and the need for fluid replacement
      1) Trauma, including burns and head injury, may increase need for fluids and electrolytes
      2) Patients undergoing surgery have specific needs requiring consideration

VI. INTRAVENOUS SOLUTIONS

A. Categorization of Intravenous Solutions

1. Tonicity
2. Maintenance vs. replacement
3. Crystalloid or colloid

B. Sodium Chloride Solutions

1. Description
   a. Crystalloid solutions
   b. Available in a variety of concentrations
2. 0.45% sodium chloride solution
   a. Hypotonic solution containing equal amounts of sodium and chloride (77 mEq/L) and free water
   b. Used to replace hypotonic fluid losses, sodium, and chloride
   c. No calories provided
   d. Dilution and depletion of electrolytes and calories possible with continuous infusion
3. 0.9% sodium chloride solution
   a. Isotonic solution containing equal amounts of sodium and chloride (154 mEq/L)
   b. Variety of uses
      1) Sodium and chloride replacement
      2) In conjunction with blood transfusion
      3) Treatment of metabolic alkalosis
      4) Diluent for medications
   c. Calories, other electrolytes, or free water not provided
   d. Sodium excess, fluid volume overload, and depletion of calories and other electrolytes possible with continuous or rapid administration
4. 3% and 5% sodium chloride solutions
   a. Hypertonic solutions containing equal amounts of sodium and chloride
      1) 3% solution contains 257 mEq/500 ml
      2) 5% solution contains 428 mEq/500 ml
   b. Replacement for severe sodium deficits
   c. Slow and careful administration is required to prevent fluid volume overload or pulmonary edema

C. Dextrose Solutions

1. Description
   a. Crystalloid solutions available in a variety of concentrations
   b. Water and calories are provided
2. 5% dextrose in water
   a. Isotonic solution given peripherally

1) Provides 5 grams of dextrose per 100 ml (170 calories/L)
2) Metabolized quickly, leaving only the water for distribution as needed within the appropriate fluid compartment
3) Contains no electrolytes

b. Generally used for initial hydration or as a vehicle for administering medications

c. Water excess or intoxication is possible with prolonged use

d. Not used for blood administration; dextrose causes the red blood cells to clump in the tubing

3. 10% dextrose in water
a. Hypertonic solution
1) Contains 10 grams of dextrose per 100 ml (240 calories/L)
2) Provides calories and free water

b. The highest percent of dextrose solution given peripherally

c. Electrolyte depletion is possible with continuous administration as electrolytes are not found in the solution

4. Concentrated dextrose in water (20%, 40%, 50%, 60%, and 70% dextrose in water)
a. Hypertonic solutions
b. Major use as a source of calories
c. Usually added to amino acid solutions administered via a central line to provide total nutrition
d. With administration, possible tolerance to glucose is compromised by sepsis, stress, and hepatic and renal failure
e. Some medications such as steroids or diuretics may affect glucose tolerance
f. Hypertonic dextrose solutions, mainly 50%, are used to correct blood sugar levels related to hypoglycemia
g. Complications may occur as a result of hypertonic glucose solutions
1) Hyperglycemia (if given rapidly)
   • Subsequent osmotic diuresis
   • May result in loss of fluids and electrolytes possibly leading to hyperosmolar coma
2) Sudden demand for increased insulin production (hyperinsulinism) from excessive amounts of hypertonic dextrose
   • Weakness
   • Diaphoresis
   • Confusion
3) Vein irritation, damage, and thrombosis may occur unless hypertonic solutions are diluted before peripheral administration

D. Dextrose/Saline Solutions

1. Description
a. Variety of dextrose/saline combination solutions are available

  b. Calories, free water, sodium, and chloride are provided (with the amounts depending on the concentration of the particular fluid)

  c. Used to replace deficits in fluid volume as they contain free water

  d. Calories are supplemented by dextrose; concentration is based on individual patient needs

  e. Electrolytes, sodium, and chloride are also provided; concentration selected is dependent on the patient's serum electrolyte levels

  f. Complications include any of those discussed under the sections related to dextrose solutions and saline solutions

   1) Also sodium excess

   2) Fluid overload possible from sodium excess or administration of excessive volume

   3) Fluid overload possible, leading to dilution or depletion of other electrolytes

 2. 5% dextrose in 0.225% sodium chloride (hypertonic)

 3. 5% dextrose in 0.33% sodium chloride (hypertonic)

 4. 5% dextrose in 0.45% sodium chloride (hypertonic)

 5. 5% dextrose in 0.9% sodium chloride (hypertonic)

 6. 2.5% dextrose in 0.45% sodium chloride (isotonic)

 7. 10% dextrose in 0.225% sodium chloride (hypertonic)

 8. 10% dextrose in 0.45% sodium chloride (hypertonic)

 9. 10% dextrose in 0.9% sodium chloride (hypertonic)

E. Electrolyte Solutions

 1. Description

  a. Crystalloid solutions

  b. Variety of electrolyte combinations are available

   1) May or may not contain dextrose

   2) Vary slightly among different manufacturers

  c. Patient history, signs and symptoms, and diagnostic findings determine formulation needed

 2. Ringer's injection

  a. Isotonic solution containing sodium, potassium, calcium, and chloride

  b. Content approximates the electrolyte content found in the plasma

  c. Used to replace electrolytes

   1) Provides a water source for hydration

   2) Replaces ECF losses

  d. Complications may result from continuous administration of Ringer's solutions only

   1) Even though solution contains several electrolytes, volume of some is not adequate when intake or losses are abnormal

   2) Rapid administration may lead to excessive amounts of electrolytes

3) With no calorie source, using only Ringer's injection may lead to caloric depletion

4) Excessive amounts may cause fluid overload and dilution of some or all the serum electrolytes

3. 5% dextrose in Ringer's injection

   a. Hypertonic solution provides electrolytes and calories

   b. Similar applications as for Ringer's injection with the ability to provide calories

   c. Complications similar to Ringer's injection

      1) Possible electrolyte depletion if no other source of intake or abnormal losses present

      2) Rapid or excessive administration leads to abnormally high serum electrolyte levels

      3) An excessive volume may result in hypervolemia with possible dilution of serum electrolytes

   d. Caution required when administering dextrose-containing solutions to patients with diabetes mellitus

4. Lactated Ringer's injection (Hartmann's solution)

   a. Electrolyte content similar to that found in plasma

   b. Isotonic solution providing sodium, potassium, calcium, chloride, and lactate

      1) Lactate added as a buffer

      2) Lactate metabolized to produce bicarbonate normally found in the ECF

   c. Used to treat hypovolemia and provide electrolytes

   d. With little or no intake or abnormal losses, inadequate electrolyte content provided for maintenance therapy

   e. Complications include overhydration, electrolyte excess, electrolyte dilution, caloric depletion, and a magnesium deficit

   f. Metabolic alkalosis from excessive volume

   g. Contraindicated in hepatic disorders as lactate is metabolized by the liver

   h. Not used when lactic acidosis is present because of possible overload of the buffering system

5. 5% dextrose in lactated Ringer's

   a. Hypertonic solution

   b. Similar to lactated Ringer's solution, plus calories are provided

   c. Uses and complications are similar to those for lactated Ringer's

6. Other electrolyte solutions

   a. Large number of specialty electrolyte solutions are available, with some containing dextrose

   b. Mostly isotonic until dextrose is added; then hypertonic

   c. Uses determined by patient history, clinical signs and symptoms, and laboratory findings

   d. Precautions and complications are dependent on the fluid content and flow rate

F. Plasma Expanders

1. Description
   a. Plasma expanders are colloids
   b. Act osmotically to expand the intravascular space
   c. Do not expand the intracellular or interstitial spaces
   d. Used to rapidly increase the intravascular volume in emergency situations
   e. Include blood components and albumin and synthetic colloids such as dextran and mannitol
2. Dextran
   a. Plasma expander available in two forms, low molecular weight and high molecular weight
   b. Dextran 6%, high molecular weight, is available in 5% dextrose and 0.9% sodium chloride solutions
      1) Increased volume dependent on amount of solution administered and on preadministration fluid status and renal status
      2) Maximum effect occurs approximately 1 hour after completion of administration; lasts for approximately 24 hours
      3) Used in treatment of shock or anticipated shock related to trauma, burns, or hemorrhage
      4) Not substitutes for blood or blood products
      5) May be used on short notice when time does not allow for a blood type and cross match
      6) Complications
         • Severe anaphylactoid reactions
         • Wheezing
         • Tightness in chest
         • Gastrointestinal disturbances
      7) Blood samples for typing and cross matching drawn before administering dextran because of possible interference with laboratory testing
      8) Fluid overload possible
         • Lowered hematocrit
         • Decreased plasma protein levels
         • Diluted serum electrolyte levels
      9) Contraindicated in patients with renal diseases, congestive heart failure, bleeding disorders, and known dextran hypersensitivity
   c. 10% Dextran, low molecular weight, is available in 5% dextrose and 0.9% sodium chloride solutions
      1) Maximum volume expansion occurs shortly after completion of administration
      2) Excreted by renal system within 24 hours
      3) Volume expansion relative to volume delivered, pre-existing fluid status, and excretion rate

4) May be used to treat shock related to vascular volume loss
- Burns
- Surgery
- Hemorrhage
- Trauma

5) Also used to help prevent venous thrombosis and pulmonary embolism prophylactically during surgical procedures

6) Complications possible
- Anaphylactoid reactions
- Dilution of electrolytes
- Circulatory overload with possible hematocrit and plasma protein dilution
- Increased bleeding time

7) Blood samples drawn before giving this solution to eliminate any interference with laboratory testing

3. Mannitol
a. A sugar alcohol substance available in a variety of concentrations from 5% to 25%
b. Osmotic pull of fluid into the intravascular space is created
c. Majority of the fluid is excreted by the kidneys within 3 hours
d. Used to promote fluid loss
1) Diuresis in the oliguria phase of acute renal failure
2) Excretion of toxic substances
3) Treatment of intracranial pressure and cerebral edema
4) Reduction of cerebrospinal fluid and intraocular pressure
e. Complications
1) Fluid and electrolyte imbalances
2) Fluid overload
3) Cellular dehydration
4) Nervous system toxicity
5) Extravasation leads to skin irritation and tissue necrosis
f. When administering concentrated solutions, such as 20%, there is a potential for crystal formation; a filter and cautious administration are necessary

4. Hetastarch (Hespan)
a. Synthetic polymer with colloidal properties similar to albumin
b. Available as a 6% concentration in 0.9% sodium chloride solution
c. Fluids are pulled from the cells into the intravascular space
d. Maximum volume is reached shortly following the completion of the infusion
e. Volume and duration are dependent on the volume delivered, pre-administration fluid status, and renal function
f. Used for fluid replacement in the treatment of shock related to a decreased intravascular volume
1) Trauma

2) Burns

3) Hemorrhage

4) Surgery

g. Complications

1) Anaphylactoid reactions

2) Increased bleeding times

3) Altered platelet function

4) Fluid volume overload

5) Electrolyte and fluid imbalances

6) Decreased hematocrit and plasma protein from increased fluid volume

5. Albumin

a. Natural plasma protein prepared from human blood and blood-related products

b. Available in 5% and 25% concentrations

c. Osmotic pressure allows fluid to be pulled into the intravascular space, increasing the fluid volume and possibly the plasma protein volume

d. 5% solution is isotonic; 25% solution is hypertonic

e. Used for volume expansion in treating shock or impending shock related to circulatory volume deficit

f. Used for providing protein or for its ability to bind bilirubin

g. Complications

1) Fluid volume overload

2) Anemia

3) Increased bleeding

4) Dilution or depletion of electrolytes

5) Allergic reactions

6) Decreased hematocrit and plasma protein levels from increased fluid volumes

7) Altered laboratory findings possible

G. Other Solutions

1. Alkalinizing solutions: 5% sodium bicarbonate

a. Neutralize excess acids and restore homeostasis

1) Excessive depletion of bicarbonate

2) Retention of ketone bodies or organic salts[28]

b. Dissociates to provide the bicarbonate ion, the principal buffer in the ECF

c. Maintains osmotic pressure and acid-base balance

d. Used to treat metabolic acidosis and severe hyperkalemia

e. Complications

1) Metabolic alkalosis

2) Hypocalcemia

3) Hypokalemia

4) Sodium retention

5) Hypervolemia, which may result in electrolyte imbalances

6) Extravasation possibly resulting in chemical cellulitis, necrosis, ulceration, and/or sloughing

2. Alcohol solutions

a. Hypertonic solution containing 5% ethyl alcohol in 5% dextrose in water

b. Metabolized primarily in the liver to acetaldehyde or acetate

c. Used to replace water and provide calories

d. Complications often related to continuous or rapid administration

1) Hypervolemia

2) Intoxication

3) Dilution of electrolytes

4) Acid-base imbalances

e. Care required to prevent extravasation, which may result in phlebitis and tissue necrosis

f. Caution necessary in the presence of impairment, shock, and diabetes mellitus because of potential complications

g. Not used when there is a history of alcoholism

3. Premixed solutions

a. Wide variety of premixed large-volume intravenous solutions and medications available

b. Greater assurance that the proper medication, diluent, base solution, and pH of the solution have been used

c. Longer expiration dating as a result of the sterilization process being completed following the admixture procedure

d. General disadvantages

1) Potential increased costs

2) Accidental delivery of a medication not ordered

3) Incorrect dose when several concentrations of the same medication stocked

e. Potential complications are related to the individual solution and medication; viewed on an individual basis before administration

VII. ACID-BASE BALANCE AND IMBALANCE

A. Overview

1. Acid-base balance is necessary to maintain homeostasis

2. Acids are substances that give up hydrogen ions

3. Bases accept hydrogen ions

4. Acid-base balance is regulated through the chemical buffering system, the kidneys, and the lungs

a. These buffers are present in all body fluids, tissue, and bone

b. Bicarbonate-carbonic acid is the major extracellular buffer

c. Organic and inorganic phosphates and proteins are intracellular buffers[29]

5. The renal system helps to maintain balance through the reabsorption and regeneration of bicarbonate and the secretion of hydrogen
6. The lungs regulate carbon dioxide by adjusting the rate and depth of ventilation
7. Acid-base imbalances may be classified as metabolic or respiratory and further subdivided as acidosis or alkalosis
8. Acid-base balance is determined through the use of ABGs
   a. The pH measures the hydrogen ion (H+) concentration
   b. The $PaCO_2$ is the respiratory component of acid-base balance and is related to the partial pressure of CO_2 in arterial blood
   c. Bicarbonate is the major extracellular buffer
   d. The PaO_2 is the partial pressure of arterial oxygen
   e. The normal values include:[30]
      1) pH: 7.35–7.45
      2) Partial pressure of arterial blood ($PaCO_2$): 35–45 mm Hg
      3) Bicarbonate (HCO_3): 22–26 mEq/L
      4) Arterial oxygen pressure (PaO_2): 80–100 mm Hg

B. Metabolic Acidosis

1. Description
   a. Indicated by a decreased bicarbonate level
   b. May be caused by an increased loss of bicarbonate or fixed acids as a result of increased production or decreased excretion by the kidneys
   c. Imbalance may be chronic or acute
      1) Chronic imbalance is usually related to chronic renal disease; correction usually not required for adults
      2) Acute metabolic acidosis
         • Generally occurs from bicarbonate losses due to diarrhea or decreased renal excretion
         • May be caused by an excessive amount of hydrogen ions due to decreased renal excretion, increased production, lactic acidosis, ketoacidosis, or ingestion of acids such as methanol or salicylates
2. Signs and symptoms (usually directly related to the cause)
   a. Increased rate and depth of respirations
   b. Decreased blood pressure
   c. Headaches
   d. Weakness
   e. Confusion
   f. Nausea
   g. Vomiting
   h. Cardiac response becomes limited, leading to vasodilation exhibited as warm, dry, and flushed skin (in severe cases)
3. Laboratory findings
   a. pH: less than 7.35
   b. Bicarbonate level: less than 22 mEq/L

    c. Urine pH: acidic (with normal renal function)

    d. Serum potassium level: frequently increased

4. Treatment (correct the cause)

    a. Initiation of an intravenous line as very low arterial pH levels could be life-threatening

    b. Administration of sodium bicarbonate and potassium

      1) Add to a parenteral solution

      2) Administer by intravenous drip

      3) Sodium bicarbonate may be given by intravenous push for cardiac arrest

5. Complications

    a. Fluid overload with dilution or depletion of electrolytes

    b. Dilution of the hematocrit and plasma protein

    c. Overcorrection of acidosis may lead to alkalosis

6. Nursing interventions

    a. Monitor related signs and symptoms and diagnostic findings

    b. Document all observations, medications, and procedures

    c. Notify physician of any abnormal findings

C. Metabolic Alkalosis

1. Description

    a. Results from an excess of sodium bicarbonate due to a bicarbonate gain or a hydrogen ion loss; occurs in two forms (acute and chronic)

    b. Acute

      1) Primarily from hydrogen ion, extracellular volume, and potassium chloride depletion

        • Vomiting

        • Gastric suctioning

        • Diuretics

      2) Signs and symptoms (generally related to hypovolemia and hypokalemia)

        • Hyperactive reflexes

        • Mental confusion

        • Depressed respirations

        • Tetany from decreased calcium levels

        • Cardiac dysfunction from hypokalemia

      3) Diagnostic findings (acute and chronic)

        • Arterial bicarbonate level: elevated (greater than 26 mEq/L)

        • pH level: exceeding 7.45

        • Sodium, potassium, and phosphorus levels: underlying cause may reveal deficits

        • Calcium level: increased or decreased

        • ECG: reveals an increased heart rate and prolonged QT intervals

      4) Treatment (varies with underlying cause)

- No treatment necessary unless imbalance is severe
- 0.9% or 0.45% sodium chloride solutions for more severe imbalances resulting from gastric and urinary losses
- Potassium chloride when alkalosis is related to hypokalemia
- Acidifying agents, histamine H^2 receptor antagonists, and acetazolamide (Diamox) are used

5) Nursing interventions (acute and chronic)
- Monitor signs and symptoms and laboratory data
- Initiate an intravenous line
- Provide routine monitoring
- Document all observations and procedures
- Notify physician of abnormal findings

c. Chronic
1) Results when acute form not corrected
- Long-term diuretic therapy (thiazides, furosemide); hydrogen ion loss
- Excretion of bicarbonate related to mineralocorticoid effect[31]
2) Shift of hydrogen ions into cells due to hypokalemia, bicarbonate retention, administration of excess parenteral alkalotic solutions
3) Signs and symptoms
- Few to none
- Possible manifestations of potassium depletion
4) Diagnostic findings (see Acute)
5) Treatment (related to negating the underlying cause)
- 0.9% sodium chloride solutions for correction of volume depletion (often unsuccessful in correcting chronic alkalosis)
- Oral or intravenous potassium chloride administration (most often successful)
- Diuretics (acetazolamide [Diamox], potassium-sparing)
6) Nursing interventions (see Acute)

D. Respiratory Acidosis

1. Description
a. Inability of the lungs to eliminate carbon dioxide equal to the amount produced
b. Level is controlled through the rate and depth of respirations
c. Occurs as acute and chronic
d. Inability to control rate and depth of respirations in acute respiratory acidosis is related to:
1) Medications (sedatives)
2) Cerebral injury (cardiac arrest)
3) Disease (pneumonia)
e. Chronic respiratory acidosis occurs when the amount of carbon dioxide produced exceeds the amount eliminated over an extended period of time

        1) Emphysema
        2) Cystic fibrosis
        3) Bronchial asthma
  2. Signs and symptoms
    a. Usually directly related to the cause, not the acidosis
    b. Often as a result of the effects on the central nervous system
        1) Restlessness
        2) Confusion
        3) Nausea
        4) Vomiting
        5) Muscular twitching
        6) Convulsions
    c. Cardiac indicators
        1) Increased pulse and respiratory rates
        2) Increased blood pressure
        3) Warm, flushed skin
        4) Weakness with a dull headache when the arterial baseline level increases rapidly
  3. Laboratory findings
    a. Serum pH: less than 7.35
    b. $PaCO_2$ level: greater than 42 mm Hg
  4. Treatment
    a. Correction of the underlying cause
    b. Restoration of the carbon dioxide level
        1) Oxygen therapy
        2) Intubation and mechanical ventilation
        3) Bronchodilators and antibiotics if indicated (chronic form)
        4) Avoidance of narcotics and sedatives unless patient intubated and mechanically ventilated (because of respiratory depression associated with chronic form)

E. Respiratory Alkalosis

  1. Description
    a. Result of increased ventilation
    b. More carbon dioxide is eliminated than produced (hyperventilation)
        1) Hypoxemia
        2) High fever
        3) Excessive mechanical ventilation
        4) Salicylate intoxication
  2. Signs and symptoms
    a. Lightheadedness
    b. Tinnitus
    c. Sweating
    d. Increased respiratory rate and depth
    e. Numbness and tingling of extremities

3. Treatment (directly related to correcting the underlying cause)
   a. Oxygen therapy if hypoxemia is the causative factor
   b. Rebreathing CO_2 therapy in severe cases
   c. Reassurance to help the patient gain control and slow respirations (if caused by anxiety)
   d. Sedative and/or tranquilizer for anxiety-related respiratory alkalosis

VIII. DISEASE STATES AND CONDITIONS AFFECTING FLUID AND ELECTROLYTE BALANCE

A. Cardiac System

1. Helps in the control of fluids and electrolytes
2. The heart is affected by fluids and electrolytes
   a. Regulation of fluids and electrolytes is dependent on the heart pumping plasma through the kidneys
   b. Fluid volume is controlled by stretch receptors located in the heart and blood vessels
      1) Fluid volume deficit causes weak, rapid pulse
      2) Fluid excess leads to bounding, full pulse
3. Potassium affects impulse conduction and contractibility
4. Sodium influences the cardiovascular system by causing changes in blood volume
5. Calcium helps to regulate contraction and relaxation of the heart muscle
6. Magnesium produces vasodilation
   a. May lead to a drop in blood pressure and possibly precipitate cardiac arrest
   b. Imbalances may lead to cardiac arrhythmias including premature ventricular contractions, supraventricular tachycardia, and ventricular fibrillation

B. Renal System

1. The kidneys play a major role in maintaining fluid and electrolyte balance by excreting or retaining water, electrolytes, and organic materials
2. Thirst, hormones, and the heart and blood vessels affect renal function
   a. The hypothalamus manufactures ADH, which is stored in the posterior pituitary
   b. When released, ADH causes the kidney tubules to reabsorb more water from the distal renal tubule and collecting duct
3. Laboratory tests, such as BUN and creatinine, help evaluate the renal system
4. Improper functioning of the renal system may lead to acute or chronic renal failure

5. Potassium is one of the major electrolytes excreted by the kidneys; any malfunction of the kidneys will impact the balance

C. Endocrine System

1. Plays a major role in regulating fluids and electrolytes
2. ADH is secreted by the hypothalamus and stored in the posterior pituitary
3. Syndrome of inappropriate antidiuretic hormone (SIADH) results in water retention and hyponatremia
   a. Correction of the underlying cause and the excessive water retention
   b. Close monitoring of sodium and fluid levels
4. The thyroid and parathyroid glands secrete hormones that affect calcium, magnesium, and phosphorus levels
5. Two forms of diabetes: diabetes insipidus and diabetes mellitus
   a. Diabetes insipidus is a disorder related to water imbalance as a result of a lack of ADH or failure of the kidney to respond to ADH
      1) Central diabetes insipidus may be caused by head trauma or metastatic tumors
      2) Clinical indicators include intense thirst, polyuria, increased serum sodium, and increased osmolality
      3) Treatment involves replacing the ADH and use of intravenous fluids and electrolytes
   b. Diabetes mellitus results from a reduced secretion or utilization of insulin
      1) Hyperglycemia and diabetic ketoacidosis may result; evident by high blood glucose levels and high urine glucose readings
      2) Imbalances related to diabetes mellitus include decreased serum carbon dioxide level, hypokalemia, and fluid volume level
      3) Treatment may include insulin and fluid replacement
         • 0.9% sodium chloride
         • Lactated Ringer's injection
         • 0.45% sodium chloride
         • Electrolytes

D. Hepatic System

1. Normally, aldosterone is inactivated by the liver
2. An impaired liver is unable to carry out this function
   a. Excess levels of aldosterone cause sodium to be retained, resulting in water retention
   b. Other imbalances occur
      1) Hypokalemia
      2) Hyperkalemia (related to secondary kidney failure)
      3) Hypomagnesemia
      4) Hypocalcemia
      5) Hypophosphatemia
      6) Acid-base imbalances

c. Treatment is related to eliminating fluid excess and correcting electrolyte imbalances

E. Burns

1. Traumatize the skin and allow loss of fluid and electrolytes
2. Severity of the imbalances is related to the depth of the burns and the percent of the body surface area affected
   a. For the first 24 hours following more severe burns, intravascular water, proteins, and electrolytes are lost through the damaged capillaries and cells
   b. After this period, the capillary walls start to seal and the compensatory changes begin
   c. By the second or third day, the fluid causing the edema starts to shift from the interstitial space to the vascular space
      1) Blood volume increases
      2) Results in increased urinary output
3. Treatment includes the administration of intravenous solutions
   a. Caution must be exercised to prevent fluid volume overload as the fluid shift occurs
   b. Electrolyte levels must be monitored to ensure electrolyte balance, particularly potassium levels because of its loss from traumatized cells

F. Pregnancy-induced Hypertension (toxemia of pregnancy)

1. Pregnancy has a great effect on fluid and electrolyte balance
   a. Increased fluid volume
   b. Changes in the renal function
   c. Reduction in serum calcium
   d. Alterations in the acid-base balance with respiratory alkalosis as a normal finding
2. Pregnancy-induced hypertension is characterized by edema, hypertension, proteinuria, and convulsions
3. When the condition becomes severe, magnesium sulfate may be used for its anticonvulsant effect[33]
4. Serum magnesium levels must be monitored closely to prevent hypermagnesemia

REFERENCES

1. Terry J. *Intravenous Therapy: Clinical Principles and Practice.* Philadelphia, PA: Saunders, 1995:114–115.
2. Horne MM, et al. Fluid, electrolyte and acid-base balance. *Pocket Guide Series,* 3rd ed. St. Louis, MO: Mosby-Year Book, 1997:6.
3. Ibid, p. 4.
4. Ibid, p. 6.
5. Ibid, p. 6.

6. Paradisco C. *Fluids and Electrolytes,* 2nd ed. Philadelphia, PA: Lippincott, 1999:119.
7. Ibid, p. 21–22.
8. Metheny NM. *Fluid and Electrolyte Balance: Nursing Considerations,* 3rd ed. Philadelphia, PA: Lippincott-Raven, 1996:429–433.
9. Cavanaugh BM. *Nurse's Manual of Laboratory Tests and Diagnostic Procedures,* 3rd ed. Philadephia, PA: FA Davis Company, 1999:164–165.
10. Ibid, p. 313.
11. Metheny NM. *Fluid and Electrolyte Balance: Nursing Considerations,* 3rd ed. Philadelphia, PA: Lippincott-Raven, 1996:40.
12. Ibid, p. 17.
13. Ibid, p. 428.
14. Ibid, p. 412.
15. Ibid, p. 32.
16. Ibid, p. 17.
17. Horne MM, et al. Fluid, electrolyte and acid-base balance. *Pocket Guide Series,* 3rd ed. St. Louis, MO: Mosby-Year Book, 1997:33–34.
18. Metheny NM. *Fluid and Electrolyte Balance: Nursing Considerations,* 3rd ed. Philadelphia, PA: Lippincott-Raven, 1996:98.
19. Ibid, p. 96.
20. McEvoy GK. AHFS Drug Information 98. Bethesda, MD. *American Society of Hospital Pharmacists* 1998:2142.
21. Horne MM. *Fluid, Electrolyte, and Acid-Base Balance: Pocket Guide Series,* 3rd ed. St. Louis, MO: Mosby-Year Book, 1997:104.
22. Metheny NM. *Fluid and Electrolyte Balance: Nursing Considerations,* 3rd ed. Philadelphia, PA: Lippincott-Raven, 1996:115.
23. Horne MM, et al. Fluid, electrolyte and acid-base balance. *Pocket Guide Series,* 3rd ed. St. Louis, MO: Mosby-Year Book, 1997:113.
24. Paradisco C. *Fluids and Electrolytes,* 2nd ed. Philadelphia, PA: Lippincott, 1999:98.
25. Metheny NM. *Fluid and Electrolyte Balance: Nursing Considerations,* 3rd ed. Philadelphia, PA: Lippincott-Raven, 1996:138.
26. Ibid, p. 384.
27. *Nurse Manual of Laboratory Diagnostic Tests,* 3rd ed. Philadelphia, PA: FA Davis Company, 1999:274–275.
28. McEvoy GK. *AHFS Drug Information 98.* Bethesda, MD: American Society of Health-System Pharmacists, 1998:2113–2119.
29. Metheny MM. *Fluid and Electrolyte Balance: Nursing Considerations,* 3rd ed. Philadelphia, PA: Lippincott-Raven, 1996:160.
30. Metheny NM. *Fluid and Electrolyte Balance: Nursing Considerations,* 3rd ed. Philadelphia, PA: Lippincott-Raven, 1996:161.
31. Horne MM, et al. Fluid, electrolyte and acid-base balance. *Pocket Guide Series,* 3rd ed. St. Louis, MO: Mosby-Year Book, 1997:183.
32. Metheny NM. *Fluid and Electrolyte Balance: Nursing Considerations,* 3rd. ed. Philadelphia, PA: Lippincott-Raven, 1996:136.
33. Ibid, p. 400.

CHAPTER 3

Pharmacology

Sharon M. Weinstein, MS, CRNI

I. OVERVIEW

A. Resources Available

1. The professional nurse should use all available resources in determining the appropriateness of therapy
2. Physician's written order: the order to initiate therapy should include solution/medication, dosage, volume, rate, frequency, and route
3. Hospital/institutional/agency policy
   a. The hospital, agency, and other institutions should provide written policies and procedures relevant to intravenous drug administration[1]
   b. Approved drug listing: a list of drugs for intravenous administration by nurses should be developed and approved by appropriate institutional committees
4. Applicable *Intravenous Nursing Standards of Practice*
   a. Intravenous medication administration[2]
      1) Responsibilities before, during, and after drug administration
   b. Compatibility[3]
      1) Determined before admixing and administering intravenous medications
   c. Laminar flow hood:[4] minimizes the potential for airborne contamination during admixing
   d. Admixing[5]: the preparation and/or compounding of medications in a designated, clean area under the direction of the pharmacy
   e. Expiration dates[6]: shelf life, drug stability, and optimum temperature should be considered
   f. Administration of investigational agents[7]
      1) Federal and state laws must be considered
      2) Signed, informed patient consent is required
      3) Investigational protocols may be continued in the alternative care setting if all guidelines for disposal, documentation, care, and handling have been met

5. State Nurse Practice Act[8]: determines the scope of practice for professional nursing within a given geographical area
6. Joint Policy Statements: those issued by licensing boards to address specific areas of clinical practice
7. Package inserts

B. Equipment

1. Preparation
   a. Parenteral solutions[9]: the nurse should know whether the parenteral solution is hypertonic, hypotonic, or isotonic, and whether it is appropriate for the prescribed route
   b. Syringes: a wide selection of products is available; the intravenous nurse should use the appropriate sized syringe for the volume of drug to be withdrawn
   c. Needles: the nurse should select the appropriate sized needle for withdrawing solution from a vial or ampule
   d. Filters and filter needles: add-on or integral devices are used to prevent passage of undesirable substances into the vascular system and to eliminate introduction of extraneous particles (e.g., rubber stoppers or other materials)
      1) Particulate-matter filters of 1 to 5 microns appropriate when preparing intravenous medications
   e. Medications
   f. Diluent (a substance used to attenuate or dilute another product): various diluents are available; the type recommended in a package insert should be used
      1) Bacteriostatic water for injection, United States Pharmacopeia (U.S.P.)
      2) Sterile water for injection, U.S.P.
      3) 0.9% sodium chloride for injection, U.S.P.
   g. Preservatives/buffering agents: substances used to offset reaction of an agent administered in conjunction with it (e.g., Neut [neutralizing agent])
   h. Hazardous waste disposal: products are available to facilitate disposal of supplies and materials used to prepare antineoplastic agents
2. Drug forms
   a. Powders: require reconstitution
   b. Liquids: in the appropriate liquid form
   c. Premixed: drugs may be premixed with intravenous additives
   d. Prefilled syringes: minimize errors in calculation, and ensure drug preparation in the correct volume of diluent
3. Drug containers
   a. Vials include double-compartment, pump-action, and additive piggyback

1) Single-use vial: hermetically sealed with rubber stopper and intended for one-time use
2) Multiple-dose vial: hermetically sealed with rubber stopper and designed to be entered more than once
   b. Ampules: a hermetically sealed glass medication container in which the neck of the container must be broken to access the medication

C. Compatibility[3]

1. Capability of being mixed and administered without undergoing undesirable chemical and/or physical changes or loss of therapeutic action
2. Factors affecting compatibility
   a. Concentration of drug
   b. Length of time drugs are in contact with other additives or diluent
   c. pH of admixture and presence of buffers
      1) pH: symbol for degree of concentration of hydrogen ions or acidity of solution
      2) Addition of buffers may minimize potential for development of phlebitis

D. Incompatibilities[3,6]

1. Chemical: a change, which may or may not be visually observed, in the molecular structure or pharmacological properties of a substance (e.g., penicillin and ascorbic acid, lowering the pH)
2. Physical: an undesirable change that is physically observed (e.g., sodium bicarbonate and calcium chloride, forming an insoluble precipitate)
3. Therapeutic: an undesirable reaction resulting from the overlapping effects of two drugs given together or closely together (e.g., penicillin and tetracycline, inhibiting the bactericidal effect of penicillin)

E. Drug Stability

1. Factors affecting drug stability and safety
   a. Parenteral solutions: tonicity may affect stability
   b. Additive drugs: presence may affect pH
   c. Buffers: used to stabilize the drug in solution
   d. Preservatives: to prolong shelf life
   e. Amount of diluent: may affect stability
   f. Time in solution: some drugs require admixing immediately before administration
   g. Order of mixing: end product may be affected; consult manufacturer's recommendations
   h. Light
   i. Temperature

F. Drug Calculations[10]

1. Dosage
   a. Dosage calculations are an inherent part of clinical practice, regardless of the clinical setting
   b. Body surface area is frequently used to calculate dosage (surface area of the body determined by a nomogram)
      1) To calculate body surface area, draw straight line between point representing patient's height on left vertical scale to point representing patient's weight on right vertical scale
      2) The point at which this line intersects the middle vertical scale represents patient's surface area in square meters
2. Percent solutions[10]: alligation applies to calculation of desired concentration and final volume
3. Conversions[10]: required conversions include microgram/kilogram; units/hour; milligrams/minute

II. PATIENT ASSESSMENT[10]

A. Nursing History (sequence and length are modified[10] consistent with type of therapy ordered, acuity level of patient, and clinical setting in which care is delivered)

1. Health status: question patient concerning present and past health history, including disease-specific conditions such as diabetes, cardiac disease, cirrhosis, and surgeries
2. Allergies: specific to foods and drugs; other allergies and type[10] of reaction and severity
3. Medication history: for specific illness (e.g., diuretics, insulin, anticoagulants, aspirin, over-the-counter drugs)
4. Patient care plan[10]: an individualized plan of care relative to medication administration should be developed

B. Laboratory Data (certain medications require monitoring of laboratory data to determine either therapeutic or adverse response)

1. Chemistry/hematology
   a. Prothrombin time (PT)
   b. Partial thromboplastin time (PTT)
   c. Complete blood count (CBC)
   d. Blood urea nitrogen (BUN)
   e. Chemistry panel: a comprehensive measurement of the body's chemical constituents found in the blood, including electrolytes, enzymes, hepatic and renal function, and blood sugar
2. Urine: determines various properties of urine; analysis of drug excretion is often measured

3. Therapeutic drug monitoring ensures appropriate dosing regimens
   a. Required for patients:
      1) On combination therapies
      2) With renal dysfunction
      3) With third-spacing
      4) In whom therapeutic failure would prove catastrophic
      5) Who fail to respond to therapy despite appropriate dosing
   b. Test samples
      1) Peak: maximum drug concentration achieved following administration of single dose
      2) Trough: minimum drug concentration following administration of single dose
4. Sensitivities: a screen used in determining sensitivity or resistance of bacteria to specific drugs
5. Toxicology screens

C. Clinical Assessment Parameters

1. Age
2. Weight: such as percent loss in comparison with usual body weight and time span involved (30 days, 90 days)
3. Height
4. Body temperature
5. Skin
   a. Tissue turgor: skin elasticity is dependent on interstitial fluid volume; turgor is measured by pinching the skin over the sternum, inner aspects of the thighs, or forehead
   b. Appearance: skin should be dry and intact
   c. Presence or absence of rash: assessment of any rash should be documented and reported
   d. Lesions: presence of lesions may inhibit ability to administer drug therapy
   e. Petechiae: presence may inhibit the ability to administer drug therapy
6. Edema
7. Other sources of fluid loss, such as fistulas, vomiting, diarrhea, and drains
   a. Assessment will facilitate determination of true fluid loss and anticipated replacement
8. Sensorium
9. Related therapies may affect the ability to maintain patency of the intravenous line; for example, hydrotherapy may limit the use of hand veins for infusion purposes, and hyperbaric medicine may necessitate removal of a flush solution from an intermittent infusion device before treatment

III. LEGAL CONSIDERATIONS

A. Applicable Torts

1. Assault: an intentional or indirect action by one person directed at another, placing him in apprehension (fear) of immediate bodily harm or offensive contact
2. Battery: intentional infliction of offensive bodily touching
3. Negligence: negligent conduct by a professional person
4. Personal liability: each individual is responsible for his own actions

B. Medication Errors

1. Prevention
2. Classification/reporting

C. Documentation

1. A recording in written or printed form, containing original, official, or legal information
   a. Drug
   b. Dosage
   c. Rate of administration as given
   d. Time of actual administration
   e. Route of administration
   f. Patient's response to treatment

D. Investigational Drugs[10]

1. State and federal regulations must be considered
2. Hospital protocols may be continued in alternative care settings
3. Informed consent is required
4. Policies and procedures[11] must be established
   a. Information concerning the protocol should be kept in the clinical record
   b. Institutional Review Board (IRB) approval should be on file
   c. Principal investigator
      1) Name of the licensed physician should be made available to nurse and patient

E. Significance of Clinical Environment

1. Hospital: institutional policy required for intravenous administration
2. Home: agencies should address all concerns of inpatient settings; additional liability for autonomous practice is applicable
3. Alternative sites
   a. Intravenous drugs may be administered in outpatient and infusion centers, walk-in clinics, and physician's offices

b. Nurses practicing in those settings are required to provide the same standard of intravenous nursing

IV. DRUG CLASSIFICATIONS

A. Responsibility

1. Knowledge of drug classifications and nursing considerations in administration of drugs is an inherent component of intravenous nursing practice

B. Antibiotics

1. Aminoglycosides
   a. Amikacin sulfate (Amikin)
      1) Indications: gram-negative organisms
      2) Usual dose: up to 15 mg/kg/24 hours in 2 to 3 divided doses
      3) Mode of administration: intermittent
      4) Major side effects: ototoxicity, nephrotoxicity, hypotension, paresthesia, tinnitus
      5) Nursing considerations: monitor serum peak and trough levels to avoid peak serum concentrations above 35 µg/ml and trough concentrations above 10 µg/ml
      6) Patient/caregiver education: instruct patient to report hearing difficulties or flank pain[12]
   b. Gentamicin sulfate (Garamycin)
      1) Indications: specific gram-negative and gram-positive bacilli, including *Escherichia coli, Klebsiella, Pseudomonas,* and *Proteus*
      2) Usual dose: 3 mg/kg/24 hours in 3 to 4 divided doses
      3) Mode of administration: intermittent
      4) Major side effects: ototoxicity, tinnitus, nephrotoxicity, hypotension, rash
      5) Nursing considerations: monitor BUN and serum creatinine, peak/trough levels
      6) Patient/caregiver education: instruct patient to report hearing difficulties
   c. Kanamycin sulfate (Kantrex)
      1) Indications: short-term treatment of gram-negative infection
      2) Usual dose: up to 15 mg/kg/24 hours in 2 to 4 divided doses
      3) Mode of administration: intermittent
      4) Major side effects: nephrotoxicity, ototoxicity, vertigo, tinnitus, paresthesia, skin rash
      5) Nursing considerations: reduce daily dose in renal impairment; monitor urine output, BUN, serum creatinine, creatinine clearance
      6) Patient/caregiver education: instruct patient to recognize and report side effects of all drugs

d. Netilmicin sulfate (Netromycin)[13]
1) Indications: short-term treatment of specific gram-negative and gram-positive bacilli, including *Escherichia coli, Klebsiella, Pseudomonas, Proteus;* treatment of staphylococcal infections when other antibiotics contraindicated or ineffective
2) Usual dose: up to 3.25 mg/kg/24 hours in 2 to 4 divided doses
3) Mode of administration: intermittent
4) Major side effects: ototoxicity, tinnitus, vertigo, numbness, tingling, nausea, vomiting, nephrotoxicity, purpura, pain, irritation at site, leukemoid reaction
5) Nursing considerations: monitor BUN and serum creatinine, peak/trough levels
6) Patient/caregiver education: instruct patient to report hearing difficulties
e. Tobramycin sulfate (Nebcin)[14]
1) Indications: gram-negative and gram-positive bacilli
2) Usual dose: 3 mg/kg/24 hours in 3 to 4 divided doses
3) Mode of administration: intermittent
4) Major side effects: thrombocytopenia, granulocytopenia, ototoxicity, nephrotoxicity
5) Nursing considerations: monitor for nephrotoxicity; may lead to renal failure; draw peak 6 to 8 hours after infusion
6) Patient/caregiver education: instruct patient to report hearing difficulties
2. Cephalosporins
a. Cefamandole nafate (Mandol)
1) Indications: second-generation cephalosporin used to treat gram-positive, gram-negative, and some anaerobic infections
2) Usual dose: 0.5 g to 2 g every 4 to 8 hours
3) Mode of administration: push, intermittent
4) Major side effects: nephrotoxicity, neutropenia, pain and induration at site, thrombophlebitis, hypersensitivity
5) Nursing considerations: monitor renal function and intravenous site
6) Patient/caregiver education: instruct patient in self-administration and the need to report pain and induration at intravenous site or a skin reaction
b. Cefazolin sodium (Kefzol)
1) Indications: first-generation cephalosporin used to treat gram-positive and gram-negative infections
2) Usual dose: 250 mg to 1.5 g every 6 to 8 hours
3) Mode of administration: push, intermittent
4) Major side effects: nephrotoxicity, leukopenia, pain and induration at site
5) Nursing considerations: in a patient with a penicillin allergy,

cefazolin may cause cross-sensitivity (similarity in chemical structure); monitor infusion site for pain and induration

    6) Patient/caregiver education: instruct patient in recognizing and reporting change at intravenous site and flank pain

c. Cefepime hydrochloride ((Maxipime)[15]

    1) Indications: used to treat serious bacterial infections

    2) Usual dose: 0.5 to 2 g every 12 hours

    3) Mode of administration: push, intermittent

    4) Major side effects: anaphylaxis, bleeding, pain at site

    5) Nursing considerations: monitor renal and hepatic function

    6) Patient/caregiver education: instruct patient to avoid breast-feeding; teach signs and symptoms of allergic reaction

d. Cefonicid sodium (Monocid)

    1) Indications: second-generation cephalosporin used to treat lower respiratory and urinary infections; septicemia

    2) Usual dose: 500 mg to 2 g every 24 hours

    3) Mode of administration: push, intermittent

    4) Major side effects: diarrhea, elevated platelet count, alkaline phosphatase, serum glutamic-oxaloacetic transaminase (SGOT), serum glutamic-pyruvic transaminase (SGPT), lactic acid dehydrogenase

    5) Nursing considerations: do not mix with aminoglycosides in same infusion

    6) Patient/caregiver education: instruct patient in self-administration

e. Cefmetazole sodium (Zefazone)[16]

    1) Indications: used to treat gram-negative infections, including serious urinary tract infections

    2) Usual dose: 2 g every 6 to 12 hours

    3) Mode of administration: push, intermittent

    4) Major side effects: anaphylaxis, pseudomembranous colitis, urticaria, shortness of breath

    5) Nursing considerations: monitor liver, renal, hematopoietic function

    6) Patient/caregiver education: instruct patient to monitor signs of superinfection (vaginitis, bloody diarrhea) and report unusual fatigue

f. Cefoperazone sodium (Cefobid)

    1) Indications: third-generation cephalosporin used to treat respiratory, gynecological, and skin infections; septicemia

    2) Usual dose: 2 to 4 g every 24 hours

    3) Mode of administration: push, intermittent

    4) Major side effects: colitis, diarrhea, abnormal bleeding, dyspnea, phlebitis, nephrotoxicity

    5) Nursing considerations: select intravenous site carefully to avoid phlebitis

6) Patient/caregiver education: instruct patient in self-administration; instruct patient to report changes in bowel and bladder habits, induration at the intravenous site, and flank pain

g. Cefotaxime sodium (Claforan)
1) Indications: third-generation cephalosporin used to treat respiratory, urinary, skin, bone, and joint infections
2) Usual dose: 1 to 2 g every 4 to 8 hours
3) Mode of administration: push, intermittent
4) Major side effects: decreased prothrombin time, platelet function, lactic acid dehydrogenase and BUN; transient neutropenia, diarrhea
5) Nursing considerations: watch for early signs of allergic reaction; administer within 24 hours of preparation or within 5 days if refrigerated; monitor intravenous site for induration
6) Patient/caregiver education: instruct patient in self-administration; instruct patient to report skin rash, change in bowel habits

h. Cefotetan disodium (Cefotan)
1) Indications: third-generation cephalosporin used to treat gram-negative, gram-positive, and anaerobic infections
2) Usual dose: 1 to 2 g every 12 hours for 5 to 10 days
3) Mode of administration: push, intermittent
4) Major side effects: bleeding, diarrhea, nausea, colitis
5) Nursing considerations: administer within 24 hours of preparation or within 96 hours if refrigerated; slight yellowing does not affect potency
6) Patient/caregiver education: instruct patient in self-administration; instruct patient to report bleeding episodes or changes in bowel habits

i. Cefoxitin sodium (Mefoxin)
1) Indications: third-generation cephalosporin used to treat respiratory, genitourinary, bone, and skin infections
2) Usual dose: 1 to 2 g every 6 to 8 hours
3) Mode of administration: push, intermittent
4) Major side effects: nausea, vomiting, leukopenia, neutropenia, thrombophlebitis
5) Nursing considerations: administer within 24 hours of preparation; monitor intravenous site for induration
6) Patient/caregiver education: instruct patient in self-administration; instruct patient to report change in eating habits or pain at intravenous site

j. Ceftazidime (Fortaz)
1) Indications: third-generation cephalosporin used to treat gram-positive, gram-negative, and anaerobic infections
2) Usual dose: 1 g every 8 to 12 hours
3) Mode of administration: push, intermittent

4) Major side effects: nausea, vomiting, diarrhea, colitis, elevated alkaline phosphatase, BUN

5) Nursing considerations: solution may be light yellow and is safe for use

6) Patient education: instruct patient in self -administration; instruct patient to report change in eating and elimination habits

k. Ceftizoxime sodium (Cefizox)

1) Indications: third-generation cephalosporin used to treat respiratory, urinary, skin, bone, and joint infections

2) Usual dose: 500 mg to 4 g every 8 to 12 hours

3) Mode of administration: push, intermittent

4) Major side effects: decreased prothrombin time and platelet function, leukopenia, oral thrush, diarrhea

5) Nursing considerations: may cause phlebitis; administer oral care

6) Patient/caregiver education: instruct patient to report redness, induration, swelling at intravenous site

l. Ceftriaxone sodium (Rocephin)

1) Indications: third-generation cephalosporin used to treat gram-positive, gram-negative, and anaerobic infections

2) Usual dose: 1 to 2 g every 24 hours

3) Mode of administration: push, intermittent

4) Major side effects: bleeding, diarrhea, prolonged prothrombin time

5) Nursing considerations: monitor prothrombin time and serum electrolytes

6) Patient/caregiver education: instruct patient in self-administration; instruct patient to report signs of bleeding and to avoid injury

m. Cefuroxime sodium (Kefurox)

1) Indications: second-generation cephalosporin used to treat gram-positive, gram-negative, and anaerobic infections

2) Usual dose: 750 mg to 3 g every 8 hours for 5 to 10 days

3) Mode of administration: push, intermittent

4) Major side effects: leukopenia, neutropenia, vomiting, oral thrush, diarrhea

5) Nursing considerations: may cause phlebitis; administer oral care

6) Patient/caregiver education: instruct patient to report changes in bowel habits or signs of bleeding

n. Cephalothin sodium (Keflin)[17]

1) Indications: used to treat gram-positive infections

2) Usual dose: 500 mg to 2 g every 4 to 6 hours

3) Mode of administration: push, intermittent, continuous

4) Major side effects: anaphylaxis, anemia, diarrhea, leukopenia, pain at site

5) Nursing considerations: monitor renal and hepatic function; assess for penicillin/cephalosporin sensitivity

6) Patient/caregiver education: instruct patient to report unusual fatigue, rash, bleeding

o. Cephapirin sodium (Cefadyl)[18]

1) Indications: used to treat gram-positive cocci infections

2) Usual dose: 500 mg to 2 g every 4 to 6 hours

3) Mode of administration: push, intermittent, continuous

4) Major side effects: anaphylaxis, anemia, diarrhea, leukopenia, phlebitis

5) Nursing considerations: monitor renal, hepatic function; assess vital signs

6) Patient/caregiver education: instruct patient to monitor signs of allergic reaction and to identify signs of superinfection

3. Penicillins

a. Ampicillin sodium (Omnipen-N)

1) Indications: gram-positive and gram-negative organisms, except penicillinase-producing *staphylococci*

2) Usual dose: 1 to 12 g every 24 hours in 4 divided doses

3) Mode of administration: push, intermittent

4) Major side effects: dermatitis, rash, urticaria, anemia

5) Nursing considerations: stability is concentration-dependent and decreases as concentration of drug increases; drug is especially susceptible to inactivation in dextrose solutions

6) Patient/caregiver education: instruct patient to report skin rash, previous sensitivities

b. Methicillin sodium (Staphcillin)

1) Indications: gram-positive organisms

2) Usual dose: 4 to 12 g every 24 hours in 6 to 8 divided doses

3) Mode of administration: push, intermittent

4) Major side effects: anemia, neutropenia, oral thrush, rash

5) Nursing considerations: monitor carefully for signs of sensitivity; those with history of allergic reactions to penicillin are prone to cross-sensitivity reactions

6) Patient/caregiver education: instruct patient to report hypersensitivity reaction

c. Mezlocillin sodium (Mezlin)

1) Indications: gram-positive, gram-negative organisms

2) Usual dose: 200 to 300 mg/kg every 24 hours

3) Mode of administration: push, intermittent

4) Major side effects: nausea, vomiting, thrombocytopenia, neutropenia

5) Nursing considerations: confirm patency of vein and avoid extravasation or intra-arterial injection; may result in sloughing

6) Patient/caregiver education: instruct patient to recognize and report signs of bleeding; report pain at intravenous site

d. Nafcillin sodium (Unipen)
   1) Indication: infection caused by penicillinase-producing staphylococci
   2) Usual dose: 500 to 1000 mg every 4 hours
   3) Mode of administration: push, intermittent
   4) Major side effects: bleeding, nausea, rash
   5) Nursing considerations: monitor renal, hepatic, and hematopoietic functions
   6) Patient/caregiver education: instruct patient to recognize and report bleeding

e. Oxacillin sodium (Prostaphlin)
   1) Indications: infection caused by penicillinase-producing organisms
   2) Usual dose: 250 to 1000 mg every 4 to 6 hours
   3) Mode of administration: push, intermittent
   4) Major side effects: diarrhea, vomiting, skin rash
   5) Nursing considerations: may potentiate anticoagulants
   6) Patient/caregiver education: instruct patient to report side effects, especially related to bleeding

f. Penicillin G potassium/sodium
   1) Indications: used to treat severe gram-positive, gram-negative, and anaerobic infections, Vincent's gingivitis, spirochetal infections, meningitis, endocarditis
   2) Usual dose: 1,000,000 to 20,000,000 units every 24 hours
   3) Mode of administration: intermittent, continuous
   4) Major side effects: chills, edema, fever, urticaria
   5) Nursing considerations: may potentiate anticoagulants; monitor electrolyte balance because of sodium or potassium base
   6) Patient/caregiver education: instruct patient to report venous pain

g. Piperacillin sodium (Pipracil)
   1) Indications: respiratory, urinary, skin, bone, and joint infections
   2) Usual dose: 3 to 4 g in divided doses every 4 to 12 hours
   3) Mode of administration: push, intermittent
   4) Major side effects: vertigo, nausea, neutropenia, pruritus
   5) Nursing considerations: evaluate renal, hepatic, and hematopoietic systems
   6) Patient/caregiver education: instruct patient to report skin rash

h. Ticarcillin disodium (Ticar)
   1) Indications: extended-spectrum penicillin for bacterial septicemia

2) Usual dose: 150 to 300 mg/kg every 24 hours in divided doses
3) Mode of administration: intermittent
4) Major side effects: abnormal clotting time and prothrombin time, anemia, leukopenia, nausea, pruritus, urticaria
5) Nursing considerations: administer slowly to avoid pain
6) Patient/caregiver education: instruct patient to report venous pain

4. Tetracyclines
   a. Doxycycline hyclate (Vibramycin Hyclate Intravenous)
      1) Indications: broad-spectrum against gram-negative and gram-positive organisms
      2) Usual dose: 200 mg in 1 to 2 infusions, followed by 100 to 200 mg every 24 hours
      3) Mode of administration: intermittent
      4) Major side effects: anorexia, diarrhea, skin rashes, blood dyscrasias, photosensitivity, thrombophlebitis
      5) May potentiate digoxin; phlebitis may occur because doxycycline is inhibited by alkalinizing agents
      6) Patient/caregiver education: instruct patient to avoid exposure to sun when taking this medication and to recognize and report induration at the intravenous site

5. Antifungals
   a. Amphotericin B (Fungizone)
      1) Indications: treatment of systemic fungal infections such as cryptococcosis, blastomycosis, moniliasis, coccidioidomycosis, histoplasmosis, and others
      2) Usual dose: 10 mg/250 ml over 4 hours
      3) Mode of administration: slow infusion at concentrations of 0.1 mg/ml
      4) Major side effects: headache, convulsions, fever, chills, nephrotoxicity, anorexia, thrombophlebitis, cardiac disturbances, anemia, coagulation defects
      5) Nursing considerations: alternate-day administration may decrease incidence of side effects; before administration, a test dose of 1 mg is required; initially prepare with 10 ml of preservative-free sterile water, then further dilute with 5% dextrose in water; use a 1-micron or larger filter; drug is light-sensitive and should be protected during administration
      6) Patient/caregiver education: instruct patient to report bleeding
   b. Fluconazole (Diflucan)[19]
      1) Indications: antifungal agent used to treat candidiasis, cryptococcal meningitis, systemic infections
      2) Usual dose: initially administer 400 mg followed by 200 mg daily for 28 days
      3) Mode of administration: single daily dose not to exceed 200 mg/hour

       4) Major side effects: abdominal pain, diarrhea, dry mouth, taste perversion, loss of balance

       5) Nursing considerations: in impaired renal function, monitor creatinine clearance; monitor liver function

       6) Patient/caregiver education: instruct patient regarding mouth care

  c. Miconazole (Monistat IV)[20]

       1) Indications: antifungal agent used to treat *Candida, Cryptococcus neoformans, Aspergillus fumigatus*

       2) Usual dose: 200 to 3600 mg/day every 8 hours in 3 divided doses

       3) Mode of administration: intermittent

       4) Major side effects: phlebitis at site, nausea, fever and chills, pruritus, anaphylaxis

       5) Nursing considerations: administer test dose; monitor intake and output

       6) Patient/caregiver education: instruct patient to report fever, chills, dizziness, flushing during infusion

6. Anti-Infectives

  a. Acyclovir sodium (Zovirax)

       1) Indications: initial and recurrent mucosal and cutaneous herpes simplex infections

       2) Usual dose: 5 mg/kg every 8 hours for 7 days

       3) Mode of administration: intermittent

       4) Major side effects: agitation, confusion, headache, hypotension, acute renal failure, phlebitis, nausea

       5) Nursing considerations: use with caution in impaired renal function; maintain adequate hydration before and during administration; use of electronic infusion device is recommended

       6) Patient/caregiver education: instruct patient to report change in sensorium

  b. Co-trimoxazole (Bactrim I.V. Infusion)

       1) Indications: severe urinary tract infections

       2) Usual dose: 8 to 10 mg/kg every 6, 8, or 12 hours

       3) Mode of administration: intermittent

       4) Major side effects: nausea, vomiting, tremors

       5) Nursing considerations: maintain adequate hydration to prevent crystalluria and stone formation

       6) Patient/caregiver education: instruct patient concerning hydration

  c. Foscarnet sodium (Foscavir)[21]

       1) Indications: used to treat viral infections caused by cytomegalovirus (CMV), acyclovir-resistant herpes

       2) Usual dose: 60 mg/kg every 8 hours for 14 to 21 days

       3) Mode of administration: intermittent

        4) Major side effects: renal dysfunction, anemia, diarrhea, hypocalcemia, hypomagnesemia, hypokalemia

        5) Nursing considerations: use of electronic infusion device is recommended; assess for signs of renal impairment, monitor chemistry panel

        6) Patient/caregiver education: instruct patient on importance of prehydration; instruct patient to report tingling or numbness of extremities

    d. Ganciclovir sodium (Cytovene, DHPG)[22]

        1) Indications: used to treat CMV retinitis, herpes virus, Epstein-Barr virus

        2) Usual dose: 5 mg/kg every 12 hours for 14 to 21 days

        3) Mode of administration: intermittent

        4) Major side effects: granulocytopenia, phlebitis

        5) Nursing considerations: assess renal function and output before and during therapy; monitor liver function and CBC; flush tubing before and after with 0.9% sodium chloride; maintain hydration level

        6) Patient/caregiver education: instruct patient to have regular ophthalmic examinations and effective birth control throughout treatment to avoid birth defects

    e. Metronidazole hydrochloride (Flagyl I.V.)

        1) Indications: serious infections of skin, bone, and joints

        2) Usual dose: 15 mg/kg loading dose; follow with 7.5 mg/kg every 6 hours thereafter

        3) Mode of administration: intermittent, continuous

        4) Major side effects: diarrhea, vomiting, nausea, neutropenia, pruritus, thrombophlebitis

        5) Nursing considerations: protect from light during storage; monitor intravenous site

        6) Patient/caregiver education: instruct patient concerning home storage of drug

    f. Pentamidine isethionate (Pentam 300)

        1) Indications: treatment of *Pneumocystis carinii* pneumonia; used investigationally for treatment of trypanosomiasis and visceral leishmaniasis

        2) Usual dose: 4 mg/kg once daily for 14 days

        3) Mode of administration: single daily dose over 60 minutes

        4) Major side effects: anemia, leukopenia, thrombocytopenia, nausea, bad taste in mouth, hyperkalemia, hypoglycemia, hypotension

        5) Nursing considerations: side effects may be life-threatening; monitor blood pressure (BP) before, during, and after infusion; keep patient in supine position; monitor chemistry panel

        6) Patient/caregiver education: instruct patient to report bleeding

    g. Vidarabine (Vir-A)

        1) Indication: herpes simplex virus

        2) Usual dose: 15 mg/kg for 10 days

3) Mode of administration: continuous

4) Major side effects: tremors, malaise, vertigo, confusion, rash, nausea

5) Nursing considerations: administer by slow infusion only; use of electronic infusion device recommended; use of in-line filter less than 0.45 microns required

6) Patient/caregiver education: instruct patient to avoid injury

h. Zidovudine (AZT, Retrovir)[23]

1) Indications: used to treat Human Immunodeficiency Virus (HIV) infection

2) Usual dose: 1 to 2 mg/kg every 4 hours

3) Mode of administration: intermittent

4) Major side effects: anaphylaxis, anorexia, granulocytopenia, gastrointestinal pain, headache, fatigue

5) Nursing considerations: assess central nervous system, monitor liver and renal studies; monitor CBC

6) Patient/caregiver education: instruct patient not to breastfeed; teach patient to recognize and report signs of granulocytopenia

7. Other

a. Chloramphenicol sodium succinate (Chloromycetin)

1) Indications: treatment of bacteremia, Rocky Mountain spotted fever, cystic fibrosis regimens

2) Usual dose: 50 mg/kg every 24 hours

3) Mode of administration: push, intermittent

4) Major side effects: aplastic anemia, bone marrow depression, granulocytopenia, thrombocytopenia, diarrhea

5) Nursing considerations: obtain baseline CBC and then every 2 to 3 days during therapy

6) Patient/caregiver education: instruct patient to report bleeding

b. Vancomycin hydrochloride (Vancocin HCL IntraVenous)

1) Indications: gram-positive cocci, endocarditis

2) Usual dose: 500 mg every 6 hours or 1 g every 12 hours

3) Mode of administration: intermittent

4) Major side effects: ototoxicity, nephrotoxicity, chills, fever, hypotension, thrombophlebitis, tinnitus, pain at injection site, red-man syndrome characterized by red blotching of the face, neck, chest, and extremities

5) Nursing considerations: monitor intake and output; total daily dose should be reduced if renal function is impaired; increase diluent and slow rate of infusion for pain at injection site

6) Patient/caregiver education: instruct patient to report pain during infusion and any hearing difficulties

c. Imipenem-cilastatin sodium (Primaxin)

1) Indications: respiratory, urinary, bone, and joint infections

2) Usual dose: 250 mg to 1 g every 6 to 8 hours

3) Mode of administration: intermittent

4) Major side effects: diarrhea, glossitis, heartburn, hemorrhagic colitis, tinnitus

5) Nursing considerations: monitor intake and output; reduce rate of infusion if nausea develops; monitor intravenous site

6) Patient/caregiver education: instruct patient to report decreased urine output

d. Clindamycin phosphate (Cleocin phosphate)

1) Indications: used to treat anaerobic or aerobic bacterial infections

2) Usual dose: 600 mg to 2.7 g every 24 hours in 2 to 4 divided doses

3) Mode of administration: intermittent

4) Major side effects: abdominal pain, diarrhea, thrombophlebitis, colitis

5) Nursing considerations: observe for diarrhea because fatal colitis may occur; each milliliter contains 9.45 mg benzyl alcohol and too rapid an injection may cause severe hypotension and cardiac arrest; monitor infusion rate and intravenous site

6) Patient/caregiver education: instruct patient to report change in bowel habits, change in sensorium, pain at intravenous site

e. Erythromycin lactobionate (Erythrocin Lactobionate-I.V.)

1) Indications for use: staphylococci, pneumococci, and streptococci infections

2) Usual dose: 15 to 20 mg/kg every 24 hours

3) Mode of administration: intermittent, continuous

4) Major side effects: urticaria, pain along vein

5) Nursing considerations: monitor intravenous site for signs of phlebitis; reduce rate of infusion for pain at intravenous site

6) Patient/caregiver education: instruct patient to report pain or induration at intravenous site

C. Autonomic Drugs

1. Dopamine hydrochloride (Intropin)

a. Indications: hypotension

b. Usual dose: initially, 2 to 5 μg/kg; 5 to 10 μg/kg may be required in the critically ill patient; gradually increase by 5 to 10 μg/kg/minute at 10- to 30-minute intervals until optimum response is attained; average dose is 20 μg/kg

c. Mode of administration: continuous

d. Major side effects: ectopic beats, hypertension, hypotension, vasoconstriction, widened QRS complex, aberrant conduction, tissue necrosis following extravasation

e. Nursing considerations: monitor urine output continuously; monitor BP and central venous pressure; ensure patency of venous access; use large veins to provide adequate hemodilution of drug; avoid extravasation; antidote is injection of 5 to 10 mg of phentolamine mesylate (Regitine) diluted in 10 to 15 ml 0.9% sodium chloride; continue to monitor for hypotension following Regitine; use electronic infusion device

    f. Patient/caregiver education: instruct patient to notify nurse of pain at intravenous site

2. Norepinephrine bitartrate (Levophed)
    a. Indications: hypotension
    b. Usual dose: 8 to 12 μg initial dose; then adjust to maintain BP
    c. Mode of administration: continuous
    d. Major side effects: bradycardia, chest pain, vomiting, photophobia, pallor, tissue necrosis following extravasation
    e. Nursing considerations: monitor BP every 2 minutes until stable, and every 5 minutes thereafter; monitor intravenous flow rate and injection site carefully; avoid extravasation; antidote is injection of 5 to 10 mg phentolamine mesylate (Regitine) diluted in 10 to 15 ml 0.9% sodium chloride; use electronic infusion device
    f. Patient/caregiver education: instruct patient to report pain at infusion site

3. Atropine sulfate
    a. Indications: sinus bradycardia, atrioventricular block
    b. Usual dose: varies with condition being treated
    c. Mode of administration: push
    d. Major side effects: blurred vision, dilation of pupils, postural hypotension, urinary retention
    e. Nursing considerations: use with caution in the very young or in elderly patients
    f. Patient/caregiver education: instruct patient concerning visual changes

4. Dobutamine hydrochloride (Dobutrex)
    a. Indications: short-term inotropic support
    b. Usual dose: 2.5 to 10 μg/kg to maximum of 40 μg/kg/minute
    c. Mode of administration: continuous
    d. Major side effects: anginal pain, chest pain, palpitations, headache, nausea
    e. Nursing considerations: monitor patient's heart rate, BP, urine output; use electronic infusion device
    f. Patient/caregiver education: instruct patient to report changes in urine output, headache, or nausea

5. Epinephrine hydrochloride (Adrenalin chloride)
    a. Indications: drug of choice for anaphylactic shock and antidote of choice for histamine overdose and allergic reactions
    b. Usual dose: 0.2 to 0.5 mg of 1:10,000 solution
    c. Mode of administration: push
    d. Major side effects: anxiety, vertigo, palpitations
    e. Nursing considerations: administer with extreme caution; check BP every 5 minutes for 1 hour

f. Patient/caregiver education: instruct patient to report change in sensorium or anxiety level

6. Isoproterenol hydrochloride (Isuprel hydrochloride)
   a. Indications: atrioventricular heart block and cardiac standstill
   b. Usual dose: varies according to mode of administration
   c. Mode of administration: push, continuous
   d. Major side effects: angina, flushing, palpitations, sweating, nausea, vomiting
   e. Nursing considerations: monitor rate of infusion and titrate to heart rate and rhythm; do not use if pink in color; use electronic infusion control device
   f. Patient/caregiver education: instruct patient to report episodes of chest pain or flushing

7. Metaraminol bitartrate (Aramine)
   a. Indications: acute hypotensive states
   b. Usual dose: 0.5 to 5 mg in emergency situations
   c. Mode of administration: 5 mg over 1 minute
   d. Major side effects: vertigo, agitation, hypertension
   e. Nursing considerations: monitor BP every 5 minutes until desired pressure obtained; monitor intravenous site
   f. Patient/caregiver education: instruct patient to report episodes of vertigo and agitation

8. Ritodrine hydrochloride (Yutopar)
   a. Indications: arrest preterm labor
   b. Usual dose: 0.1 mg/minute initially; gradually increase by 0.05 mg/minute every 10 minutes until desired result obtained
   c. Mode of administration: continuous
   d. Major side effects: anxiety, chest pain, palpitations, vomiting
   e. Nursing considerations: ensure patient comfort; obtain maternal baseline electrocardiogram (ECG) to rule out heart disease; monitor uterine contractions, maternal pulse rate, BP, and fetal heart rate; maintain adequate hydration
   f. Patient/caregiver education: instruct patient to report vomiting, chest pain, or palpitations

D. Coagulants and Anticoagulants

1. Heparin sodium[24]
   a. Indications: prevention and treatment of thrombosis and emboli; diagnostic aid in disseminated intravascular coagulation; maintain patency of vascular catheters; produces anticoagulant effect by inhibiting the conversion of prothrombin to thrombin and fibrinogen to fibrin
   b. Usual dose: varies with use and clinical indications
   c. Mode of administration: push, intermittent, continuous
   d. Major side effects: bleeding, prolonged coagulation time, bruising, epistaxis, hematuria, pain, headache

e. Nursing considerations: use electronic infusion device; most important laboratory value for dose-regulating is the partial thromboplastin time (PTT); when administered for venous thrombosis, PTT should be maintained at 1.5 to 2 times the control value; antidote for overdose is protamine sulfate

f. Patient/caregiver education: instruct patient to watch for bruises, bleeding gums, hematuria, to avoid over-the-counter aspirin products, and to use an electric razor when shaving

2. Protamine sulfate (a heparin antagonist)

a. Indication: to neutralize the activity of heparin sodium in severe overdose

b. Usual dose: 1 mg for every 100 U.S.P. units of heparin sodium given; may repeat in 10 to 15 minutes; never exceed 50 mg in any 10-minute period; dose decreases rapidly with time elapsed after heparin sodium injection

c. Mode of administration: push

d. Major side effects: dyspnea, bradycardia, hypertension or hypotension, feeling of warmth

e. Nursing considerations: monitor PTT; potential for hypersensitivity in patients with fish allergies

f. Patient/caregiver education: instruct patient to report episodes of bleeding

3. Aminocaproic acid (Amicar Intravenous)

a. Indications: treatment of hemorrhage caused by overactivity of fibrinolytic system

b. Usual dose: initial dose 4 to 5 g; follow with 1 to 1.25 g/hour or at hourly intervals for 6 to 8 hours

c. Mode of administration: intermittent, continuous

d. Major side effects: diarrhea, nausea, tinnitus, vertigo, grand mal seizure, rash

e. Nursing considerations: rapid administration may cause hypotension, bradycardia, or dysrhythmia; monitor carefully

f. Patient/caregiver education: instruct patient to report episodes of dizziness

4. Antithrombin III (AT-III, Thrombate III)[25]

a. Indications: treatment of thrombotic episodes

b. Usual dose: varies with use and clinical indications

c. Mode of administration: push, intermittent

d. Major side effects: dyspnea, hematoma formation, shortness of breath

e. Nursing considerations: assess for viral infections; assess lungs and breathing patterns; avoid unnecessary venipunctures

f. Patient/caregiver education: instruct patient to watch for bruises, bleeding gums, hematuria, to avoid over-the-counter aspirin products, and to use an electric razor when shaving

E. Thrombolytic Agents

1. Streptokinase (Streptase)
   a. Indications: plasmin activator used to treat pulmonary emboli, acute myocardial infarction
   b. Usual dose: 250,000 IU loading dose; 100,000 IU/hour for 24 to 72 hours as maintenance dose; 1.5 million IU within 6 hours of onset of symptoms of acute myocardial infarction or 750,000 IU within 3 hours of onset of symptoms; follow with 2,000 IU/minute for 1 hour
   c. Mode of administration: push, continuous
   d. Major side effects: hypersensitivity, fever, bleeding
   e. Nursing considerations: monitor bleeding parameters and vital signs; obtain baseline creatinine phosphokinase before intravenous use; avoid invasive procedures, including intravenous and intramuscular injections, rotating tourniquets, and antiplatelet agents; use electronic infusion device
   f. Patient/caregiver education: instruct patient to report episodes of bleeding; to avoid use of straight razors, to avoid use of aspirin products

2. Urokinase (Abbokinase)
   a. Indications: restores patency of intravenous catheters; used for lysis of acute massive pulmonary emboli; acute myocardial infarction
   b. Usual dose: varies with use and clinical indications
   c. Mode of administration: push, continuous
   d. Major side effects: bleeding, bronchospasm, arrhythmias
   e. Nursing considerations: observe patient constantly; monitor bleeding parameters and vital signs; obtain creatinine phosphokinase before direct intravenous use; avoid invasive procedures, including intravenous and intramuscular injections, rotating tourniquets, and antiplatelet agents; use electronic infusion device
   f. Patient/caregiver education: instruct patient to avoid injury

3. Alteplase (Activase)
   a. Indications: lysis of acute massive pulmonary emboli; acute myocardial infarction
   b. Usual dose: varies with use and clinical indications
   c. Mode of administration: push, continuous
   d. Major side effects: bleeding, nausea, vomiting, arrhythmias
   e. Nursing considerations: obtain baseline ECG and monitor ECG continuously; monitor bleeding parameters and vital signs; obtain creatinine phosphokinase before direct intravenous use; avoid invasive procedures, including intravenous and intramuscular injections, rotating tourniquets, and antiplatelet drugs; use electronic infusion device

f. Patient/caregiver education: instruct patient to avoid injury and to report episodes of bleeding

F. Cardiovascular Drugs

1. Bretylium tosylate (Bretylol)
   a. Indications: antiarrhythmic used to treat refractory ventricular tachycardia
   b. Usual dose: 5 mg/kg increasing to 10 mg/kg for ventricular tachycardia; repeat at 15- to 30-minute intervals
   c. Mode of administration: push, intermittent, continuous
   d. Major side effects: bradycardia, hypotension, increased frequency of premature ventricular contractions (PVCs), nausea, vomiting, vertigo
   e. Nursing considerations: observe for postural hypotension; maintain supine position; monitor cardiac status; monitor for signs of dehydration or hypovolemia; may aggravate digitalis toxicity
   f. Patient/caregiver education: instruct patient to remain supine and to report episodes of angina

2. Digoxin (Lanoxin)
   a. Indications: treatment of congestive heart failure, atrial fibrillation, atrial flutter, cardiogenic shock, ventricular dysrhythmias with congestive heart failure
   b. Usual dose: 0.25 to 0.5 mg as initial dose followed by 0.25 to 0.5 mg at 4- to 6-hour intervals; maintenance dose of 0.125 to 0.5 mg daily
   c. Mode of administration: push
   d. Major side effects: partial atrioventricular block, abdominal discomfort, blurred vision, confusion, diarrhea, nausea, vomiting
   e. Nursing considerations: calcium gluconate is contraindicated in digitalis toxicity; in severe intoxication, hyperkalemia may be present; monitor electrolyte and digoxin levels; may be administered undiluted
   f. Patient/caregiver education: instruct patient to avoid injury and to report episodes of bleeding

3. Lidocaine hydrochloride (Xylocaine)
   a. Indications: treatment of ventricular arrhythmias
   b. Usual dose: 50 to 100 mg bolus, followed by infusion of 4 mg/minute
   c. Mode of administration: push, continuous
   d. Major side effects: blurred vision, vertigo, twitching, vomiting, hypotension, bradycardia
   e. Nursing considerations: use with caution in severe renal or hepatic disease, hypovolemia, shock, heart block; use electronic infusion device
   f. Patient/caregiver education: instruct patient to report visual changes

4. Verapamil hydrochloride (Isoptin)
   a. Indications: treatment of supraventricular tachyarrhythmias
   b. Usual dose: 5 to 10 mg; may repeat in 30 minutes if needed
   c. Mode of administration: push over 2 minutes
   d. Major side effects: abdominal discomfort, nausea, asystole, hypotension, vertigo, headache
   e. Nursing considerations: monitor BP and ECG during administration; protect vial from light; do not use if solution is discolored
   f. Patient/caregiver education: instruct patient to report headache

5. Amrinone lactate (Inocor Lactate)
   a. Indications: short-term management of congestive heart failure
   b. Usual dose: 0.75 mg/kg; may repeat in 30 minutes; maintenance dose of 5 to 10 μg/kg/minute
   c. Mode of administration: push, continuous
   d. Major side effects: abdominal pain, nausea, chest pain, dyspnea, pain and burning at injection site; hypotension
   e. Nursing considerations: use with caution in renal or hepatic dysfunction; monitor BP, urinary output
   f. Patient/caregiver education: instruct patient to report pain at infusion site

6. Esmolol hydrochloride (Brevibloc)
   a. Indications: treatment of supraventricular tachycardia
   b. Usual dose: individualized by titration
   c. Mode of administration: continuous
   d. Major side effects: induration at site, confusion, speech disorders, taste disorders, tissue necrosis following extravasation
   e. Nursing considerations: monitor BP, monitor patient's cardiovascular status; monitor intravenous site; use electronic infusion device
   f. Patient/caregiver education: instruct patient to report pain at infusion site

7. Labetalol hydrochloride (Normodyne)
   a. Indications: control BP in severe hypertension
   b. Usual dose: 20 to 80 mg as initial dose; continuous: 50 to 200 mg, not to exceed a 300-mg total
   c. Mode of administration: push, continuous
   d. Major side effects: diaphoresis, vertigo, moderate hypotension, numbness, severe postural hypotension
   e. Nursing considerations: keep patient supine; monitor BP before and 5 and 10 minutes after direct injection
   f. Patient/caregiver education: instruct patient to report dizziness or shortness of breath

8. Methyldopate hydrochloride (Aldomet)
   a. Indications: treatment of acute hypertensive crisis
   b. Usual dose: 250 to 500 mg/kg every 6 hours

    c. Mode of administration: intermittent

    d. Major side effects: vertigo, dry mouth, mild postural hypotension

    e. Nursing considerations: use with caution in renal or hepatic disease; monitor BP and urinary output

    f. Patient/caregiver education: instruct patient to report dry mouth

9. Propranolol hydrochloride (Inderal)

    a. Indications: management of paroxysmal atrial tachycardia, sinus tachycardia, atrial flutter and fibrillation

    b. Usual dose: 0.5 to 3 mg given 1 mg/minute

    c. Mode of administration: push

    d. Major side effects: bradycardia, cardiac failure, hypotension, vertigo, visual disturbances

    e. Nursing considerations: monitor ECG, BP, and pulmonary wedge pressure continuously

    f. Patient/caregiver education: instruct patient to report changes in vision or sensorium

10. Quinidine gluconate

    a. Indications: treatment of cardiac arrhythmias

    b. Usual dose: 200 mg; administer dose over 1 minute; repeat as needed

    c. Mode of administration: continuous at 1 ml/minute

    d. Major side effects: cramps, nausea, urge to void/defecate, apprehension, diaphoresis, rash, tinnitus

    e. Nursing considerations: use with caution in presence of heart block, liver or hepatic dysfunction; use electronic infusion device; monitor BP and heart rhythm continuously during infusion

    f. Patient/caregiver education: instruct patient to report abdominal cramping, rash, tinnitus

11. Sodium nitroprusside (Nipride)

    a. Indications: treat hypertensive emergencies, reduce preload and afterload in cardiogenic shock

    b. Usual dose: 3 μg/kg/minute; dose varies dependent on response

    c. Mode of administration: continuous

    d. Major side effects: hypotension, tissue sloughing with extravasation, acidosis

    e. Nursing considerations: 5% dextrose in water is the only compatible infusate; monitor intravenous site; use electronic infusion device

    f. Patient/caregiver education: instruct patient to report pain at intravenous site

12. Nitroglycerin (Tridil)

    a. Indications: control of BP in perioperative hypertension; congestive heart failure associated with acute myocardial infarction

b. Usual dose: 5 μg/minute initially; titrate to obtain response

c. Mode of administration: continuous infusion

d. Major side effects: headache, tachycardia, abdominal pain, nausea, vertigo

e. Nursing considerations: use glass containers and nonPVC administration sets; use with caution in patients with liver or renal disease; monitor BP and heart rhythm; use electronic infusion device

f. Patient/caregiver education: instruct patient to report headache, dizziness, abdominal pain

13. Adenosine (Adenocard)[26]
   a. Indications: vasodilator used to restore normal sinus rhythm
   b. Usual dose: varies with use and clinical indications
   c. Mode of administration: push over 1 to 2 seconds
   d. Major side effects: shortness of breath, transient facial flushing, chest pain, hypotension, asystole
   e. Nursing considerations: monitor heart rate every 15 to 30 seconds; monitor ECG continuously; monitor BP throughout treatment
   f. Patient/caregiver education: instruct patient to report facial flushing, shortness of breath, dizziness

14. Ibutilide fumarate (Corvert)[27]
   a. Indications: used to treat atrial fibrillation flutter
   b. Usual dose: varies with use and clinical indications
   c. Mode of administration: push over 10 minutes
   d. Major side effects: prolonged QT, hypertension, nausea, vomiting, palpitations
   e. Nursing considerations: assess baseline ECG and QT interval; assess weight to determine dosage
   f. Patient/caregiver education: instruct patient to report faintness, difficulty breathing, chest discomfort

15. Procainamide hydrochloride (Pronestyl)[28]
   a. Indications: used to treat wide-complex tachycardias and when lidocaine is contraindicated
   b. Usual dose: varies with use and clinical indications
   c. Mode of administration: push, intermittent, continuous
   d. Major side effects: drug-induced systemic lupus syndrome, hypotension, ventricular arrhythmias, asystole
   e. Nursing considerations: use electronic infusion device; monitor ECG continuously and vital signs frequently; monitor renal function
   f. Patient/caregiver education: instruct patient to report dizziness

16. Hydralazine hydrochloride (Apresoline)[29]
   a. Indications: potent antihypertensive agent; vasodilator in cardiogenic shock
   b. Usual dose: 5 to 20 mg

      c. Mode of administration: push

      d. Major side effects: headache, tachycardia, sodium retention, drug-induced lupus syndrome

      e. Nursing considerations: assess renal and hepatic function, monitor CBC and chemistry panel

      f. Patient/caregiver education: instruct patient to report drowsiness, muscle or joint pain, chest pain, tingling

17. Methyldopate hydrochloride (Aldomet)[30]

      a. Indications: used to treat moderate to severe hypertension

      b. Usual dose: 250 to 1000 mg every 6 hours

      c. Mode of administration: intermittent

      d. Major side effects: sedation, orthostatic hypotension, bradycardia, myocarditis, hepatitis

      e. Nursing considerations: use electronic infusion device; assess for signs and symptoms of sodium retention

      f. Patient/caregiver education: inform patient that urine may darken; educate patient to change position often, monitor intake and output

G. Central Nervous System Drugs

1. Morphine sulfate

      a. Indications: relief of severe, acute pain or moderate to severe chronic pain

      b. Usual dose: varies with use and clinical response

      c. Mode of administration: push, continuous

      d. Major side effects: respiratory depression, circulatory depression, hypersensitivity

      e. Nursing considerations: do not administer to patients with bronchial asthma; use with caution in head injury, increased intracranial pressure; use electronic infusion device; intrathecal dose is one-tenth the epidural dose; monitor respiratory rate and level of consciousness; naloxone hydrochloride (Narcan) should be readily available

      f. Patient/caregiver education: instruct patient to report breathing difficulties

2. Diazepam (Valium)

      a. Indications: treatment of moderate to severe psychoneurotic reactions, acute alcohol withdrawal, acute stress reactions

      b. Usual dose: 2 to 10 mg every 3 to 4 hours; may repeat in 1 hour up to maximum of 30 mg in 8 hours

      c. Mode of administration: push

      d. Major side effects: apnea, bradycardia, ataxia, blurred vision, confusion, depression, venous thrombosis, phlebitis, respiratory depression, drowsiness

      e. Nursing considerations: administer directly into the vein; avoid smaller veins; inject into intravenous tubing closest to vein site only when direct intravenous injection is not feasible; flush before and immediately following injection with 0.9% sodium chloride

    f. Patient/caregiver education: instruct patient to report pain at intravenous site

3. Phenytoin sodium (Dilantin)
   a. Indications: control of grand mal and psychomotor seizures; treatment of choice in status epilepticus
   b. Usual dose: 100 to 250 mg initially as an anticonvulsant
   c. Mode of administration: push, intermittent
   d. Major side effects: ataxia, confusion, vertigo, tremors, visual disturbances, cardiac arrhythmias, tissue necrosis following extravasation
   e. Nursing considerations: observe for crystals in solution or in the intravenous line during administration; flush with 0.9% sodium chloride before and after administration; monitor site for induration; use 0.22-micron filter
   f. Patient education: instruct patient to report pain at intravenous site and any visual disturbances

4. Buprenorphine hydrochloride (Buprenex)
   a. Indication: relief of moderate to severe pain
   b. Usual dose: 0.3 mg/ml
   c. Mode of administration: push
   d. Major side effects: hypersedation, vertigo
   e. Nursing considerations: monitor vital signs
   f. Patient education: instruct patient to report change in sensorium

5. Chlordiazepoxide hydrochloride (Librium)
   a. Indications: treatment of acute or severe agitation; tremors, alcohol withdrawal
   b. Usual dose: 50 to 100 mg
   c. Mode of administration: push
   d. Major side effects: blood dyscrasias, skin eruption, nausea, hypotension
   e. Nursing considerations: use only freshly prepared solution and discard unused portion; observe patient for up to 3 hours following administration for respiratory or cardiac complications
   f. Patient/caregiver education: instruct patient to report changes in skin

6. Droperidol (Inapsine)
   a. Indications: preoperative sedation, antiemetic
   b. Usual dose: varies with clinical indications
   c. Mode of administration: push
   d. Major side effects: vertigo, tremors, hypotension
   e. Nursing considerations: monitor vital signs and response to treatment; monitor level of consciousness
   f. Patient education: instruct patient to report change in sensorium

7. Hydromorphone hydrochloride (Dilaudid)
    a. Indications: treatment of moderate to severe pain
    b. Usual dose: 1 to 4 mg every 4 to 6 hours
    c. Mode of administration: push, continuous
    d. Major side effects: nausea, vomiting, vertigo, hypotension, respiratory depression
    e. Nursing considerations: monitor vital signs frequently; keep patient supine; orthostatic hypotension and fainting may occur; naloxone hydrochloride (Narcan) and oxygen should be readily available
    f. Patient/caregiver education: instruct patient to avoid injury
8. Lorazepam (Ativan)
    a. Indications: preanesthetic medication; antiemetic
    b. Usual dose: 2 mg
    c. Mode of administration: push
    d. Major side effects: apnea, confusion, delirium, excessive drowsiness
    e. Nursing considerations: remain at bedrest after injection for 3 to 5 hours following administration; may require assistance for up to 8 hours; monitor intravenous site
    f. Patient/caregiver education: instruct patient to avoid injury
9. Magnesium sulfate
    a. Indications: treatment of convulsive states; electrolyte replacement; toxemia
    b. Usual dose: varies with clinical indication
    c. Mode of administration: push
    d. Major side effects: flaccid paralysis, respiratory depression, sweating, CNS depression
    e. Nursing considerations: monitor respirations before each dose; monitor serum magnesium; do not administer within 2 hours preceding delivery of pregnancy-induced hypersensitive to avoid injury to fetus
    f. Patient/caregiver education: instruct patient to avoid injury
10. Naloxone hydrochloride (Narcan)
    a. Indications: narcotic-induced depression
    b. Usual dose: 0.4 to 2.0 mg
    c. Mode of administration: push
    d. Major side effects: nausea, vomiting, hypotension or hypertension, reversal of analgesia
    e. Nursing considerations: monitor respiratory rate; duration of narcotic action may exceed that of naloxone hydrochloride
    f. Patient/caregiver education: instruct patient to report nausea
11. Meperidine hydrochloride (Demerol)
    a. Indications: moderate to severe pain relief
    b. Usual dose: varies with indication and clinical response
    c. Mode of administration: push, intermittent, continuous

   d. Major side effects: agitation, sedation
   e. Nursing considerations: monitor BP, pulse, respiratory rate, level of consciousness
   f. Patient/caregiver education: instruct patient to report ongoing pain not relieved by medication

12. Fentanyl citrate
   a. Indication: pain control
   b. Usual dose: varies with indication and clinical response
   c. Mode of administration: epidural or intrathecal; push, continuous
   d. Major side effects: pruritus, urinary retention, respiratory depression
   e. Nursing considerations: drug preparation must be preservative-free; naloxone hydrochloride (Narcan) should be readily available
   f. Patient/caregiver education: instruct patient to report change in sensorium

13. Bupivacaine hydrochloride (Marcaine)
   a. Indication: pain control
   b. Usual dose: varies with indication and clinical response, degree of anesthesia required
   c. Mode of administration: epidural or intrathecal
   d. Major side effects: central nervous and cardiovascular system reactions
   e. Nursing considerations: drug preparation must be preservative-free; resuscitative equipment and drugs that may be required for treatment of adverse reactions should be immediately available[18]
   f. Patient/caregiver education: instruct patient to report prolonged episodes of pain not relieved by medication

H. Electrolyte and Water Balance Agents

1. Calcium chloride
   a. Indications: treatment of tetany associated with hypocalcemia
   b. Usual dose: varies with clinical indication
   c. Mode of administration: push
   d. Major side effects: bradycardia, cardiac arrest, tingling sensation, tissue necrosis following extravasation
   e. Nursing considerations: monitor serum calcium, vital signs, intravenous site for pain and induration
   f. Patient/caregiver education: instruct patient to report pain at intravenous site

2. Calcium gluconate
   a. Indications: to treat calcium deficiency caused by vitamin D deficiency; antidote for magnesium sulfate toxicity; electrolyte replacement
   b. Usual dose: varies with clinical indication

    c. Mode of administration: push, continuous

    d. Major side effects: bradycardia, cardiac arrest, flushing, tingling sensation, tissue necrosis following extravasation

    e. Nursing considerations: monitor serum calcium, vital signs, intravenous site for pain and induration

    f. Patient/caregiver education: instruct patient to report pain at intravenous site

3. Ammonium chloride

    a. Indications: metabolic alkalosis caused by chloride loss

    b. Usual dose: varies with patient condition and tolerance

    c. Mode of administration: continuous

    d. Major side effects: bradycardia, hypokalemia, hyperglycemia, metabolic acidosis, pallor, pain along intravenous site

    e. Nursing considerations: monitor respirations and serum electrolytes

    f. Patient/caregiver education: instruct patient to report palpitations

4. Bumetanide (Bumex)

    a. Indications: congestive heart failure

    b. Usual dose: 0.5 to 1.0 mg

    c. Mode of administration: push

    d. Major side effects: excessive diuresis, electrolyte imbalances, impaired hearing

    e. Nursing considerations: monitor serum electrolytes, intake and output

    f. Patient/caregiver education: instruct patient to report hearing loss

5. Chlorothiazide sodium (Diuril)

    a. Indications: treatment of edema, toxemia of pregnancy

    b. Usual dose: 500 mg to 1.0 g once or twice daily

    c. Mode of administration: push

    d. Major side effects: diarrhea, nausea, vertigo, photosensitivity, tissue necrosis following extravasation

    e. Nursing considerations: determine patency of vein before administration; monitor BP, serum electrolytes, intake and output, intravenous site for pain and induration

    f. Patient/caregiver education: instruct patient to avoid injury

6. Ethacrynate sodium (Sodium edecrin)

    a. Indications: treatment of congestive heart failure

    b. Usual dose: 0.5 to 1.0 mg/kg

    c. Mode of administration: push, intermittent

    d. Major side effects: anorexia, thirst, vomiting, electrolyte imbalance

    e. Nursing considerations: monitor serum electrolytes, intake and output

    f. Patient/caregiver education: instruct patient to avoid injury

7. Hetastarch (Hespan)
   a. Indications: adjunctive therapy in shock
   b. Usual dose: depends on degree of fluid loss
   c. Mode of administration: continuous
   d. Major side effects: vomiting, peripheral edema
   e. Nursing considerations: maintain adequate hydration, monitor pulse, BP, intake and output, CBC, serum electrolytes, observe for increased bleeding
   f. Patient/caregiver education: instruct patient to report changes in skin
8. Potassium chloride/acetate
   a. Indications: prophylaxis or treatment of deficiency
   b. Usual dose: varies with clinical condition
   c. Mode of administration: intermittent, continuous
   d. Major side effects: bradycardia, ECG changes, voluntary muscle paralysis, weakness, pain along intravenous site
   e. Nursing considerations: monitor cardiac status for dose in excess of 10 mEq/hour, serum potassium
   f. Patient/caregiver education: instruct patient to report pain at intravenous site
9. Sodium chloride
   a. Indications: replacement of sodium and chloride ions
   b. Usual dose: varies with clinical indication
   c. Mode of administration: continuous
   d. Major side effects: anorexia, dehydration, disorientation, distention, edema, hypertension
   e. Nursing considerations: monitor intake and output, vital signs, serum electrolytes
   f. Patient/caregiver education: instruct patient to report change in sensorium
10. Dextran
    a. Indications: adjunctive therapy in treatment of shock
    b. Usual dose: 20 ml/kg body weight over first 24 hours; 10 ml/kg over each succeeding 24 hours
    c. Mode of administration: continuous
    d. Major side effects: hypotension, anaphylaxis
    e. Nursing considerations: monitor BP, pulse, urinary output every 5 to 15 minutes for the first hour and hourly thereafter
    f. Patient/caregiver education: instruct patient to report change in sensorium
11. Furosemide (Lasix)
    a. Indications: treatment of congestive heart failure, acute pulmonary edema, hypercalcemia
    b. Usual dose: varies with clinical indication
    c. Mode of administration: continuous
    d. Major side effects: anemia, leukopenia, vomiting, anorexia, tinnitus, leg cramps, paresthesias, blurring of vision, hypokalemia

    e. Nursing considerations: monitor intake and output, serum electrolytes status, BP

    f. Patient/caregiver education: instruct patient to report dizziness, blurring of vision, tingling sensations

12. Mannitol (Osmitrol)

    a. Indications: cerebral edema, decreased intraocular pressure, oliguric phase of acute renal failure

    b. Usual dose: varies with clinical indication

    c. Mode of administration: intermittent; give 200 mg/kg to produce 40 ml of urine in 1 hour

    d. Major side effects: convulsions, blurred vision, vertigo, headache, urinary retention, polyuria followed by oliguria, chills, chest pain, edema, fluid and electrolyte imbalance

    e. Nursing considerations: administer test dose over 3 to 5 min; monitor for increased urine output, serum electrolytes, intravenous site; maintain hydration; crystals must be dissolved before administration; use a 170-micron in-line filter

    f. Patient/caregiver education: instruct patient to report changes in sensorium

13. Sodium bicarbonate

    a. Indications: status asthmaticus, barbiturate intoxication, metabolic acidosis

    b. Usual dose: adjusted consistent with pH, $PaCO_2$, calculated base deficit, fluid limitations

    c. Mode of administration: push, continuous

    d. Major side effects: hyperexcitability, tetany, headache, distention, nausea, alkalosis, tissue necrosis following extravasation, hypokalemia

    e. Nursing considerations: monitor intravenous site, serum electrolytes, arterial blood gases

    f. Patient/caregiver education: instruct patient to report pain at intravenous site

I. Gastrointestinal Drugs

1. Ranitidine (Zantac)

    a. Indications: pathologic hypersecretory conditions

    b. Usual dose: varies with mode of administration and clinical indication

    c. Mode of administration: push, intermittent, continuous

    d. Major side effects: abdominal discomfort, diarrhea, nausea, vomiting, headache

    e. Nursing considerations: rapid administration may precipitate bradycardia or PVCs; slight darkening of solution does not affect potency; increase frequency of dose not amount, if necessary, for pain relief

    f. Patient/caregiver education: instruct patient to report abdominal discomfort

2. Cimetidine hydrochloride (Tagamet hydrochloride)
   a. Indications: ulcers, pathologic hypersecretory conditions
   b. Usual dose: varies with mode of administration and clinical indication
   c. Mode of administration: push, intermittent, continuous
   d. Major side effects: bradycardia, hypotension, fever, vertigo, delirium, confusion
   e. Nursing considerations: monitor prothrombin time; may potentiate warfarin anticoagulants; maximum dose 2.4 g/day
   f. Patient/caregiver education: instruct patient to avoid injury
3. Famotidine (Pepcid IV)
   a. Indications: ulcers, pathologic hypersecretory conditions
   b. Usual dose: 20 mg every 12 hours
   c. Mode of administration: push, intermittent
   d. Major side effects: constipation, diarrhea, nausea, headache, vertigo
   e. Nursing considerations: increase frequency of dose not amount, if necessary, for pain relief
   f. Patient/caregiver education: instruct patient to report change in sensorium
4. Metoclopramide hydrochloride (Reglan)
   a. Indication: antiemetic
   b. Usual dose: 2 mg/kg/30 minutes
   c. Mode of administration: intermittent
   d. Major side effects: restlessness, drowsiness, fatigue, lassitude
   e. Nursing considerations; too rapid an injection may increase anxiety; given 30 minutes pre- and post-administration of antineoplastics
   f. Patient/caregiver education: instruct patient to avoid injury
5. Ondansetron (Zofran)
   a. Indications: antiemetic
   b. Usual dose: varies with clinical indication
   c. Mode of administration: push, intermittent
   d. Major side effects: headache, diarrhea, or constipation
   e. Nursing considerations: none
   f. Patient/caregiver education: instruct patient to report any changes in bowel habits

J. Hormone and Synthetic Substitutes

1. Insulin (regular)
   a. Indications: diabetic coma, ketoacidosis, short-term use for treatment of hyperkalemia
   b. Usual dose: based on serum glucose level
   c. Mode of administration: push, continuous
   d. Major side effects: nausea, hunger, fatigue, clammy skin, nervousness, sweating, convulsions, hypokalemia

   e. Nursing considerations: regular insulin is the only type appropriate for intravenous administration; monitor serum glucose levels
   f. Patient/caregiver education: instruct patient regarding signs and symptoms of hypoglycemia, hyperglycemia
2. Glucagon hydrochloride
   a. Indications: hypoglycemia
   b. Usual dose: 0.5 to 1 mg
   c. Mode of administration: push
   d. Major side effects: nausea, vomiting, anaphylaxis
   e. Nursing considerations: monitor serum glucose levels
   f. Patient/caregiver education: instruct patient on prevention of hypoglycemia

K. Vitamin Preparations[31]

1. Folic acid (Folvite)
   a. Indications: megaloblastic anemias of malnutrition
   b. Usual dose: 1 mg daily
   c. Mode of administration: continuous
   d. Major side effects: rare
   e. Nursing considerations: none
   f. Patient/caregiver education: none
2. Multivitamins (M.V.I.-12)
   a. Indication: vitamin deficiency
   b. Usual dose: one 5- to 10-ml dose every 24 hours; varies according to manufacturer's recommendations
   c. Mode of administration: continuous
   d. Major side effects: rare
   e. Nursing considerations: never use undiluted; do not use if crystals are present
   f. Patient/caregiver education: instruct patient regarding vitamin supplementation
3. Pyridoxine hydrochloride (Hexa-Betalin)
   a. Indications: Vitamin B_6 deficiency
   b. Usual dose: 10 to 100 mg every 24 hours
   c. Mode of administration: push, continuous
   d. Major side effects: rare
   e. Nursing considerations: deteriorates when exposed to excessive heat
   f. Patient/caregiver education: instruct patient to report change in body temperature, flushing
4. Thiamine hydrochloride (Betalin S)
   a. Indication: thiamine deficiency syndromes
   b. Usual dose: varies with clinical indication and response
   c. Mode of administration: 100 mg or fraction thereof over 5 minutes, continuous
   d. Major side effects: hypersensitivity reaction

   e. Nursing considerations: none
   f. Patient/caregiver education: instruct patient to report unusual signs and symptoms
5. Vitamin K_1–phytonadione (Aquamephyton)
   a. Indications: anticoagulant-induced prothrombin deficiency; hemorrhagic disease of newborn; hypothrombinemia resulting from obstructive jaundice, ulcerative colitis, biliary disease
   b. Usual dose: 2.5 to 25 mg
   c. Mode of administration: 1 mg or fraction thereof over 1 minute; continuous
   d. Major side effects: cyanosis, diaphoresis, vertigo, hypotension, change in taste
   e. Nursing considerations: monitor prothrombin time; administer with caution because of potential for anaphylactic reaction
   f. Patient/caregiver education: instruct patient to report unusual signs and symptoms

L. Respiratory Smooth Muscle Relaxant

1. Theophylline ethylenediamine (Aminophylline)
   a. Indications: bronchial asthma, reversible bronchospasm of chronic bronchitis or emphysema
   b. Usual dose: varies with clinical indication and response
   c. Mode of administration: push, continuous
   d. Major side effects: nausea, vomiting, delirium, vertigo, anxiety, ventricular fibrillation, palpitations, headache
   e. Nursing considerations: avoid rapid administration; monitor serum levels; 500 mg aminophylline is equivalent to 400 mg theophylline; monitor respiratory rate
   f. Patient/caregiver education: instruct patient to report changes in sensorium and to avoid injury

M. Miscellaneous Drugs

1. Oxytocin (Pitocin)
   a. Indications: induce or stimulate labor, postdelivery to stimulate contractions to decrease bleeding
   b. Usual dose: varies with clinical indications
   c. Mode of administration: continuous
   d. Major side effects
      1) maternal: uterine rupture, fluid retention, hypertension
      2) fetal: central nervous system or brain damage, arrhythmias
   e. Nursing considerations: monitor BP, fetal heart, strength and timing of contractions, fluid intake
   f. Patient/caregiver education: instruct patient concerning uterine cramping

2. Immune globulin IV (Sandoglobulin)
   a. Indications: maintain and treat those unable to produce adequate amounts of IgG antibodies
   b. Usual dose: varies with clinical indication and manufacturer's recommendations
   c. Mode of administration: continuous
   d. Major side effects: angioedema, fever, hypotension, erythema, urticaria
   e. Nursing considerations: monitor vital signs, may cause hypotensive reaction; initiate infusion slowly; emergency equipment should be readily available
   f. Patient/caregiver education: instruct patient to report any feelings of lightheadedness

V. RESPONSE TO THERAPY

A. Factors Affecting Patient's Response[32]

1. Age: pediatric and geriatric dosing regimens and other variables
2. Size
3. Sex
4. Genetics
5. Presence of other disease process
6. Route of administration
7. Rate of administration: consideration of pediatric and geriatric variables
8. Other treatment protocols
9. Drug interactions

B. Therapeutic Response (occurs when the desired clinical response is obtained)

C. Absence of Associated Pain, Redness, Swelling

1. Associated pain, redness, swelling require immediate nursing intervention

D. Presence of Associated Pain, Redness, Swelling

1. Requires immediate attention, especially in case of irritant and vesicant drug agents

E. Complications[32]

1. Extravasation: inadvertent administration of vesicant solution/medication into surrounding tissue
   a. Vesicant: an agent capable of causing or forming a blister or causing tissue destruction; knowledge base concerning antidotes necessary

b. Irritant: an agent capable of producing venous pain at the site or along the wall of the vein, with or without inflammatory reaction[32]

2. Infiltration: the inadvertent administration of a nonvesicant solution/medication into surrounding tissue

3. Therapeutic incompatibilities[9]: an undesirable reaction resulting from the overlapping effects of two drugs given together or closely together

   a. Antagonism: cross reaction in which a drug's action is inhibited by the action of another drug

   b. Synergism: harmonious action of two drug agents producing an effect that neither could produce alone or an effect that is greater than the total effects of each agent operating by itself

   c. Potentiation: synergistic action of two substances in which the total effects are greater than the sum of the independent effects of the two substances

4. Anaphylaxis: a hypersensitive state of the body to a foreign protein or drug, induced by a preliminary injection

5. Speed shock: systemic reaction to a substance rapidly injected into the bloodstream

6. Phlebitis: inflammation of the vein wall, evidenced by pain, erythema, edema, and/or a palpable cord

   a. Bacterial: attributed to contamination of intravenous equipment, drugs or infusates, or poor site care

   b. Chemical: attributed to hypertonic solutions, pH, or drug particulates

   c. Mechanical: attributed to poor site selection, loose cannula or 'needle hub, injury during cannulation, or particulate matter in solutions

REFERENCES

1. Weinstein SM. *Plumer's Principles and Practice of Infusion Therapy*, 6th ed. Philadelphia, PA: Lippincott-Raven, 1997:589.
2. Intravenous Nurses Society. Intravenous Nursing Standards of Practice (revised 1998). *Journal of Intravenous Nursing* 1998;21(1):suppl.
3. Ibid, Compatibility, p. S38, 39.
4. Ibid, Laminar Flow, p. S37.
5. Ibid, Admixing, p. S38.
6. Weinstein SM. *Plumer's Principles and Practice of Infusion Therapy*, 6th ed. Philadelphia, PA: Lippincott-Raven, 1997:436.
7. Karch AM. *1999 Lippincott's Nursing Drug Guide.* Philadelphia, PA: Lippincott-Raven, 1999:1321.
8. Intravenous Nurses Society. Position paper: The intravenous nurse specialist's role in the evolving healthcare environment. *Journal of Intravenous Nursing* 1997;20(3):119–120.
9. Trissel LA. *Handbook on Injectable Drugs*, 9th ed., Bethesda, MD: American Society of Health-System Pharmacists, 1998.

10. Intravenous Nurses Society. Intravenous Nursing Standards of Practice (revised 1998). *Journal of Intravenous Nursing* 1998;21(1):suppl.

11. Intravenous Nurses Society. Intravenous Nursing Standards of Practice (revised 1998). *Journal of Intravenous Nursing* 1998;21(1):suppl.

12. Phillips LD, Kuhn MA. *Manual of IV Medications,* 2nd ed. Philadelphia, PA: Lippincott-Raven, 1999:28–31.

13. Ibid, p. 145–147.

14. Karch AM. *1999 Lippincott's Nursing Drug Guide.* Philadelphia, PA: Lippincott-Raven, 1999:1136–1137.

15. Phillips LD, Kuhn MA. *Manual of IV Medications,* 2nd ed. Philadelphia, PA: Lippincott-Raven, 1999:47–48.

16. Ibid, p. 49–51.

17. Ibid, p. 73–75.

18. Ibid, p. 75–77.

19. Ibid, p. 88–90.

20. Ibid, p. 114.

21. Ibid, p. 91.

22. Ibid, p. 93.

23. Ibid, p. 155–156.

24. Ibid, p. 313–316.

25. Ibid, p. 297.

26. Ibid, p. 338.

27. Ibid, p. 378.

28. Ibid, p. 404.

29. Ibid, p. 376.

30. Ibid, p. 387.

31. American Hospital Formulary Service. *AHFS Drug Information 98.* Bethesda, MD: American Society of Health-System Pharmacists. 1998:2233.

32. Weinstein S. *Plumer's Principles and Practice of Intravenous Therapy,* 7th ed. Philadelphia, PA: Lippincott-Raven, 1999. In progress.

CHAPTER 4

Infection Control

Roxanne R. Perucca, MSN, CRNI

I. EPIDEMIOLOGY/HOST DEFENSE

A. Overview

1. Epidemiology and host defense are concerned with defining and explaining the interrelationship of the host, agent, and environment in the prevention and control of disease
2. Principles of infection control provide a foundation for the delivery of intravenous therapy
3. Initiation of an intravenous cannula breaks the transcutaneous skin barrier, which is the first line of host defense

B. Immune System

1. Provides host defense by a complex system of interdependent components
2. One missing element can cause the entire immune system to be ineffective
3. Leukocytes are important components of the immune system
   a. Normal white blood cell count ranges from 4,500 to 11,000/mm^{3}[1]
4. Differential white blood cell count provides more specific information related to infection and disease processes
   a. Granulocytes
      1) Neutrophils or polymorphonuclear leukocytes (bands and segments)
         • Provide the foundation for the body's nonspecific immune response
         • Are the most numerous circulating white blood cell
         • Rapidly respond to inflammatory and tissue injury sites
      2) Eosinophils
         • Increase during allergic reactions and parasitic conditions
         • Decrease when steroids are increased during stress or by parenteral administration
      3) Basophils
         • Increase during the healing process
         • Decrease when steroids are increased during stress or by parenteral administration

b. Agranulocytes
1) Monocytes
2) Lymphocytes

C. Nonspecific Immune Response

1. Provided by granulocytes and monocytes
2. Neutrophils and monocytes are macrophages responsible for engulfing and partially digesting or phagocytizing invading antigens
   a. Neutrophils (bands and segments) predominate in the first hours of injury
      1) Segments are mature neutrophils
      2) Bands are less mature cells of a neutrophil that multiply quickly during acute infection
   b. Monocytes respond late during the acute phase of infection
      1) Stronger action than neutrophils
      2) Can ingest larger particles of debris

D. Specific Immune Response

1. Formed by the B lymphocytes and T lymphocytes
2. Lymphocytes have specific antigen recognition
   a. Neutralize bacterial endotoxins
   b. Phagocytize invading bacteria and viruses
   c. Increase with the occurrence of chronic and viral infections

E. Risk Factors for Developing an Intravascular Device-related Infection

1. Immunosuppression and immunodeficiency
2. Severe underlying chronic illness
3. Administration of multiple infusions
4. Extended hospitalization
5. Leukopenia (an abnormal decrease of white blood corpuscles usually below 5000/mm^3)
6. Presence of a concurrent infection
7. Age (infants younger than 1 year or persons older than 60 years)
8. Burns

II. MEANS OF CONTAMINATION

A. Extrinsic

1. Occurs after the manufacturing process, during clinical use
2. Most prevalent means of contamination
3. Primary causes
   a. Inadequate hand washing by healthcare personnel

   b. Compounding of admixtures
      1) Improper use of laminar flow hoods
      2) Use of malfunctioning laminar flow hoods
      3) Incorrect use of admixing equipment, such as needles, syringes, or calibration devices that contaminate products
      4) Failure to refrigerate admixed fluid containers
   c. Venipuncture procedure
      1) Improper site preparation
      2) Touch contamination of cannula/equipment
      3) Use of contaminated skin-prepping agents
      4) Improper application of dressing
      5) Failure to rotate cannula insertion sites
   d. Intravenous infusion system
      1) Change of intravenous administration sets
      2) Flashback of blood into the administration set
      3) Withdrawal of blood for laboratory specimens
      4) Accidental disconnection of the administration set
      5) Failure to maintain sterile, closed infusion system
      6) Use of external devices to calibrate pressure monitoring systems
   e. Medication administration
      1) Addition of medications to the intravenous container
      2) Injections into the injection ports of intravenous administration sets
      3) Administration of intermittent medication infusions
      4) Use of multidose vials increase potential for contamination
4. Primary causative organisms (not limited to the following):
   a. Tribe *Klebsielleae* (*Enterobacter cloacae, Enterobacter agglomerans, Serratia marcescens, Klebsiella* species)
   b. *Staphylococcus aureus*
   c. Coagulase-negative staphylococci
   d. *Candida* species
   e. *Corynebacterium* species
   f. *Mycobacterium* species
   g. *Malassezia furfur*
5. Preventive strategies
   a. Proper hand washing
   b. Correct storage and use of admixture equipment/supplies
   c. Close inspection of intravenous fluids/equipment
   d. Maintenance of aseptic technique
   e. Routine rotation of cannula insertion sites
   f. Proper skin preparation of cannula insertion site
   g. Routine change of cannula, dressing, and administration set
   h. Maintenance of dry, intact dressing on cannula insertion site
   i. Maintenance of sterile, closed infusion system

B. Intrinsic

1. Occurs during the manufacturing process
   a. Continuously monitored by industry and regulatory agencies
   b. Sampling procedures devised to detect ongoing problems resulting in low levels of contamination
   c. Sequential sampling procedures to monitor the production process
      1) Rejection of products contaminated at unacceptable frequencies
      2) Consideration of previous sterility testing results to determine the acceptability of current tests
2. Low rate of occurrence
   a. An epidemic of infusion-related bacteremias possibly related to:
      1) Mass production of large volumes of intravenous solutions
      2) Microorganisms present in solution containers that proliferate during storage
   b. Nearly all reported septicemias are associated with contaminated infusate by aerobic gram-negative bacilli[2]
3. Primary causative organisms (not limited to the following):
   a. Tribe *Klebsielleae* (*Enterobacter cloacae, Enterobacter agglomerans, Serratia marcescens, Klebsiella* species)
   b. *Pseudomonas*
   c. *Xanthomonas maltophilia*
   d. *Pseudomonas acidovorans*
   e. *Pseudomonas pickettii*
   f. *Citrobacter freundii*
   g. *Flavobacterium* species
   h. *Candida tropicalis*
4. Preventive strategies
   a. Stringent quality control during the manufacturing process
   b. Inspection of administration equipment before use
      1) Discoloration
      2) Torn packages
      3) Missing or improperly fitting port covers
      4) Expiration date
   c. Inspection of intravenous solutions before use
      1) Clarity
      2) Particulate matter
      3) Puncture holes or cracks in container
      4) Loss of vacuum
      5) Damage to bag or bottle closures
      6) Expiration date
5. Documentation and reporting mechanisms for contamination
   a. If potential contamination is suspected, report promptly to the following:

1) Infusion therapy manager
2) Pharmacist
3) Materials management
4) Risk management
5) Physician
b. Immediate notification of regulatory agencies
1) Local, state, and federal authorities
2) Centers for Disease Control and Prevention (CDC)
3) Food and Drug Administration (FDA)

C. Exogenous Contamination

1. Caused by transmission of organisms from sources other than the patient; can be caused by intrinsic or extrinsic contamination
2. Frequent occurrences
3. Primary causative organisms (not limited to the following):
   a. *Staphylococcus aureus*
   b. Coagulase-negative staphylococci
4. Preventive strategies
   a. Proper hand washing
   b. Using aseptic technique

D. Endogenous Contamination

1. Caused by patient's own microflora
   a. Patients who are immunocompromised are more susceptible
   b. Variety of microorganisms associated with the flora of the skin are commonly involved
   c. Normal microflora of the skin can be altered by antimicrobial therapy
   d. Intravenous cannula can become colonized by microorganisms from a distant site of infection
   e. Current studies focus on the ability of microorganisms to translocate across the gastrointestinal tract to normally sterile tissues such as the mesenteric lymph nodes, spleen, liver, and blood[3]
2. Most frequent occurrences are in high-risk, severely ill patients
3. Primary causative organisms (not limited to the following):
   a. *Staphylococcus aureus*
   b. Coagulase-negative staphylococci
   c. *Escherichia coli*
   d. *Klebsiella pneumoniae*
   e. *Pseudomonas aeruginosa*
   f. *Candida albicans*
4. Preventive strategies
   a. Proper site preparation
   b. Using aseptic technique
   c. Rotation of cannula insertion sites

III. MICROORGANISMS COMMONLY INVOLVED IN INTRAVASCULAR-RELATED INFECTIONS (refer to Table 4-1)

A. Gram-Negative Bacteria

1. Infusate
   a. Tribe *Klebsielleae*
      1) *Enterobacter cloacae*
      2) *Enterobacter agglomerans*
      3) *Serratia marcescens*
      4) *Klebsiella* species
   b. *Pseudomonas* species

TABLE 4-1 *Infusion-related Infections: Microorganisms and Source*

Microorganism	Source
Tribe *Klebsielleae*	Infusate
Enterobacter cloacae	
Enterobacter agglomerans	
Serratia marcescens	
Klebsiella species	
Candida albicans	
Candida tropicalis	
Enterobacter cloacae	Blood products
Serratia marcescens	
Pseudomonas species	
Klebsiella species	Peripheral cannula
Enterobacter species	
Pseudomonas species	
Staphylococcus aureus	
Staphylococcus epidermidis	
Coagulase-negative staphylococcus	
Candida albicans	
Klebsiella species	Central venous catheter
Enterobacter species	
Staphylococcus aureus	
Staphylococcus epidermidis	
Coagulase-negative staphylococcus	
Candida albicans	

2. Blood products
   a. *Enterobacter cloacae*
   b. *Serratia marcescens*
   c. *Pseudomonas* species
3. Peripheral cannula
   a. *Klebsiella* species
   b. *Enterobacter* species
   c. *Pseudomonas* species
4. Central venous catheters
   a. *Klebsiella* species
   b. *Enterobacter* species

B. Gram-Positive Bacteria

1. Peripheral cannula
   a. *Staphylococcus aureus*
   b. Coagulase-negative staphylococci
2. Central venous catheters
   a. *Staphylococcus aureus*
   b. Coagulase-negative staphylococci

C. Fungi

1. Infusate
   a. *Candida tropicalis*
   b. *Candida albicans*
2. Peripheral cannula
   a. *Candida albicans*
3. Central venous catheters
   a. *Candida albicans*

IV. MICROORGANISM LIFESPAN/MULTIPLICATION IN INTRAVENOUS SOLUTIONS[4]

A. Rapid Growth in 5% Dextrose in Water Mainly Limited To:

1. Tribe *Klebsielleae*
   a. *Enterobacter cloacae*
   b. *Enterobacter agglomerans*
   c. *Serratia marcescens*
   d. *Klebsiella* species
2. *Pseudomonas cepacia*

B. Rapid Growth in Lactated Ringer's Solution Mainly Limited To:

1. *Pseudomonas aeruginosa*
2. *Enterobacter* species
3. *Serratia* species

C. 0.9% Sodium Chloride Allows Growth of Most Bacteria

D. Crystalline Amino Acid and 25% Dextrose Solutions

1. Very slow growth of *Candida tropicalis*
2. Inhibition of most bacteria

E. Lipid Emulsion

1. Rapid growth of most organisms
2. Rapid multiplication of *Candida* species

V. CATHETER-RELATED INFECTION

A. Predisposing Factors

1. Improper aseptic technique during cannula insertion
   a. Inadequate barrier protection
   b. Inadvertent contamination
2. Migration of bacteria through the subcutaneous catheter tract
3. Contamination of infusion system
4. Hematogenous seeding from a distant focus such as with translocation of bacteria

B. Factors That May Cause Catheter-related Infections

1. Presence of a fibrin sheath around the intravascular portion of the catheter may promote bacterial adherence and replication around the catheter[5]
2. Longer catheter dwell time may increase colonization of microorganisms
3. Catheters with multiple lumens have numerous connection manipulations possibly resulting in greater risk of contamination
4. Colonization of microorganisms on the catheter hub[6]
5. Greater tissue injury with large-gauge catheters increasing the risk of infection
6. Long-term antimicrobial therapy alters the normal flora of the skin

C. Microorganisms Frequently Associated with Catheter-related Infections

1. Gram-positive microorganisms (associated with approximately two-thirds of intravenous-related infections)[7]
   a. *Staphylococcus aureus*
   b. Coagulase-negative staphylococci
   c. *Enterococcus* species
2. Gram-negative microorganisms
   a. *Pseudomonas aeruginosa*
   b. *Proteus*

    c. *Klebsiella* species
    d. *Escherichia coli*
  3. Fungus
    a. *Candida albicans*

VI. CONTAMINATION AT THE INSERTION SITE

A. Predisposing Conditions

1. Colonization of microorganisms at the insertion site is associated with the highest incidence of catheter-related infections
2. Often related to microorganisms on the skin
3. Microorganisms of the skin are classified as resident or transient flora
  a. Resident flora is referred to as colonizing flora
    1) Considered to be permanent residents of the skin
    2) Not readily removed by mechanical friction
    3) Organisms involved (not limited to the following):[8]
      • Coagulase-negative staphylococci
      • *Corynebacterium* (commonly referred to as diphtheroids or coryneforms)
      • *Propionibacterium*
      • *Acinetobacter* species
      • Probably certain members of the *Klebsiella-Enterobacter* group
  b. Transient flora is referred to as contaminating or noncolonizing flora
    1) Microorganisms not consistently present on the majority of persons
    2) Loosely attached to the skin, varying from day to day
    3) Readily transmitted by the hands of healthcare workers
    4) Removed when hands are properly washed with soap and water using mechanical friction

B. Site-associated Risk Factors

1. Peripheral
  a. Average concentration of 10 colony-forming units (CFUs) is found on the arm or wrist[9]
  b. Cooler core body temperature is present on extremities
  c. Emergency-inserted cannula is suspected of contamination because of improper site preparation and compromised aseptic technique
    1) Discontinue as soon as patient is stable or at least within 24 hours of cannula insertion
    2) Replace with a cannula inserted in a new location
  d. Cut down sites are associated with a higher risk of infection and sepsis

2. Central
   a. Subclavian site
      1) As many as 1,000–10,000 CFUs can be found on the chest or neck of long-term patients
      2) Warmer core body temperature on trunk of body resulting in greater potential for microbial growth
      3) Easy to maintain sterile occlusive dressing
   b. Jugular site
      1) Difficult to maintain sterile occlusive dressing
      2) Possible limitation of patient mobility and comfort
   c. Femoral site
      1) Difficultly maintaining sterile occlusive dressing
      2) Greater amount of CFUs found on the skin
3. Arterial
   a. Peripheral arterial catheter[10]
      1) Inflammation present at the insertion site
      2) Catheter dwell time greater than 4 days
      3) Catheter inserted by cutdown
   b. Central arterial catheter (Swan-Ganz catheter)
      1) Length of catheter dwell time
      2) Introducer (with or without catheter) left in place longer than 5 days[11]
4. Intraspinal
   a. Long-term catheters are associated with increased risk for infection
   b. Failure to maintain sterile occlusive dressing
5. Intraventricular: increased risk for infection related to the absence of leukocytes
6. Intraosseous: increased risk for osteomyelitis and sepsis if the cannula is left in place longer than 24 hours[12]
7. Umbilical
   a. Risk of infection is greater with the venous catheter[13]
   b. Risk is increased if the catheter is left in place longer than 24 hours[14]

VII. PERSONAL PROTECTIVE EQUIPMENT

A. Gloves

1. Worn to prevent broken skin transmission of bloodborne infections
2. Worn for all tasks in which contact with blood or body fluids may occur
3. Nonsterile gloves: worn with insertion of a peripheral cannula
4. Sterile gloves: worn during placement and administration of site care to an arterial or central venous catheter, and during insertion

of a peripheral venous cannula in a severely immunocompromised patient

B. Face Masks

1. Used to protect the mucous membranes of nose and mouth
2. Worn when blood or body fluid could splash, splatter, or spray
3. Worn when within 2 to 3 feet of a sterile area to prevent breathing of colonized nasal bacteria onto the sterile field

C. Long-sleeve Clothing (such as a disposable gown)

1. Provides protection when infectious materials are splashed or sprayed
2. Prevents shedding epithelial cells from falling onto the sterile field

D. Eyewear

1. Used to protect mucous membranes of the eye
2. Worn when the splashing of blood or body fluids is possible, such as with the use of a breakaway needle

VIII. INSERTION PREPARATION TECHNIQUE

A. Hand Washing

1. Use antimicrobial soap; liquid soap preferred over bar soap
2. Lather hands and wrists for a minimum of 15 to 20 seconds
3. Paper towels are preferred over reusable cloth towels
4. Use a towel to turn off the faucet; prevents recontamination of hands

B. Hair Removal

1. Excessive hair at the site of an intravenous catheter should be clipped
2. Shaving can cause microabrasions, which increase the risk of infection
3. Depilatories are not recommended because of the risk for allergic reactions
4. Surgical clippers with disposable clipper heads are acceptable to prevent cross contamination; clipper heads are to be changed after each patient use

C. Insertion Site Cleansing

1. Clean intended insertion site with soap and water if the extremity is excessively dirty

IX. RECOMMENDED ANTIMICROBIAL PREPARATIONS

A. 70% Isopropyl Alcohol

1. Inexpensive
2. Rapidly reduces microbial counts on skin by denaturing protein
3. Apply with friction for a minimum of 30 seconds or until the final applicator is visually clean

B. Povidone-Iodine

1. Iodophors consist of iodine and a carrier substance; the amount of free iodine is decreased to lessen skin irritation
2. Tincture of iodine has the combined effect of isopropyl alcohol and iodine and can cause skin irritation
3. Iodine and iodophors penetrate the cell wall, substituting the microbial contents with free iodine
4. Iodophors require approximately 2 minutes of skin contact time to allow the release of free iodine
   a. Have the ability to kill gram-negative and gram-positive organisms, fungi, and yeast
   b. Are rapidly neutralized in the presence of blood, serum, and other protein-rich materials
5. Application of 70% isopropyl alcohol after povidone-iodine preparation negates the effect of the iodophor

C. Chlorhexidine Gluconate

1. Presently unavailable as commercially prepared single-use packages in the United States
2. Chemically bonds to the protein in the bacterial cell wall
3. Has a residual antibacterial activity persisting for hours after application[15]

D. Aqueous Benzalkonium-like Compounds and Hexachlorophene

1. Are not used to prepare the cannula insertion site[16]

E. Acetone

1. Cleansing with acetone is associated with an increased potential for local inflammation at the insertion site and increased skin irritation
2. Exhibits no decrease in the incidence of catheter-related infection[17]

X. ANTIMICROBIAL APPLICATION

A. Antimicrobial Solutions

1. Single-use containers are recommended
2. Apply in a circular motion, beginning at the insertion site and working outward to the periphery

a. Work from "clean to dirty"
b. For peripheral cannula insertion, clean an area 2 to 3 inches in diameter (acceptable)
c. Apply generous amounts
d. Allow to air dry
e. Do not fan, blot, or blow on the area
f. If the patient is allergic to iodine, use 70% isopropyl alcohol
   1) Preferred prepping solution
   2) Apply until the final applicator is visually clean

B. Antibiotic/Antimicrobial Ointment

1. Clinical trials regarding its usage are not conclusive[18,19]
2. Use is not generally recommended under a transparent semipermeable membrane (TSM) dressing
3. Application is at the skin-cannula junction

XI. CANNULA CARE

A. General Considerations

1. Anchor cannula securely to eliminate any to-and-fro motion
2. Chevron taping may be used to stabilize the cannula
3. Tape may be placed to secure the cannula hub but it should not cover the insertion site
4. Cover skin-cannula junction site with sterile dressing
   a. Transparent semipermeable membrane (TSM) dressing
      1) Optimal time period for routine changing of TSM dressings is unknown[20]
      2) Peripheral-short catheters with TSM dressings are changed at the time of site rotation
      3) TSM dressings used on all sites other than short peripheral catheters are changed at least every 3 to 7 days
      4) Change dressing immediately if it is damp, soiled, or no longer intact
   b. Gauze dressing
      1) Should be changed in accordance with the *Intravenous Nursing Standards of Practice*
      2) If gauze is placed under a TSM, the dressing is considered a gauze dressing
      3) All edges of the gauze should be securely taped
      4) If the edges are no longer closed or intact, or if the gauze is damp or soiled, it should be changed immediately
5. A nonocclusive type Band-Aid dressing is not recommended

B. Dressing Protocols

1. Specific to the type of central venous catheter

2. Percutaneously inserted central catheters require a sterile dressing change protocol requiring the use of a mask and sterile gloves
3. Tunneled catheters require a sterile dressing change
   a. Until exit site has healed
   b. With severely immunocompromised patients
   c. Aseptic technique is used with nonimmunocompromised patients once the exit site has healed
4. Implantable ports require a dressing change only while port remains accessed
   a. Change dressing when noncoring needle is changed
   b. If the dressing becomes soiled, damp, or no longer intact change immediately using sterile technique
5. Arterial cannulas require sterile dressing change daily
   a. Five-fold increased catheter-related bacteremia rate with transparent dressing is reported, versus that with gauze and tape[21]
   b. Change immediately if the dressing is soiled, damp, or no longer intact

C. Evaluation of Insertion Site

1. Minimizes potential risk of complications
2. Frequency
   a. At the time of each dressing change
   b. Before removal of the cannula
   c. At regular intervals as established in policies and procedures
3. Varies according to:
   a. Type of vascular access device
   b. Therapy being administered
   c. Patient's age and condition
   d. Practice setting
4. Assessment parameters include (but are not limited to) indications of:
   a. Infiltration
   b. Phlebitis
   c. Infection
   d. Occlusion

XII. PREVENTION OF CATHETER-RELATED INFECTIONS
A. Recommendations

1. Establish intravenous catheter care policies and procedures based on specific recommendations
   a. The *Intravenous Nursing Standards of Practice*[22]
   b. The *Guidelines for Prevention of Intravascular Device-Related Infections* published by the Centers for Disease Control and Prevention[23]
2. Employment of a specialized team of nurses administering and monitoring intravenous care[24]

B. Nursing Considerations

1. Perform stringent hand washing with antiseptic soap before and after palpating, inserting, or dressing an intravenous device
2. Adhere to the principles of aseptic and sterile technique
3. Use maximum sterile barriers (hair cover, mask, sterile gloves, gown, and wide sterile draping) during the insertion of catheters with extended dwell times
4. Carefully inspect all equipment before use
5. Establish routine inspections and scheduled dressing changes of cannula insertion sites
6. Maintain a sterile, dry, and intact dressing on the cannula insertion site
7. Designate a time interval for peripheral cannula site rotations
8. Maintain a closed sterile system
   a. Limit tubing junctions
   b. Use Luer-Lok connections
   c. Reduce manipulation of the system
9. Use a dedicated line for the administration of total parenteral nutrition
10. Maintain catheter tip placement of central venous catheters in the distal superior vena cava
11. Follow pharmacy-directed admixture program
12. Change solution containers every 24 hours[25]

XIII. COMPLICATIONS OF INTRAVENOUS THERAPY

A. Phlebitis

1. Inflammation of the vein, and may be accompanied by pain, erythema, edema, streak formation, and/or palpable cord
2. Possible precursor to sepsis
3. Measure in accordance with the *Intravenous Nursing Standards of Practice* phlebitis scale
4. Types
   a. Chemical
   b. Mechanical
   c. Bacterial(or septic)
5. Causes
   a. Chemical
      1) Increased osmolarity of intravenous solution
      2) Acidic or alkaline intravenous solution
      3) Particulate matter
   b. Mechanical
      1) Frequent manipulation of the cannula
      2) Improper cannula stabilization

        3) Insertion of a large-gauge cannula into a small vein

        4) Insertion in an area of flexion

    c. Bacterial or septic

        1) Inadequate hand washing

        2) Contamination during admixture of solution or medications

        3) Improper site preparation

        4) Improper cleansing of injection sites before medication administration

        5) Frequent entries into the administration system

        6) Contamination during the manufacturing process

        7) Failure to inspect solution containers for cracks and leaks

        8) Noncompliance of established recommendations for changing administration equipment

6. Preventive measures

    a. Perform proper hand washing

    b. Adhere to the aseptic technique, avoiding touch contamination

    c. Rotate peripheral cannula according to an established schedule

    d. Use smallest gauge and shortest length cannula to administer prescribed therapy

    e. Stabilize cannula to prevent any to-and-fro motion

    f. Know that the amount and type of solutions used to administer or dilute medications alters the pH

    g. Understand that neutral solutions cause less venous irritation

    h. Use a 0.2-micron air-eliminating, bacteria-retentive filter

    i. Infuse solution and medication according to the recommended administration rate

B. Thrombosis

1. Formation of a blood clot within a vein in the neck, chest, or arms
2. Vessel wall injury and stasis may be related to a catheter-related infection

C. Thrombophlebitis

1. Inflammation of the vein with clot formation
2. Tenderness and edema may precede pus formation
3. Purulent drainage can be life-threatening and may be a precursor to sepsis

D. Localized Inflammation at the Insertion Site (may be accompanied by the following)

1. Redness
2. Edema
3. Tenderness
4. Purulent drainage at the insertion or exit site, tunnel, or portal pocket
5. Fever
6. Leukocytosis

E. Bacteremia

1. Occurs when bacteria colonizes the skin around the catheter insertion site, migrates along the surface of the catheter and enters the bloodstream to cause a bloodstream infection
2. Considered catheter-related when the same microorganisms are isolated from both the catheter surface and the blood
3. Bloodstream infection is identified by positive blood cultures
   a. Primary bacteremia
      1) No underlying source
      2) Usually associated with intravenous device
   b. Secondary bacteremia
      1) Developed from an existing site of infection, such as pneumonia or urinary tract infection
      2) Increased risk for patients with burns, cardiovascular infection, or intra-abdominal wound infections
4. Clinical manifestation:
   a. Fever
   b. Chills
   c. Hypotension

F. Septicemia

1. Systemic infection in the circulating blood caused by the presence of pathogenic microorganisms or their toxins in the body
2. Difficult to interpret current data
   a. Many cases of sepsis go unreported
   b. Frequently, appropriate cultures of blood, cannula, and intravenous fluids are not obtained
3. Considered catheter-related when the source of the infection is identified as the indwelling vascular cannula
4. When caused by fluid contamination, it may be clinically indistinguishable from other causes of sepsis
   a. Identification facilitated with the presentation of signs/symptoms
      1) Occurs within a few hours after initiation of intravenous infusion
      2) Occurs in a stable patient without underlying causes
5. Defined as catheter-related with a positive semi-quantitative culture of greater than 15 CFUs and a positive blood culture for the same organism
6. Clinical manifestations, possibly with abrupt onset
   a. Fever and chills
   b. Tachycardia
   c. Tachypnea
   d. Alterations in mentation
   e. Gastrointestinal disturbances: nausea, vomiting, diarrhea
   f. Hypotension

g. Oliguria
h. Respiratory failure
i. Shock
j. Vascular collapse
k. Death

XIV. DIAGNOSTIC METHODS

A. Solution/Infusate

1. Culture of intravenous solution, fluid container, administration set, and blood
2. Sample of fluid is aspirated from the administration set and cultured quantitatively
3. Change entire intravenous system, including the cannula

B. Cannula

1. Perform a semi-quantitative culture of the cannula tip
2. Obtain blood cultures

C. Site Drainage

1. Perform a swab culture of the drainage
2. Obtain a gram stain

D. Blood Cultures

1. Isolate causative organisms
2. Identify source of organisms
3. Draw two or three separate 10-ml blood cultures from peripheral veins by separate venipunctures[27]
4. Isolate blood into aerobic and anaerobic media
5. If the patient is on antimicrobial therapy, obtain blood cultures immediately before a dose is due, possibly providing a higher yield

E. Gram-stained Culture

1. Perform if drainage can be expressed from the insertion site

F. Semi-quantitative Culture

1. Catheter colonization is confirmed
2. Cannula insertion site is disinfected with 70% isopropyl alcohol (preferred over iodine-containing compounds) and allowed to air dry[28]
3. For short indwelling cannulas, the entire length of the cannula from the skin-junction site is cut with sterile scissors into a sterile specimen container
4. For central catheters, a 2-inch segment of the catheter tip and

intracutaneous segment is cut with sterile scissors into two separate sterile specimen containers
5. Semi-quantitative culture results indicate infection
   a. Negative, if less than 15 CFUs are present
   b. Catheter-related infection is confirmed, if greater than 15 CFUs are present[29]

G. Quantitative Culture

1. Useful in determining if infection is catheter-related
2. Blood cultures are drawn peripherally from two separate sites
3. To rule out central catheter-related infection, one set of cultures is drawn peripherally and one set is drawn through the catheter
4. Concentration of organisms in the catheter is compared with the peripheral sample
5. Results showing a greater than tenfold increase in concentration of organisms in the catheter blood sample than in the peripheral blood sample are considered significant for catheter-related infection; catheter removal is necessary[30]

XV. ANTIMICROBIAL THERAPY RELATED TO CATHETER INFECTIONS

A. General Considerations

1. Broad-spectrum therapy initiated to target the majority of microorganisms present
2. Antimicrobial therapy adjusted against the microorganisms isolated

B. Host Factors Affecting Selection

1. Pre-existing disease states
2. Renal function
3. Liver function
4. Sites of infection
5. Age
6. Immune status

C. Drug Factors Affecting Selection

1. Toxicity
2. Drug interactions
3. Compatibilities
4. Cost
5. Pharmacokinetics
   a. Dose
   b. Route
   c. Frequency

1) Intermittent administration of drugs results in fluctuating blood concentration levels
2) Drug concentration levels monitored by laboratory analysis
   • Maximum level (peak) obtained just following a dose
   • Lowest level (trough) determined just before administering dose

REFERENCES

1. Chernecky CC, Berger BJ. *Laboratory Tests and Diagnostic Procedures.* Philadelphia, PA: Saunders, 1997:451.
2. Maki DG. Infections due to infusion therapy. In *Hospital Infections,* 4th ed., edited by Bennett JV, Brachman PS. Philadelphia, PA: Lippincott-Raven, 1998:701.
3. O'Boyle CJ, MacFie J, Johnstone D, Sagar PM, et al. Microbiology of bacterial translocations in humans. *Gut* 1998;42(1):29–35.
4. Maki DG. Infections due to infusion therapy. In *Hospital Infections,* 4th ed., edited by Bennett JV, Brachman PS. Philadelphia, PA: Lippincott-Raven, 1998:702.
5. Cunha BA. Intravenous line infections. *Critical Care Clinics* 1998;14(2):339–346.
6. Stiges-Serra A, Pi-Suner T, Garces JM, Segura M. Pathogenesis and prevention of catheter-related septicemia. *American Journal of Infection Control* 1995;23(5):310–316.
7. Green JN. Catheter-related complications of cancer therapy. *Infectious Disease Clinics of North America* 1996;10(2):255–294.
8. Larson EL. APIC guidelines for hand washing and hand antisepsis in health care settings. *American Journal of Infection Control* 1995;23(40:247–269.
9. Beam TR, Goodman EL, Maki DG, et al. Preventing central venous catheter-related complications. *Infection in Surgery* 1990:1–13.
10. U.S. Department of Health and Human Services. Public Health Services. Centers for Disease Control and Prevention. Guideline for prevention of intravascular device-related infections. *American Journal of Infection Control* 1996;24:262–293.
11. Maki DG, Stolz SS, Wheeler S, Mermel LA. A prospective, randomized trial of gauze and two polyurethane dressings for site care of pulmonary artery catheters: Implications for catheter management. *Critical Care Medicine* 1992;22:1729–1737.
12. Wheeler C. Intravenous therapy in children. In *Intravenous Therapy: Clinical Principles and Practice,* edited by Terry J, Barnanowski L, Lonsway RA, and Hedrick D. Philadelphia, PA: Saunders, 1995:491–492.
13. Wheeler C. Intravenous therapy in children. In *Intravenous Therapy: Clinical Principles and Practice,* edited by Terry J, Barnanowski L, Lonsway RA, and Hedrick D. Philadelphia, PA: Saunders, 1995:490–491.
14. Intravenous Nurses Society. Intravenous Nursing Standards of Practice (revised 1998). *Journal of Intravenous Nursing* 1998;21(1): suppl.
15. Maki DG, Ringer M, Alvarado CJ. Prospective randomized trial of povidone-iodine, alcohol, and chlorhexidine for prevention of infection associated with central venous and arterial catheters. *Lancet* 1991;338:339–343.
16. Intravenous Nurses Society. Intravenous Nursing Standards of Practice (revised 1998). *Journal of Intravenous Nursing* 1998;21(1):suppl.
17. Maki DG, McCormack KN. Defatting catheter insertion sites in total parenteral nutrition is of no value as an infection control measure. *American Journal of Medicine* 1987;83:833–840.

18. Intravenous Nurses Society. Intravenous Nursing Standards of Practice (revised 1998). *Journal of Intravenous Nursing* 1998;21(1):suppl.

19. Jones GA. A practical guide to evaluation and treatment of infections in patients with central venous catheters. *Journal of Intravenous Nursing* 1998;21(5): S134–S142.

20. Clemence MA, Walker D, Farr BM. Central venous catheter practices: Results of a survey. *American Journal of Infection Control* 1995;23(1):5–12.

21. Maki DG. Infections due to infusion therapy. In *Hospital Infections*, 4th ed., edited by Bennett JV, Brachman PS. Philadelphia, PA: Lippincott-Raven, 1998:712.

22. Intravenous Nurses Society. Intravenous Nursing Standards of Practice (revised 1998). *Journal of Intravenous Nursing* 1998;21(1):suppl.

23. U.S. Department of Health and Human Services. Public Health Service. Centers for Disease Control and Prevention: Guideline for prevention of intravascular device-related infections. *American Journal of Infection Control* 1996;24:262–293.

24. Miller JM, Goetz AM, Squier C, Muder RR. Reduction in nosocomial intravenous device-related bacteremias after institution of an intravenous therapy team. *Journal of Intravenous Nursing* 1996;19(2):103–106.

25. U.S. Department of Health and Human Services. Public Health Service. Centers for Disease Control and Prevention: Guideline for prevention of intravascular device-related infections. *American Journal of Infection Control* 1996;24:262–293.

26. Intravenous Nurses Society. Intravenous Nursing Standards of Practice (revised 1998). *Journal of Intravenous Nursing* 1998;21(1): suppl.

27. Maki DG. Infections due to infusion therapy. In *Hospital Infections*, 4th ed., edited by Bennett JV, Brachman PS. Philadelphia, PA: Lippincott-Raven, 1998:693.

28. Intravenous Nurses Society. Intravenous Nursing Standards of Practice (revised 1998). *Journal of Intravenous Nursing* 1998;21(1):suppl.

29. Maki DG. Infections due to infusion therapy. In *Hospital Infections*, 4th ed., edited by Bennett JV, Brachman PS. Philadelphia, PA: Lippincott-Raven, 1998:694.

30. U.S. Department of Health and Human Services. Public Health Service. Centers for Disease Control and Prevention: Guideline for prevention of intravascular device-related infections. *American Journal of Infection Control* 1996;24:262–293.

CHAPTER 5

Pediatrics

Viki Patch Shutak, ASN, BSN, MS(c), CRNI

I. GROWTH AND DEVELOPMENT

A. Physiological Development

1. Premature neonate (less than 37 weeks; also called preterm or premature infant)
   a. Body water content
      1) Total body water (TBW) estimated to be 94% of body weight during third month of fetal life
      2) By 24 weeks the TBW is approximately 86%
         - Up to 50% of body water is contained in the extracellular fluid (ECF) compartment
         - With continued growth and development, this proportion decreases as intracellular fluid and cell solids increase
   b. Body surface area (BSA)
      1) Approximately five times greater in relationship to body weight
      2) Gastrointestinal tract is relatively larger at this age and considered an extension of BSA
         - Gastrointestinal tract is potential source of proportionally greater fluid loss
         - BSA is important factor in metabolism and heat production, possibly influencing fluid loss by skin and gastrointestinal membranes
   c. Acid-base regulation
      1) Significantly larger BSA affects route of metabolism by increasing production of metabolic waste that must be excreted by the kidneys
      2) Buffers help to maintain a constant pH by removing or releasing hydrogen ions
      3) Buffers act immediately to correct an abnormal pH
         - Premature neonates have less homeostatic buffering mechanisms
         - Bicarbonate deficit (a slightly lower pH at 7.30 to 7.35) is more common because of high metabolic acid production and renal immaturity (metabolic acidosis)

    d. Renal function
      1) Kidneys functionally immature
      2) Inefficient in ability to maintain fluid balance, excrete metabolic products, concentrate or dilute urine, retain or excrete sodium, and acidify urine
    e. Electrolyte balance
      1) Regulation of fluid volume and solute concentration (electrolytes) closely interrelated
      2) Plasma sodium concentration changes little from birth to adulthood
      3) Potassium concentration higher in first few months of life than at any other time, as is plasma chloride concentration
      4) Low magnesium and calcium levels
        • Inability of premature neonate to regulate calcium, combined with high level of serum phosphate (6.5 to 7.5 mg/dL), may contribute to hypocalcemia-associated tetany
        • This condition may be associated with an immature parathyroid or vitamin D deficiency
  2. Neonate (term infant at birth to 28 days)
    a. Body water content
      1) Estimated to be approximately 70 to 80% of body weight by term (first day of week 38 through last day of week 42)
      2) Largest proportion of body water (40 to 50%) contained in the ECF compartment
      3) Circulating blood volume is approximately 85 to 90 ml/kg of body weight
    b. BSA
      1) Estimated to be two to three times as great as that of an adult
      2) Gastrointestinal membranes remain larger in proportion to an adult and are considered in BSA calculations
    c. Acid-base regulation
      1) Immature renal function and high metabolic acid production cause a tendency toward mild acidosis (pH 7.30 to 7.35)
    d. Renal function
      1) Immature and inefficient kidneys lead to excretion of larger quantities of solute-free water than found in older pediatric patients
    e. Electrolyte balance
      1) Similar to the premature neonate
  3. Infant (1 month to 1 year)
    a. Body water content
      1) Approximately 75% of infant's body is water
      2) During first year, percentage of ECF decreases from 45 to 27%
        • Due to net result in changes involving increased muscle growth and organ size

- In combination with decreased secretions into the gastrointestinal tract and TBW in skin
3) Exchange up to one-half of ECF daily through urine output, respiration, and heat loss
4) At approximately 3 months, blood volume is 75 to 80 ml/kg of body weight
b. BSA
1) Remains proportionately larger than that of an adult
2) More vulnerable to fluid balance disturbances
c. Acid-base regulation
1) pH within the normal range (7.35 to 7.45)
d. Renal function
1) Remains immature and inefficient
2) Vulnerable to any change in fluid status because of limited ability to respond and regulate fluid and solutes
e. Electrolyte balance
1) Serum phosphate slightly elevated above the adult level
2) Other electrolyte concentrations within normal ranges
4. Toddler (1 to 3 years)
a. Body water content
1) After first year, TBW content is approximately 64%
- 34% in the intracellular fluid (ICF) compartment
- 30% in the ECF compartment
2) By end of second year, TBW approaches adult percentage of approximately 60%
- 36% in the ICF compartment
- 24% in the ECF compartment
3) Blood volume 70 to 75 ml/kg (approximately equal to an adult)
b. BSA
1) By end of third year, will approach proportions similar to that of an adult
c. Acid-base regulation
1) pH within normal range (7.35 to 7.45)
d. Renal function
1) Reaches full maturity at end of second year
e. Electrolyte balance
1) Serum phosphate remains slightly above adult level
2) Other electrolyte concentrations are within normal ranges
5. Preschool (3 to 6 years)
a. Body water content
1) TBW is 60%, equal to that of an adult
- 36% in the ICF compartment
- 24% in the ECF compartment
2) Blood volume approximately equal to that of an adult

b. BSA
   1) Proportionally equal to that of an adult
c. Acid-base regulation
   1) pH within normal range (7.35 to 7.45)
d. Renal function
   1) Matured kidney function
e. Electrolyte balance
   1) Serum phosphate remains slightly above the adult level until approximately age 5
   2) Other electrolyte concentrations within normal ranges

6. School age (6 to 12 years)
  a. Body water content
    1) TBW is 60%, equal between males and females until puberty
    2) Blood volume is approximately equal to an adult
  b. BSA
    1) Proportionally equal to that of an adult
  c. Acid-base regulation
    1) pH within normal range
  d. Renal function
    1) Mature kidney function
  e. Electrolyte balance
    1) Serum levels within normal ranges

7. Adolescent (12 to 18 years)
  a. Body water content
    1) From puberty to maturity, percentage of total body weight somewhat higher in the male (60%) than in the female (52%)
    2) Probably the result of differences in body composition, particularly fat and muscle content
    3) Like adults, the ICF comprises 40 to 50% of total body weight, and the ECF comprises 20 to 30% of total body weight
    4) Remainder of body weight is the result of solid matter
    5) Blood volume is 65 to 70 ml/kg (equal to an adult)
  b. BSA
    1) Equal to that of an adult
  c. Acid-base regulation
    1) pH within normal range
  d. Renal function
    1) Mature kidney function
  e. Electrolyte balance
    1) Serum levels within normal ranges

B. Psychosocial Development

1. Premature neonate/neonate
  a. Social and emotional needs

1) Respond to manipulation, restraint, hunger, pain, and changes in temperature (usually cold) by generalized total body movement, tachycardia, and a brief period of crying that ceases with decreased manipulation, warmth, or feeding
2) Do not associate objects or persons with prior painful experiences

b. Preparation for procedures
   1) Decrease manipulation
   2) During procedure use sensory soothing measures such as a pacifier, talking softly, or avoiding sudden moves
   3) Anticipate the need for restraining during procedures
   4) Undress only the body area needed, and/or perform procedures in an isolette or use a radiant heat warmer or heat lamp to conserve neonate's energy, maintain body temperature, and promote vasodilation
   5) Use a flashlight or vein light to enhance venous visualization

2. Infant
   a. Social and emotional needs
      1) A sense of trust (or mistrust) develops
      2) Major fears are separation and stranger anxiety
      3) Desire pleasure and seek to avoid unpleasant situations
      4) Response to pain is similar to a neonate's
         • At approximately 3 to 6 months, able to localize pain and purposefully withdraw the extremity
         • At approximately 6 months, a response to pain is influenced by the recall of past painful experiences associated with objects or persons
      5) Fearful of sudden loud noises and bright light

   b. Preparation for procedures
      1) Response to procedures is related to separation from the primary caregiver
      2) Provide consistent caretakers and minimize separation from parents
      3) Immobilize as necessary during procedures
      4) Coordinate procedures before or sufficiently after feedings to prevent vomiting
      5) Perform invasive or painful procedures in a separate "safe" room, not in a crib (or bed)
      6) During procedures, use sensory soothing measures such as stroking the skin, talking softly, offering a pacifier, and topical or intradermal analgesics to control discomfort
      7) Keep harmful objects out of reach
      8) Comfort and cuddle infants following procedures

3. Toddler
   a. Social and emotional needs

        1) Major fears are separation anxiety (from parents or primary caregivers viewed as their protectors) and loss of control

        2) Egocentric (inability to recognize views of others), use magical thinking, and have little concept of time or body integrity

        3) Increasingly mobile and are striving for independence

   b. Preparation for procedures

        1) Can be very strong and resistant to procedures

        2) Just before procedures, briefly and simply explain what they will see, hear, taste, smell, and feel using a positive, firm, and direct approach

        3) Allow the toddler to play with equipment or role-play with a doll

        4) Explain aspects of the procedure that will require cooperation
- Employ distraction or diversion techniques during procedure
- Explain when procedure is completed

        5) Reassure through verbal and touch stimulation

        6) Give permission to cry, yell, or use other means to verbally express discomfort

        7) Always be honest and *NEVER* tell a child the procedure will not hurt when it will

        8) Restrain as necessary and use more than one assistant

        9) Provide a reward or surprise after the procedure to end the experience on a positive note

  4. Preschooler

   a. Social and emotional needs

        1) Major fears are bodily injury and mutilation, loss of control, fear of the unknown, the dark, or being left alone

        2) Developing a sense of initiative and desire to please people

        3) Difficulty differentiating a "good" hurt (beneficial treatment) from a "bad" hurt (illness or injury)

        4) Are beginning to view themselves separately from their parents

   b. Preparation for procedures

        1) Implement same approaches as for toddler

        2) Involve in care and give choices whenever possible, but avoid excessive delays

        3) Explain why procedures are performed

        4) Directly state that the child has not done something wrong and that the procedure is not a form of punishment

        5) Begin to prepare with conversations about intravenous procedures days in advance of major events (hours for minor ones)

        6) Reassure the child that the room will not be dark and they will not be left alone (parents may come)

       7) Provide a great deal of reassurance and clear explanations

       8) Their questions frequently address "why" and "what will happen next"

5. School age

  a. Social and emotional needs

       1) Major fears are bodily injury and mutilation, loss of control, not being able to live up to expectations of important others, and death

       2) Developing a sense of self-esteem and are interested in helping and pleasing

       3) Capable of following directions and can be involved in their treatment

       4) Becoming increasingly independent and may seek more privacy

  b. Preparation for procedures

       1) Can comprehend more detailed explanations

       2) Explain procedures using correct scientific/medical terminology, simple diagrams of anatomy and physiology, and demonstrating equipment

       3) Allow time before, during, and after procedure for questions and discussion

       4) Can view themselves separately from their parents and may prefer privacy (from parents and peers) during procedures

       5) Encourage cooperation through praise and flattery

       6) Include in decision-making, such as time of day to perform procedures or the preferred intravenous site

6. Adolescent

  a. Social and emotional needs

       1) Increasingly capable of abstract thought and reasoning

       2) Very conscious of body image and appearance and are fearful of something happening that will make them different from their peers

       3) Take more responsibility for decisions regarding their own healthcare needs

       4) Mood swings and regression in coping mechanisms are possible

       5) While striving for independence, may have difficulty in accepting new authority figures and may resist complying with procedures

       6) May prefer solitary activities

  b. Preparation for procedures

       1) Provide and guard privacy

       2) Include and encourage them to participate in discussions regarding their condition and care

       3) Expect occasional noncompliance or lack of interest

4) Answer questions honestly, do not talk down to them, and explain consequences of decisions or procedures

II. CLINICAL ASSESSMENT

A. Patient History

1. Assessment of functional health patterns
   a. A parent/caregiver report is used until the child can answer
   b. Studies have reported that 60% of medical conditions in children can be diagnosed by history alone
2. Health perception/health management
   a. Immunization status
   b. Exposure to communicable diseases
   c. Reason for previous and present hospitalization
   d. Onset and frequency of symptoms
   e. Any methods of treatment given before hospitalization (include fluid mixtures and medications prescribed, as well as over-the-counter and home remedies)
   f. Information to obtain for all children under 2 years of age (and when appropriate because of related developmental disabilities or complications of prematurity)
      1) Maternal prenatal care
      2) Medications taken by mother during pregnancy
      3) Complications during pregnancy for this child
      4) Length of gestation, birth weight and length, and any complications with the neonate during the first month of life
3. Nutritional metabolic pattern
   a. Typical and current appetite
      1) Frequency
      2) Amount
   b. Infant feeding patterns
      1) Method (breast or bottle, cup, parenteral, or enteral)
      2) Formula type
      3) Solid foods
      4) Fluids
   c. Any difficulties perceived with diet or feeding behavior
   d. Any vomiting in relationship to feedings
      1) Frequency
      2) Amount and characteristic of emesis
      3) Projectile (possibly indicative of pyloric stenosis or a possible bowel obstruction)
   e. Food restrictions or special diet intolerance
   f. Other health problems or religious practices
   g. Vitamins and/or supplements
   h. Information for the child less than 1 years old: pattern of introduction of new foods

4. Medication history
  a. Dosages and frequency of medications taken in the last 2 months
5. Allergies
  a. Food or medication
  b. Potential allergic reactions associated with, but not limited to: intravenous medications, topical antimicrobial solutions or ointments, tape, and latex
  c. Reports of severe, immediate-type allergic reactions after latex exposure (have appeared in the past 10 years)
  d. Maternal allergies, especially for the newborn
6. Bowel elimination pattern
  a. Frequency, color, amount, odor, and consistency
  b. Diarrhea (dehydration occurs rapidly in an infant experiencing diarrhea)
  c. Toilet training and age when achieved
  d. Presence of colostomy/ileostomy
  e. Need for laxatives, enemas, or suppositories
7. Bladder elimination
  a. Frequency, color, odor of the urine
  b. Problems associated with urination
    1) Bed wetting
    2) Burning or other dysuria
    3) Dribbling
    4) Oliguria
    5) Polyuria
    6) Urinary retention
    7) Need for catheterization or presence of a stoma
  c. Toilet training (during daytime and/or nighttime) and any accidents
  d. If not toilet trained, the number of wet diapers in the last 24 hours and frequency of checking the diaper during this time (normally an infant will have at least 6 to 7 wet diapers per day)
8. Skin integrity
  a. Moisture
  b. Texture
  c. Itching
  d. Swelling
  e. Rashes
  f. Sores
  g. Bruises
  h. Acne or open areas
  i. Color
  j. Turgor (elasticity)
  k. Temperature changes

9. Activity-exercise pattern
   a. Gross and fine motor skills
   b. Self-care activity information appropriate to the child's age and developmental abilities
   c. Normal effect
   d. Effect of symptoms or complaints on activity patterns
10. Cognitive-perceptual pattern
    a. Any sensory perception deficits (hearing, smell, sight, touch)
11. Self-perception pattern
    a. Impact of illness on how the child feels about himself or herself
12. Role-relationship pattern
    a. Questions appropriate for child's age and developmental abilities
    b. Primary language spoken
    c. Language development or characteristics of speech
    d. Any concerns related to communication
13. Coping/stress management
    a. Reactions to and coping methods for stress
    b. Any losses or changes in the child's life in the past year
    c. Person turned to for comfort
14. Family history
    a. Significant medical histories of immediate family members to identify genetic traits or diseases with familial tendencies
    b. Diseases or conditions possibly influencing child's health
       1) Heart disease
       2) Diabetes
       3) Hypertension
       4) Cancer
       5) Obesity
       6) Congenital anomalies (e.g., heart defects)
       7) Growth abnormalities
       8) Allergies
       9) Asthma
       10) Tuberculosis
       11) Coagulation disorders
       12) Sickle cell disease
       13) Mental retardation
       14) Convulsions
       15) Genetic problems such as cystic fibrosis
       16) Mental or other emotional problems
       17) Syphilis
       18) Rheumatic fever

B. Physical Examination

1. Growth measurements
   a. Crown-to-heel recumbent length (children less than 24 months)
      1) Place supine with head in midline
      2) Grasp knees and gently push toward table to fully extend legs

       3) Measure from vertex (top) of head to heels of feet (toes pointing upward)

       4) Record admission length for BSA calculations on growth chart

       5) Obtain height weekly when less than 1 year of age

   b. Standing height/stature (children older than 24 months)

       1) Have child stand as tall as possible

       2) Measure from top of head to standing surface in one-eighth-inch increments or to the nearest centimeter

       3) Obtain height monthly when the child is older than 1 year

       4) Record admission height on growth chart

   c. Weight (mass)

       1) Weigh infants nude on platform-type scale measuring to the nearest 10 gram or half ounce

         • Record admission and all subsequent weights in kilograms on growth chart

         • Attempt to weigh each time under similar circumstances such as before or after feedings, same time of day, same scale

         • Obtain a daily weight if the child is receiving solutions or medications based on kilogram weight

       2) Weigh toddlers and older children on a standing scale measuring to the nearest one-fourth of a pound

         • Remove heavy clothing and shoes

         • Record admission and all subsequent weights in kilograms on growth chart

       3) Compare history of child's weight before onset of illness with current weight for valuable information in determining the degree of hydration

         • Weigh an ill infant daily to determine percentage of fluid loss

         • Weight loss caused by fluid volume deficit (FVD) occurs more rapidly than that caused by catabolism

       4) Assess for FVD by determining the percent of loss from normal body weight

         • Percentage of weight loss equals level of dehydration

         • < 5% loss = mild dehydration

         • 5 to 10% loss = moderate dehydration

         • 10% loss = severe dehydration

2. Temperature

   a. Following the unstable regulatory ability in the neonatal period, heat production (reflecting metabolism) steadily declines as the infant grows to an adult

   b. Temperature measurement using a mercury thermometer is taken by oral, rectal, or axillary route

   c. Recent substitutes for the mercury thermometer are the electronic thermometer (oral), the tympanic membrane sensor (opening to the auditory canal), the plastic strip (forehead), and the digital (finger) thermometer

1) Advantages for the pediatric population
- Measure temperature rapidly (1 to 60 seconds)
- Avoid oral or rectal routes

d. Axillary or tympanic temperatures are the safest and generally most accurate measurements

e. Normal body temperature registers 37.0°C (98.6°F) via the oral route by age 5

1) Subnormal temperature may be a sign of sepsis in the neonate and infant

2) Elevated temperatures are seen in children early in dehydration, and, as condition worsens, the temperature may become subnormal

3) Children less than 3 years of age tend toward rapid temperature elevation and resulting vulnerability toward febrile seizures

3. Pulse

a. In children less than 2 years old, the apical pulse is more reliable than the peripheral pulse and should be assessed for rate and rhythm for one full minute

b. In children older than 2 years, the radial pulse is satisfactory

c. During early childhood, a comparison between radial and femoral pulses should be done at least once to detect the presence of circulatory impairment, such as coarctation of the aorta (a condition in which the lower extremity pressure is less than the upper extremity pressure)

d. Tachycardia may be an early sign of fluid depletion

e. A full bounding pulse will accompany edema

4. Respirations

a. Rate, rhythm, and depth should be noted in the same manner as for the adult

b. In infants, the movements are primarily diaphragmatic and therefore observed by abdominal movement

5. Blood pressure (BP)

a. Measure in either upper arm or thigh in infants

b. Measurements of the lower extremities should be done on any child with elevated pressures in the upper extremities and at least once in childhood to detect abnormalities such as coarctation of the aorta

c. Not always a reliable sign of FVD in a young child because vessel elasticity may (initially) keep the BP stable, despite diminished blood volume

6. Skin

a. Skin color

1) Observed in natural daylight or neutral artificial light

2) Color is most reliably assessed in sclera, nail beds, earlobes, lips, oral membranes, palms, soles

3) Factors affecting skin color include ethnic group (genetics),

melanin production, edema, hygiene, hemoglobin level, atmospheric temperature

- Erythema (flushed or red skin) may result from increased environmental temperature, local inflammation, infection, or an increase in red blood cells as a compensatory response to chronic hypoxia (plethora)
- Pallor, or paleness, may be a sign of anemia, chronic disease, hypothermia, edema, or shock
- Jaundice is seen with an increase in bilirubin from hemolytic or liver disease
- Cyanosis may be seen in the newborn with hemoglobinopathies

b. Skin temperature
1) Evaluated symmetrically by feeling each body part, comparing upper with lower extremities
2) A child may feel cool to the touch with FVD, even though febrile, because of decreased peripheral blood flow

c. Turgor
1) Refers to the amount of elasticity in the skin, one of the best indicators of adequate hydration and nutrition
2) Best determined by grasping skin on the abdomen (or medial aspect of the thigh) between thumb and index finger, pulling taut, and quickly releasing
3) Normal tissue will not tent when gently lifted
- Brief tenting (suspension) of the skin and wrinkling are generally seen after a 3 to 5% body fluid loss
- An infant with hypernatremia will often have firm, thick-feeling skin

d. Edema
1) Swelling or puffiness of the extremities or sacral area may be a sign of fluid excess or of several systemic disorders such as heart failure, kidney disease, sepsis, or a protein deficiency
2) May normally be present in children who have been crying, sleeping, or have allergies

7. Mucous membranes
a. Dry mouth may be caused by FVD or mouth breathing
b. Dryness along the area between the cheek and gum will be a more accurate measurement of fluid status
c. Salivation or drooling in an infant may be a significant source of fluid loss or indicative of good hydration
d. The tongue of a child with FVD will appear smaller than normal
e. Absence of tearing is seen with a fluid deficit of 5% or greater

8. Fontanel
a. Anterior fontanel is easily palpated in infants, generally closes between 12 and 18 months of age
b. Assessed for size, pulsation, and tenseness

1) Depressed or sunken fontanel is apparent in a dehydrated infant

2) Will bulge or feel full with crying, increased intracranial pressure, hydrocephalus, and fluid overload

9. Urine

a. An adequate urine output for the newborn should be 0.5 to 1.0 ml/kg/hr and 1.0 to 2.0 ml/kg/hr for the infant

1) Most accurate method of measuring output for a child not toilet trained is to weigh the diaper before putting it on and weigh it again after infant has voided

2) One milliliter of urine will weigh 1 gram

3) Urine output should be measured hourly in dehydrated children

b. A urine-specific gravity value between 1.002 and 1.030 is usually an indication of fluid balance

1) High specific gravity occurs when there is protein or glucose in the urine or the urine is concentrated from FVD

2) Because the renal system of infants and young children is immature, the specific gravity is a less reliable indicator of fluid status

10. Neurological

a. Behavior

1) Early signs of hypernatremia in infants and young children may include lethargy and somnolence

2) Fluid retention and cerebral edema may cause restlessness and irritability

b. Changes in sensorium associated with fluid status may produce hypersensitivity to light and sound

c. Convulsions may be seen with fluid excess and fluid deficit

C. Laboratory Studies (normal laboratory values used to assess fluid and electrolyte balance)

1. Serum electrolytes

a. Sodium

1) Essentially equal to adult values of 135 to 145 mEq/L

b. Potassium

1) < 10 days: 3.5 to 6.0 mEq/L

2) > 10 days: 3.5 to 5.0 mEq/L

c. Calcium

1) Premature neonate < 1 week: 6 to 10 mg/dL

2) Neonate < 1 week: 9 to 10.6 mg/dL

3) > 1 week: essentially equal to adult values, 8.9 to 10.3 mg/dL

d. Chloride

1) Essentially equal to adult value of 97 to 110 mEq/L

e. Magnesium

1) Essentially equal to adult value of 1.3 to 2.1 mEq/L

f. Phosphorus/phosphate

1) Premature neonate: 6.5 to 7.5 mg/dL

2) Newborn: 4.2 to 9.0 mg/dL

3) 1 year: 3.8 to 6.2 mg/dL

4) 2 to 5 years: 3.5 to 6.8 mg/dL

5) > 5 years: 2.5 to 4.5 mg/dL

g. Bicarbonate

1) < 2 years: 20 to 25 mEq/L

2) > 2 years: 22 to 26 mEq/L

2. Hemoglobin

a. Premature neonate: possibly falling to 7 to 9 g/dL by 3 to 6 weeks of age

b. Neonate: 15 to 22 g/dL

c. 3 to 6 months: < 10 g/dL

1) Newborn hemoglobin level drops to its lowest point at approximately 3 to 6 months of age as a result of expansion of blood volume that accompanies rapid body growth

2) Creates a condition referred to as physiological anemia

d. 6 months to 12 years: 11.5 to 15.5 g/dL

e. > 12 years

1) Male: 13.5 to 18.0 g/dL

2) Female: 12.0 to 16.0 g/dL

3. Hematocrit

a. Newborn: 45 to 65%

b. 1 month: 44%

c. 6 months to 2 years: 36%

d. 2 to 6 years: 37%

e. 6 to 12 years: 40%

f. Adolescent (equal to adult values)

1) Male: 44 to 52%

2) Female: 39 to 47%

g. Elevated hematocrit is seen with dehydration

4. Serum osmolality

a. Equal to adult value of 280 to 295 mOsm/kg

5. Blood urea nitrogen (BUN)

a. 1 to 2 years: 5 to 15 mg/dL

b. > 2 years: 10 to 20 mg/dL

c. BUN possibly elevated in the presence of FVD

6. Serum glucose

a. Preterm neonate: 20 to 65 mg/dL

b. Full-term neonate: 20 to 110 mg/dL

c. 1 week to 16 years: 60 to 105 mg/dL

d. > 16 years: 70 to 110 mg/dL

7. Urine glucose

a. May be an early sign of sepsis

b. Children may have a low renal threshold for glucose and may develop glycosuria from high concentrations of glucose

8. Arterial blood gases (best method of assessing acid-base balance and quality of blood oxygenation)
   a. pH: indicates the acid-base level of the blood
      1) Premature neonate: 7.30 to 7.35
      2) Neonate (birth to 1 month): 7.09 to 7.30 to 7.29 to 7.453
      3) > 1 month: essentially equal to adult values of 7.35 to 7.45
   b. PaO_2: values indicate how much oxygen the lungs are delivering to the blood
      1) Infant: 60 to 70 mm Hg
      2) Thereafter: 80 to 100 mm Hg
   c. $PaCO_2$: value indicates how efficiently the lungs eliminate carbon dioxide
      1) Infant: 30 to 40 mm Hg
      2) Thereafter: 35 to 45 mm Hg
   d. Base excess: +2 mEq/L
   e. Oxygen saturation: 95 to 100%
9. Bilirubin
   a. During the first 3 days of life, 50% of neonates experience an elevation in plasma bilirubin, causing normal physiological hyperbilirubinemia resulting in jaundice
      1) Normal physiological jaundice usually peaks during the first week, declining as the liver is increasingly able to conjugate and excrete bilirubin
      2) In premature and breastfed neonates, increased blood levels of bilirubin can remain elevated for up to 6 weeks of life
      3) After 1 month, the unconjugated bilirubin should be 0.1 to 0.7 mg/dL
   b. Excessive amounts of unconjugated (indirect) bilirubin may deposit in the brain, causing permanent damage to the central nervous system—referred to as kernicterus (an encephalopathy)
      1) Hyperbilirubinemia is treated with phototherapy when serum bilirubin levels exceed 12 to 12.9 mg/dL
      2) Increased insensible fluid loss occurs during phototherapy and may require a 25% increase in fluid intake
      3) Bilirubin levels exceeding 20 mg/dL may be an indication for an exchange transfusion

III. DISEASE STATES AND CONDITIONS

A. Maintenance/Replacement Fluid Requirements

1. General goals
   a. To support vital functions, maintain health, and encourage adequate growth, the body must be supplied with water, electrolytes, nutrients, and vitamins (maintenance requirements)

     b. To repair or replace deficits of fluid and/or electrolytes lost via insensible fluid losses (skin, respiratory tract, perspiration, gastrointestinal tract, and urine)

  2. Requirements for a 24-hour period

    a. Based on child's weight in kilograms and are usually calculated by using the following formulas:

      1) ml/kg of body weight

        • Step 1: calculate weight of child in kilograms (kg) (2.2 lbs/kg)

        • Step 2: 100 ml/kg for first 10 kg (1 to 10 kg of body weight)

        • Step 3: 50 ml/kg for next 10 kg (11 to 20 kg of body weight)

        • Step 4: 20 ml/kg for each kg over 20

        • Step 5: divide total amount by 24 hours to obtain intravenous rate in ml/hr

    b. BSA or milliliters/meters squared (recommended for children over 10 kg of body weight)

      1) Nomograms exist that aid in calculation of BSA from height (cm/in) and weight (lb/kg)

      2) Surface area is indicated where a straight line connecting the child's height and weight intersects the surface area column

      3) Maintenance requirements

        • Water: 1200 to 1500 ml/m^2 per 24-hour period

    c. Metabolic rate to calculate fluid requirements

      1) 100 ml of water needed for every 100 calories consumed

      2) Caloric expenditure related to weight as follows:

        • 2 to 10 kg: 10 calories per kg

        • 10 to 20 kg: 50 calories for each kg over 10

        • > 20 kg: 20 calories per kg

    d. Variables increasing fluid requirements

      1) Elevated temperature: a 1°-elevation in temperature increases fluid requirements by 12%

      2) Stress

      3) Burns

      4) Surgery

B. Fluid Volume Imbalances

  1. Pediatric patients are more vulnerable to fluid volume imbalance than are adults because of proportionately more ECF to body size, larger BSA, increased metabolic rate, immature kidneys, and less homeostatic buffering capability

  2. FVD is expressed in percentage of fluid and weight loss

    a. Mild: < 5%

    b. Moderate: 5 to 10%

    c. Severe: 10 to 15%

  3. Acute loss of 15% of body weight will likely cause hypovolemic shock

  4. FVD is categorized according to sodium levels

C. FVD: Isotonic (Isonatremic) Dehydration (water and electrolytes are lost proportionately from ICF and ECF compartments)

1. Etiological factors
   a. Loss of large quantities of liquid stools
      1) Gastroenteritis most common cause
      2) Approximately 70% of children with an FVD from severe diarrhea develop isotonic dehydration
   b. Fever
   c. Excessive emesis, gastrointestinal suctioning, fistula drainage
   d. Hemorrhage
      1) Due to a small circulating volume in young children, blood loss (fluids and electrolytes) may lead to hypovolemic shock
   e. Burns
      1) Fluid and electrolytes shifting within the circulatory system may lead to shock
   f. Decreased fluid intake
   g. Polyuria
2. Clinical manifestations
   a. Thirst
   b. Acute weight loss
   c. Dry skin and mucous membranes, poor skin turgor, gray or ashen skin, and cold extremities as a result of poor peripheral profusion
   d. Subnormal temperature (unless infection is present)
   e. Lethargy
   f. Oliguria with increased specific gravity
   g. Sunken eyeballs as a result of decreased intraocular pressure
   h. Diminished tearing
      1) Seen with fluid loss greater than 5% total body weight
   i. Weak, rapid pulse
   j. Depressed fontanels in neonates and infants
   k. Longitudinal furrows on the tongue
   l. Signs of hypovolemia
   m. Serum sodium at normal levels
3. Treatment
   a. Initial treatment to restore circulating blood volume by administering blood products and/or intravenous fluids
   b. Rehydration to expand plasma volume is begun with an isotonic electrolyte solution: 0.9% sodium chloride, lactated Ringer's or 5% dextrose and 0.225% sodium chloride, administered at 20 ml/kg of body weight over a 12- to 18-hour period
   c. Mild isotonic dehydration may be treated with oral rehydration
   d. Frequent monitoring of vital signs, accurate intake and output, and daily weights

D. FVD: Hypertonic (Hypernatremic) Dehydration (resulting from a greater loss of water than electrolytes [net loss of water in excess of salt or a result of excessive solute intake])

1. Etiological factors
   a. Diarrhea
      1) Approximately 20% of children lose more water than electrolytes
   b. Neonates and infants fed high-solute replacement fluids or a concentrated formula (too little water mixed with the formula)
   c. Fever with hyperventilation (especially in small infants)
   d. Diabetes mellitus
      1) Excess glucose concentration in blood with similar effect as excess sodium concentration (hyperosmolar dehydration) causing water movement out of cells into the ECF
      2) Osmotic diuresis causes excessive fluid loss and possible elevated serum sodium
   e. Diabetes insipidus
      1) Disorder related to water imbalance caused by lack of antidiuretic hormone (ADH) or by failure of kidney to respond to ADH
      2) Copious amounts of fluid and few electrolytes lost (through polyuria, for example)
   f. History of low water intake
2. Clinical manifestations
   a. History of large quantities of liquid stools
   b. Avid thirst (hypertonic ECF drawing water from cells and causing dehydration)
   c. Serum electrolytes
      1) Elevated BUN
      2) Potassium within low normal range
      3) Sodium levels exceeding 145 mEq/L
      4) Elevated chloride
   d. Altered central nervous system
      1) Marked lethargy and extreme hyperirritability with stimulation
      2) Potential for seizures, coma, and tremors secondary to hypernatremia causing brain tissue to shrink
      3) Intracranial bleeding may occur in 10% of infants and young children, but rare in adults
   e. Muscle rigidity
   f. Nuchal rigidity (pain or stiffness in back or neck)
   g. Oliguria
   h. Decreased skin turgor (thick and firm-feeling skin)
   i. Weight loss
   j. Increased urine-specific gravity

3. Treatment
   a. Gradual replacement of water losses with a dilute sodium solution (5% dextrose and 0.225% sodium chloride with potassium chloride) over a 48-hour period
   b. Too rapid a rehydration can lead to brain swelling and resulting seizures and coma
   c. Potassium chloride is not given until adequate renal function is verified

E. FVD: Hypotonic (Hyponatremic) Dehydration (greater loss of electrolytes than of water)

1. Etiological factors
   a. Diarrheal episodes, especially when treated with electrolyte-free solutions for volume replacement
   b. Syndrome of inappropriate antidiuretic hormone (SIADH)
      1) Excessive release of ADH or similar substance
         • Excessive ADH leads to decreased water excretion
         • Results in serum sodium level and osmolality
         • Increased fluid volume with resultant increased glomerular filtration and decreased aldosterone release
         • Subsequent increased sodium elimination
         • Because intracellular concentration is greater, ECF is pulled into the cells
      2) Predisposing factors: medications, including nonsteroidal anti-inflammatory drugs; tumors, especially oat cell carcinoma; and central nervous system disorders
   c. Diuretic therapy
   d. Excessive amounts of salt-poor solutions
   e. Neonates and infants fed a formula too diluted with water
   f. Fresh-water drowning
2. Clinical manifestations
   a. Serum electrolytes
      1) Elevated BUN
      2) Potassium within high normal range
      3) Sodium levels less than 130 mEq/L
   b. Neuromuscular symptoms caused by cerebral edema
      1) Lethargy
      2) Seizures
      3) Coma
   c. Dry, sticky mucous membranes
   d. Weight loss
   e. Subnormal temperature
   f. Doughy skin
   g. Extremities cool to the touch
   h. Hypotension
   i. Rapid, thready pulse

j. Hypovolemic shock (in severe cases) caused by cardiovascular dysfunction and inadequate tissue perfusion (volume depletion)

3. Treatment
   a. Dependent on the severity of fluid and electrolytes loss
   b. Sodium, the major electrolyte in ECF; accompanying deficit is primary cause of symptoms
     1) If sodium level low and neurological changes present, hypertonic sodium solutions (5% dextrose in 0.3 % or 0.45% sodium chloride) may be necessary
     2) Rapid administration avoided to prevent shrinkage of brain tissue
     3) Hypertonic solution promoting return of fluid from the extracellular space into the intracellular space

F. Fluid Volume Excess (FVE) (result of abnormal retention of water and sodium [hypervolemia])

1. Etiological factors
   a. Overload of fluids (administered too rapidly or in excess volume)
   b. Dysfunction or immaturity of the homeostatic mechanisms for regulating fluid balance
     1) Congestive heart failure
     2) Renal failure
     3) Excess steroids
     4) Cirrhosis of liver
   c. Excessive sodium ingestion

2. Clinical manifestations
   a. Peripheral edema (excess of interstitial space fluid)
   b. Distended neck or peripheral veins
   c. Decreased BUN and hematocrit (result of plasma dilution)
   d. Decreased heart rate with full, bounding pulse (infant may experience tachycardia as a result of difficulty managing the increased intravascular volume)
   e. Pulmonary edema (if severe)
   f. Moist rales (crackles) on auscultation of lungs
   g. Decreased urine-specific gravity (urine dilute)
   h. Hypertension
   i. Polyuria (if normal renal function)
   j. Weight gain
   k. Hepatomegaly (seen in chronic fluid overload in children)

3. Treatment
   a. Monitor vital signs, intake and output, and urine-specific gravity frequently and weight daily
   b. Sodium and water intake restrictions
   c. Dialysis (if renal function is compromised)
   d. Diuretics

4. Prevention
   a. Use electronic flow control device

b. Limit the amount of fluid hung

c. Use a metered chamber set or microdrip administration sets

G. Pyloric Stenosis (hypertrophy of the circular muscle of the pylorus, leading to an obstruction of the gastric outlet and causing gastric distention and vomiting)

1. Etiological factors
    a. Causative mechanisms leading to hypertrophy are unclear
    b. Genetics appears to play a significant role
    c. Most common cause of vomiting in neonates 2 to 4 weeks of age and is seen five times more often in males than in females
    d. Complications of progressive pyloric obstruction may include dehydration, weight loss, malnutrition, and electrolyte disturbances
2. Clinical manifestations
    a. Early: neonate is alert and ravenously hungry but appears mildly dehydrated and malnourished
    b. Progressive
        1) Palpable pyloric mass: commonly referred to as an "olive"
        2) Peristaltic waves (left to right toward pylorus) possibly seen after feedings but before vomiting
        3) Projectile vomiting: prolonged and frequent emesis causing fluid and electrolyte imbalances
        4) Metabolic alkalosis: pH above 7.45
        5) Potassium deficit: level below 3.5 mEq/dL
        6) FVD is hypotonic (hyponatremia)
        7) Fretful, apathetic
        8) Loss of skin turgor
        9) Dry mucous membranes
3. Treatment
    a. Nothing by mouth (NPO)
    b. Intravenous fluids to correct fluid and electrolyte imbalances
    c. Glucose correction
    d. If the child is severely dehydrated, correction may take 24 to 48 hours
    e. Pyloromyotomy (the treatment of choice following correction of fluid, glucose, and electrolyte abnormalities); surgical procedure to relieve the obstruction caused by the hypertrophied muscle

H. Hemolytic Disease of the Newborn—Rh Incompatibility (isoimmunization)

1. Etiological factors
    a. Rh-negative mother produces anti-Rh antibodies toward fetal red cells, which possess Rh-positive antigens
    b. Maternal antibodies of the IgG class cross the placenta, resulting in a hemolytic fetal process

2. Clinical manifestations
   a. Hyperbilirubinemia and jaundice of the neonate within the first 24 hours of life
   b. Erythroblastosis fetalis (immature red blood cells [erythroblasts] in fetal circulation)
3. Treatment
   a. Maternal RhoGAM (RhIG): intramuscular administration within 72 hours of each delivery as protection for subsequent deliveries
   b. Phototherapy (mild cases not involving hemolysis)
   c. Fetal exchange transfusion (treatment of choice for hyperbilirubinemia caused by Rh incompatibility):
      1) Positive direct Coombs
      2) Cord blood hemoglobin < 12 gm/dL
      3) Bilirubin level 20 mg/dL or greater in the full-term neonate
      4) Hydrops fetalis
         • Most severe form of erythroblastosis fetalis
         • Progressive hemolysis causing fetal hypoxia, cardiac failure, anasarca (generalized edema)
         • Pericardial, pleural, and peritoneal space effusions and respiratory distress are indications for immediate exchange transfusions

I. Hemolytic Disease of the Newborn—ABO Incompatibility

1. Etiological factors
   a. Most common blood group incompatibility in the neonate is between maternal O blood group and infant A or B blood group
   b. Maternal anti-A or anti-B antibodies from the maternal circulation cross the placenta and cause hemolysis of fetal RBCs
2. Clinical manifestations
   a. Jaundice during the first 24 hours
      1) Hemolyzed agglutinated donor cells are trapped in peripheral blood vessels
   b. Serum levels of unconjugated bilirubin rise rapidly following birth
      1) 15 to 20 mg/dL or an increase of 1 mg/dL or more per hour
   c. Anemia from erythrocyte hemolysis
      1) If severe, pallor and hypovolemic shock can occur
   d. Hepatosplenomegaly
3. Treatment
   a. Fetal exchange transfusion is performed if the shape of the bilirubin curve (concentration versus time) indicates it will exceed 20 mg/dL

J. Hypoglycemia (an abnormally low level of serum blood glucose)

1. Etiological factors
   a. Inadequate intake of glucose (dextrose)
   b. Overproduction of insulin from islets of Langerhans or an overdose of exogenous insulin

    c. Abrupt discontinuation of intravenous dextrose solutions

    d. High glucose demand and low glucose stores

       1) Most commonly occurs in infants with acute illness

2. Clinical manifestations

    a. Blood glucose of less than 40 to 45 mg/dL

    b. Jitteriness, tremors, twitching

    c. Lethargy

    d. Apathy

    e. Poor feeding or sucking ability; refusal to feed

       1) Infant with low glucose may lack the energy to take oral fluids

    f. Hypotonia

       1) Decreased strength, limpness

    g. Irritability

    h. Headache

    i. Mental confusion

    j. Hallucinations

    k. Weak or high-pitched cry

    l. Prolonged or severe hypoglycemia (glucose below 40 mg/dL) leading to convulsions or seizures

    m. Increased epinephrine secretion causes tachycardia, BP elevation, sweating, and anxiety

    n. Hypothermia, especially in neonates and infants

    o. Rapid and irregular respirations or apnea may develop in infants, usually self-limiting

    p. Diaphoresis, cyanosis, pallor, congestive heart failure, and eye-rolling

3. Treatment

    a. Oral glucose, especially within the first hours of birth and every 2 to 3 hours thereafter

    b. Intravenous dextrose (most common is 10% solution, but may range up to 50%)

       1) Usually an intravenous bolus followed by a continuous infusion

       2) Required to maintain physiological requirements of blood serum glucose concentrations

       3) Infusion administered through large peripheral vein or central vein to increase hemodilution and prevent extravasation

       4) High concentrations of dextrose (such as total parenteral nutrition [TPN]) must be terminated gradually

       5) Intravenous dextrose solution interruptions minimized

          • Restart peripheral cannula in a timely manner (especially in neonates or infants)

          • Evaluate impact of dextrose solution interruption

          • If necessary, start a second intravenous site to enable dextrose solution and medications or a blood transfusion to infuse concurrently

          • Reduce energy requirements by providing a warm environment

K. Salicylate Intoxication (salicylism)

1. Etiological factors
   a. Toxic serum levels of salicylate (sources such as aspirin, methyl salicylate, sustained-release preparations, enteric-coated formulations and liniments)
   b. Maternal ingestion of toxic quantities
   c. Excessive topical application of methyl salicylate (oil of wintergreen)
   d. Therapeutic misuse of salicylates: administration too frequently, incorrect dose, ingestion of topical agent
2. Clinical manifestations
   a. Gastrointestinal: nausea, vomiting, gastric irritation
      1) Large doses of salicylates lead to decreased gastric motility
   b. Metabolic: hyperthermia, hypoglycemia (more common in children), and hypokalemia
      1) Disturbance in acid-base balance results in respiratory alkalosis and metabolic acidosis, either alone or combined
   c. Respiratory: hyperpnea, hyperventilation, pulmonary edema
   d. Dehydration: secondary to hyperventilation
   e. Neurologic: tinnitus, confusion, coma, seizures
   f. Renal: oliguria
   g. Hepatic: hepatitis, altered liver function tests
   h. Hematologic: hypoprothrombinemia, hemorrhagic (clotting) disorders
   i. Diaphoresis
   j. Serum salicylate level greater than 150 mg/kg
3. Treatment
   a. Prevent further salicylate absorption by gastric lavage or induced emesis (through the administration of activated charcoal or syrup of ipecac) or saline cathartic
   b. Administer antidote (N-acetylcysteine [NAC, Mucomyst]) for acetaminophen
   c. Establish adequate circulatory blood volume by administering an isotonic solution at a rate of 20 ml/kg/hr
      1) Lactated Ringer's solution and sodium bicarbonate may be required in children to correct metabolic acidosis and urinary alkalinization and enhance elimination
   d. Administer a minimum of 25 mEq/L of potassium to correct electrolyte deficits and to alkalinize the urine
      1) Maintaining urine pH above 7.50 will enhance salicylate excretion
   e. Include dextrose (5 gm/dL) when renal function is adequate to treat ketosis
   f. Administer calcium gluconate to treat tetany
   g. Give Vitamin K (aquaMEPHYTON) to prevent excessive bleeding

h. Give osmotic diuretics to increase urine output (monitor for FVD)

i. Monitor blood volume status, sodium, potassium, bicarbonate, urine pH, and arterial blood gases to determine appropriate intravenous fluid type, medications, and rate of administration

j. Anticipate hemodialysis for severe intoxication

L. Cystic Fibrosis

1. Overview
   a. Hereditary condition marked by accumulation of excessively thick and tenacious mucous and abnormal secretion of sweat and saliva
   b. Pancreas and bronchioles become obstructed as secretions precipitate or coagulate to form concretions in ducts or glands
   c. Bacteria stick to the mucous and cause infection
   d. Most common lethal genetic disease among white children, adolescents, and adults because of its numerous secondary complications affecting practically every organ system of the body

2. Etiological factors
   a. An inherited autosomal recessive trait with affected individuals exhibiting pancreatic deficiency and pulmonary disease

3. Clinical manifestations
   a. Sweat abnormality
      1) Sodium and chloride concentrations greater than 60 mEq/L required for diagnosis
      2) Failure to reabsorb sodium and chloride increases potential risk for abnormal salt loss, dehydration, hypochloremic and hyponatremic alkalosis, especially with high environmental temperatures or febrile episodes
      3) Infants are especially at risk because of limited fluid stores and the potential for limited salt intake with commercially prepared formulas
   b. Pulmonary (progressive chronic obstruction lung disease); most respiratory symptoms will develop by age 3
      1) Wheezing respirations, dyspnea
      2) Dry, nonproductive cough
      3) Bronchial and bronchiolar obstruction promote secondary infection and recurrent pneumonia
      4) Barrel-shaped chest: hyperaeration of functioning alveoli
      5) Cyanosis and clubbing of fingers and toes caused by impaired gas exchange
      6) Chronic sinusitis and nasal polyps
      7) Chronic hypoxia leads to pulmonary hypertension and eventual cor pulmonale
      8) Fatigue
   c. Gastrointestinal
      1) Meconium ileus: in 7 to 10% of newborns with cystic fibrosis,

thick meconium blocks the small intestine causing intestinal obstruction

2) Pain, abdominal distention, and vomiting throughout life as a result of thick intestinal secretions

3) Obstruction of pancreatic enzymes leads to excessively large, frothy, foul-smelling stools (steatorrhea)

4) Weight loss or failure to thrive despite healthy appetite and diet

5) Fat-soluble vitamin deficiency leads to bruising

6) Anemia

7) Rectal prolapse: most common gastrointestinal complication; result of large, bulky stools and lack of supportive fatpads around rectum in infancy and early childhood

4. Treatment

a. Aerosolized drugs to inhibit sodium and water reabsorption and to promote chloride secretion

b. Replacement gene therapy

c. Chest physiotherapy: postural drainage and percussion of the lungs to facilitate mucous expectoration

d. Prophylactic oral antibiotics at the time of diagnosis

e. Intravenous antibiotic therapy during acute episodes following sputum culture and sensitivity

1) Most common infections include: *Pseudomonas aeruginosa, Pseudomonas cepacia, Staphylococcus aureus,* and *Haemophilus influenzae*

f. Lung transplantation: usually performed in children with advanced pulmonary vascular disease and hypoxia

g. Oral replacement of pancreatic enzymes

h. High-protein, high-caloric diet, water-miscible forms of vitamins

i. Parenteral alimentation, if history of inability to gain weight

j. Electrolyte replacement therapy, especially during hot weather or physical exertion

M. Meningitis

1. Overview

a. Inflammation, exudation, WBC accumulation, and varying degrees of tissue damage to the meninges and subarachnoid space, including the cerebrospinal fluid

b. Children between 1 month and 5 years of age are the most frequently affected

2. Etiological factors

a. The most common route of infection is vascular dissemination (e.g., nasopharynx to underlying blood vessels to cerebral blood supply)

b. By direct implantation from penetrating wounds (e.g., skull fracture or lumbar puncture)

    c. Bacterial or pyogenic: most commonly caused by *Haemophilus influenzae*, *Streptococcus pneumoniae*, or *Neisseria meningitidis*, but also by other bacterium

    d. Aseptic (nonbacterial or viral): wide variety of causative viral agents

    e. Tuberculosis: tuberculin bacillus, resulting in a more chronic inflammation of the meninges

3. Clinical manifestations (depends on the age of the child)

    a. Abrupt onset of fever, chills, headache, vomiting

        1) In tuberculosis and meningitis, the symptoms develop gradually, taking 1 to 2 weeks to appear

        2) Early symptoms: sore throat, general soreness, and a red, spotty rash

    b. Alterations in sensorium: irritability, agitation, malaise, photophobia, seizure, delirium, hallucinations, aggressive or maniacal behavior, drowsiness, stupor, or coma

    c. Diarrhea and/or weight loss

    d. Occasionally, slower onset frequently preceded by respiratory or gastrointestinal symptoms

    e. Nuchal rigidity (neck stiffness) becomes marked; evidenced by drawing the head into extreme overextension (opisthotonos)

    f. Cold, cyanotic skin with poor peripheral perfusion

    g. Petechial or purpuric rash usually with meningococcemia

    h. Joint involvement with meningococci or *Haemophilus influenzae*

    i. Chronically draining ear with pneumococcal meningitis

    j. *Escherichia coli* usually associated with congenital dermal sinus connecting with the subarachnoid space

    k. Jaundice in neonates

    l. Full, tense bulging fontanel in infants and young children (may or may not be present until late in course of meningitis of neonates)

    m. High-pitched or poor cry

    n. Poor appetite or poor suck ability

    o. Complicated or untreated symptoms progressing to cardiovascular collapse, seizures, apnea, auditory nerve damage, blindness, weakness or paralysis of facial or other muscles of head and neck

        1) Meningococcal septicemia characterized by overwhelming septic shock, disseminated intravascular coagulation (DIC), and massive bilateral adrenal hemorrhage

    p. Lumbar puncture is positive for causative organism (protein concentration is usually increased)

    q. Elevated WBC count

    r. Blood cultures occasionally are positive when cerebrospinal fluid culture is negative

4. Treatment (primarily symptomatic for nonbacterial meningitis; medical emergency for bacterial meningitis)

a. Infection control and isolation precautions (for bacterial meningitis)
b. Acetaminophen for headache or muscle pain
c. Maintenance of optimum hydration involving correction of fluid deficits followed by low maintenance levels to prevent cerebral edema
d. Environmental stimuli kept to a minimum (decrease noise, bright lights, and other external stimuli)
e. Intravenous antibiotics: drug choice is based on the causative organism identified (usually cephalosporins for 10 days)
f. Reduction of increased intracranial pressure
g. Corticosteroid administration to reduce hearing loss associated with *Haemophilus influenzae* meningitis
h. Intravenous infusion started as soon as possible to administer antibiotics, electrolytes, anticonvulsive therapy (for seizures), and manage hypovolemic shock, as well as heparin for DIC
i. Control of extremes of temperature
j. Correction of anemia (blood administration)

N. Sickle Cell Anemia

1. Etiological factors
   a. Normal adult hemoglobin (hemoglobin A [HbA]) is partly or completely replaced by abnormal sickle hemoglobin (HbS)
   b. Inherited as an autosomal-recessive gene and is found primarily in the black race (although infrequently it affects whites, especially those of Mediterranean descent)
   c. Under conditions of dehydration, acidosis, hypoxia, and temperature elevations, HbS distorts to a crescent or sickle-shaped red blood cell
   d. As long as fetal hemoglobin persists, sickling does not occur
   e. During the first year of life, fetal hemoglobin decreases, placing the child at risk for sickle cell-related complications
2. Clinical manifestations
   a. Complications and clinical features are primarily a result of obstruction by the sickled RBCs in the microcirculation and increased destruction of RBCs
   b. Enlarged spleen, initially caused by engorgement of sickle cells
   c. Functional asplenia: functioning spleen cells are replaced by fibrotic tissue by age 5
      1) Without the spleen filtering bacteria and promoting release of phagocytic cells, child is at risk for infection
   d. Anemia and capillary obstruction cause liver failure and necrosis, with cirrhosis eventually occurring
   e. Kidney ischemia (secondary to glomerular congestion) results in hematuria, inability to concentrate urine, enuresis, and, occasionally, nephrotic syndrome

  f. Chronic ischemia of the bone results in osteoporosis, osteomyelitis, and, occasionally, aseptic necrosis of the femoral head

  g. Stroke or cerebrovascular accident is a major complication

   1) Other neurological symptoms include headache, aphasia, weakness, convulsions

   2) Visual disturbances or paralysis possibly resulting from cerebral thrombosis due to increased viscosity of blood

  h. Cardiomyopathy, decompensation, and cardiac failure

  i. Exercise intolerance, anorexia, jaundiced sclera, and gallstones

  j. Vaso-occlusion and tissue ischemia causing chronic leg ulcers in adolescents and adults

  k. Generalized effects

   1) Physical retardation (height and weight)

   2) Delayed sexual maturation

   3) Decreased fertility

   4) Sexual development and adult height usually attained if child reaches adulthood

  l. Recurrent attacks of fever, and pain in the arms, legs, and abdomen possibly beginning in early childhood

 3. Treatment

  a. Avoid sources of known infection

  b. Avoid contact sports (damage to spleen will cause massive internal hemorrhage)

  c. Bed rest to decrease cellular metabolism (minimize energy expenditure and oxygen utilization)

  d. Hydration for hemodilution (oral or intravenous)

  e. Electrolyte replacement to correct metabolic acidosis caused by hypoxia

  f. Analgesics for abdominal and joint pain

  g. Blood transfusions to treat anemia and reduce viscosity of sickled blood

  h. Antibiotics for infections as appropriate

  i. Oxygen therapy in severe crisis: continuous administration of oxygen can depress bone marrow activity, causing anemia to worsen

  j. Bone marrow transplantation and erythropoietin as potential treatment

O. Necrotizing Enterocolitis (an acute inflammatory disease of the bowel, with prematurity the most prominent risk factor)

 1. Etiological factors

  a. Exact etiology is still uncertain

  b. Appears to occur in neonates whose gastrointestinal tracts have suffered vascular compromise and stops producing protective lubricating mucous, allowing the intestinal wall to be attacked by proteolytic enzymes

      c. Intestinal ischemia of unknown etiology

      d. Immature gastrointestinal host defenses

      e. Enteric feedings of hypertonic substances (e.g., formula and hyperosmolar medications)

      f. Gastrointestinal bacterial proliferation

   2. Clinical manifestations

      a. Onset usually between 4 and 10 days after the initiation of feedings, but signs evident as early as 4 hours of age and as late as 30 days; necrotizing enterocolitis in full-term infants almost always occurs in the first 10 days of life

      b. Distended (often shining) abdomen

      c. Gastric retention

      d. Blood in stools

      e. Lethargy

      f. Poor feeding

      g. Hypotension

      h. Apnea

      i. Vomiting (often bile-stained)

      j. Decreased urine output

      k. Hypothermia

      l. Laboratory findings reveal

         1) Anemia

         2) Leukopenia

         3) Leukocytosis

         4) Metabolic acidosis

         5) Electrolyte imbalances

         6) In severe cases, DIC and/or thrombocytopenia

   3. Treatment

      a. Oral feedings withheld

      b. Abdominal decompression via nasogastric suction

      c. Intravenous antibiotic administration

      d. Correction of extravascular volume depletion, electrolyte abnormalities, acid-base imbalances, and hypoxia

      e. Surgical correction of intestinal perforation (resection and anastomosis or creation of an ostomy)

P. Human Immunodeficiency Virus (HIV) and Acquired Immunodeficiency Syndrome (AIDS)

   1. Etiological factors

      a. Virus HIV type I is the causative agent for AIDS

      b. Transmission of the virus occurs by sexual contact, parenteral exposure to blood (direct blood-to-blood contact with an individual infected with HIV), or from an HIV-infected mother to child (in utero or via breastfeeding)

      c. Immunosuppression is a result of a decreased number of CD4 T-cells

d. Abnormal B-cell function is apparent early in pediatric HIV infection

2. Clinical manifestations
   a. Majority of children with perinatally acquired AIDS are normal at birth but develop symptoms within the first 18 months of life
   b. Lymphadenopathy
   c. Recurrent bacterial infections
   d. Secondary cancers: Kaposi's sarcoma is found in less than 1% of affected children
   e. Confirmed HIV in blood or tissues
   f. CD4 T-lymphocyte counts are less than 200 cells/microliters
   g. Hepatosplenomegaly
   h. Recurrent pulmonary diseases, including *Pneumocystis carinii* pneumonia, lymphocytic interstitial pneumonitis, pulmonary lymphoid hyperplasia, and tuberculosis
   i. Failure to thrive (HIV-infected infants)
   j. Chronic diarrhea (either primary from HIV or secondary from opportunistic gastrointestinal infections)
   k. Neurologic involvement occurs in 75 to 90% of HIV-infected children
      1) Developmental delay or loss of motor skills
      2) Decreased brain growth (microencephaly or abnormal neurological examination results)
   l. Chronic candidiasis

3. Treatment
   a. Directed at slowing the progression of the virus; prevention, management, and treatment of opportunistic infections and nutritional support
   b. Intravenous gamma globulin administration for B-lymphocyte deficiency
   c. Therapy for *Pneumocystis carinii* pneumonia
      1) Trimethoprim/Sulfamethoxazole (Bactrim, Septra)
      2) Pentamidine isethionate
      3) Intravenous pentamidine, if side effects or sensitivities occur secondary to the Bactrim
   d. Nutritional support: enteral or total parenteral nutrition

Q. Hemophilia

1. Overview
   a. Hemophilia is an inherited, congenital blood dyscrasia characterized by the absence or malfunction of one of the factors necessary for blood coagulation, resulting in impaired coagulability and a tendency to bleed
   b. Factor VIII deficiency (hemophilia A or classic hemophilia) accounts for 75% of all cases

  c. Hemophilia B (Christmas disease) is factor IX (plasma-thromboplastin component) deficiency

  d. Hemophilia C is factor XI deficiency (plasma-thromboplastin antecedent)

2. Etiological factors

  a. Transmitted as an X-linked recessive disorder

  b. As many as one-third of cases may be caused by gene mutation

  c. Appears in males but is transmitted by females

3. Clinical manifestations

  a. Clinical severity varies depending on the plasma level of the coagulation factor involved

   1) Mild (patients with factor levels of 25 to 50% of normal): bleeding from severe trauma or surgery, spontaneous bleeding does not occur

   2) Moderate (patients with factor levels above 5% but less than 25% of normal): bleeding occurs from moderate trauma

   3) Severe (patients with factor levels less than 1% of normal): may have spontaneous bleeding or bleeding from minor trauma into the subcutaneous tissue, muscles, or joints (hemarthrosis)

4. Treatment

  a. Immobilization and elevation of affected area

  b. Local pressure to affected area to allow for clot formation

  c. Administration of cryoprecipitate or plasma concentrate containing the necessary factor

R. Leukemia

1. Overview

  a. Malignant disease characterized by unrestricted proliferation of immature WBCs in the bone marrow, spleen, and lymphatic tissue

  b. In children, the two forms generally recognized are acute lymphocytic leukemia and acute myelocytic leukemia

  c. The clinical course of the acute (immature cells) leukemias is similar for all types

2. Etiological factors

  a. Etiology is unknown although several factors are associated with increased incidence

   1) Exposure to radiation

   2) Infectious agents (e.g., viruses)

   3) Chemical agents (e.g., benzene)

   4) Familial predisposition and genetic influence (e.g., increased risk with Down syndrome)

   5) Chemotherapeutic agents (e.g., alkylating agents)

   6) Myeloproliferative disorders (e.g., polycythemia vera, myelofibrosis)

3. Clinical manifestations

  a. Anemia with fatigue, generalized malaise, and pallor

b. Fever or infection (secondary to granulocytopenia, neutropenia)

c. Pain in joints and bones (from rapidly expanding marrow in the bone)

d. Swelling of lymph nodes, spleen, and liver

e. Hemorrhage or petechiae from thrombocytopenia (decreased platelet count)

f. Anorexia and weight loss

g. Vague abdominal pain (intestinal tract inflammation)

h. Increased intracranial pressure from neurological complications (leukemic cells invading the central nervous system)

i. Tachycardia, intolerance to heat, dyspnea on exertion (as a result of increased metabolism)

4. Treatment

a. Central vein catheter insertion to facilitate vascular access for chemotherapy, multiple blood sampling or transfusion, and antibiotic administration

b. High-dose chemotherapy

c. Bone marrow transplantation

d. Total body irradiation

e. Monitor weight, vital signs, CBC, and chemistry values (compare with baseline values)

f. Observe for drug side effects (potential toxic side effects of chemotherapy)

g. Prevention and treatment of infections (monitor granulocytes)

h. Prevent and control bleeding (monitor platelet count)

i. Analgesics and narcotics to relieve pain

j. Adequate nutrition (enteral or parenteral)

IV. PHARMACOLOGY

A. Pediatric Dosage Formulas

1. Clark's weight rule

a. Determines the child's dose based on the child's weight in relation to the average adult body weight and dose

$$\frac{\text{Weight (lb)}}{\text{Average Adult Weight (150 lb)}} \times \text{Average Adult Dose} = \text{Child's Dose}$$

2. Fried's weight rule (by age in months)

a. Determines the infant's dose based on the infant's age in relation to the average adult body weight and dose

b. Is effective only for infants younger than 1 year

$$\frac{\text{Age (in Months)}}{\text{Average Adult Weight (150 lb)}} \times \text{Average Adult Dose} = \text{Infant's Dose}$$

3. Young's weight rule (by age in years)
   a. Determines the child's dose based on the child's age and average adult dose, divided by the child's age plus 12

$$\frac{\text{Age (in Years)}}{\text{Age (in Years)} + 12} \times \text{Average Adult Dose} = \text{Child's Dose}$$

4. Milligrams/kilogram (mg/kg)
   a. Kilograms used instead of pounds to provide more precise dosage administration
   b. Most commonly used formula:
      1) Know that 1 kilogram (kg) = 2.2 pounds (lb)
      2) Divide by 2.2 to convert body weight in pounds to kilograms
      3) Multiply number of kg by mg/kg to determine dose to be administered
5. BSA meters squared
   a. Nomograms exist that aid in the calculation of BSA from height (cm/in) and weight (lb/kg)
   b. Surface area is indicated where a straight line connecting the child's height and weight intersects with the surface area column
   c. This value represents the BSA in square meters (m^2)
   d. Most common method for calculating pediatric chemotherapy

B. Methods of Pediatric Medication Administration

1. IV push/bolus
   a. Medication administered directly into the vein (commonly over 1 to 5 minutes)
2. Intermittent
   a. Mini-bag
      1) Limited-volume solution container
   b. Volume-controlled metered chamber
   c. Syringe pump/syringe set
      1) 1 ml to 30 ml (or larger) syringe of medication attached to micro-bore tubing infused at a prescribed rate
   d. Disposable elastomeric pump
      1) Latex balloon filled with medication inside a plastic housing with attached extension tubing
         • Does not rely on gravity
         • Infuses at controlled rate
   e. Piggyback
      1) Secondary administration set/solution container attached to the primary tubing and infused at intervals over a specific period of time
   f. Continuous
      1) Constant infusion of solution or medication
   g. Retrograde

1) Specific 1-ml retrograde tubing with stopcocks on each end is attached to the primary administration set
2) Medication-filled syringe is attached to one stopcock
3) Tubing is clamped between the patient and the other stopcock while the medication is infused into the retrograde tubing
4) Tubing is unclamped and the medication is allowed to infuse at the same rate as the primary intravenous solution

V. INTRAVENOUS SUPPLIES AND EQUIPMENT

A. Special Considerations

1. Frequent assessment and monitoring of pediatric patients (include physical condition, infusion site, supplies, and equipment) for potential complications related to prescribed therapy or vascular access device (VAD)
2. Use electronic infusion devices or calibrated volume-control chamber to assure an accurate rate/volume of infusion
3. Volume of solution container appropriate for age, height, and weight, or BSA
4. Intravenous site selected readily visible; roller bandages are never used around the VAD site
5. Age-specific site selection
   a. Activities and stages of development affect the site selection for a VAD
   b. Site selected reflects the lowest risk for complications and supports the safest course of prescribed therapy
6. Growth of the child subsequent to central catheter insertion may necessitate periodic reverification of tip location or catheter replacement
7. Administer only those medications approved for pediatric use
   a. For children less than 2 years of age, use preservative-free medications

B. Infusion Devices

1. Control devices (elastomeric, controller, pump) selection criteria
   a. Flow rate: ability to administer in increments from one-tenth of a milliliter
   b. Tamper-resistant: minimizing potential for child tampering
   c. Occlusion detector
   d. Accuracy of infusion rate/volume
2. Solution containers
   a. Recommendation that containers exceeding 150 ml not be connected to children younger than 2 years, no more than 250 ml for children younger than 5 years, and no more than 500 ml for children younger than 10 years of age

3. Administration sets
   a. Drop factor
      1) Microdrip: recommended for use; delivers 60 gtts/ml
      2) Volume control metered chamber: calibrated to limit the amount of solution that can be infused; microdrip chamber delivers 60 gtts/ml
      3) Macrodrip: indicated for large-volume or rapid infusions; delivers at 10, 15, or 20 gtts/ml
   b. Lumen diameter
      1) Microbore: small-bore tubing recommended because of low priming volume
      2) Macrobore: large-bore tubing indicated for large volume or rapidly infused solutions, or transfusion therapy
4. Filters
   a. 0.2-micron filter is considered a bacterial/particulate retentive, air-eliminating filter recommended for use to decrease the potential of air emboli
   b. 1.2-micron filter for removal of bacteria (except *Pseudomonas*) and *Candida albicans;* used when pharmaceutical company recommends its use with the product and with TPN containing lipid emulsions
5. Needle/needleless systems
   a. Valved
   b. Resealing latex with blunt or beveled needle
   c. Protected needle
6. Add-on devices
   a. Limit use of these devices to reduce potential for infection due to increased manipulation or separation
   b. Secure junction points
   c. Luer-Lok configuration
   d. Includes stopcocks and extension sets

C. Vascular Access Devices (VADs)

1. Peripheral catheters
   a. Inserted into a peripheral vein or scalp veins of infants
   b. Recommended for solutions or medications with a pH ranging from 5 to 9, and a serum osmolality less than 500 mOsm
   c. Types of peripheral catheters
      1) Peripheral: short-term
         • Range in size from 26- to 18-gauge and larger
      2) Peripheral: midline
         • Catheter greater than 3 inches with the tip residing below the axilla
         • Insertion site no more than 1.5 inches above or below the antecubital fossa

2. Central
  a. Catheter whose tip resides in the superior or inferior vena cava
    1) Tunneled
    2) Implanted ports
    3) Percutaneously placed
  b. Recommended for solutions/medications with a pH less than 5 and greater than 9, and a serum osmolality greater than 500 mOsm
  c. Periodic reverification of catheter tip location is required to assess the impact of infant/child growth during long-term therapy
  d. Peripherally inserted central catheters (PICC)
    1) Peripherally inserted into one of several sites, including the basilic, cephalic, and median cubital veins of the antecubital fossa with the catheter tip terminating in the superior vena cava (SVC)
    2) In newborns or small children, other insertion sites include the large saphenous vein and the popliteal veins of the lower extremity (catheter tip termination in the IVC), the axillary vein, the superficial temporal vein, and the external jugular vein of the upper extremities and head (catheter tip termination in the SVC)
3. Intraosseous
  a. Large-bore intraosseous needle is inserted into the medullary cavity of a long bone (1 inch away from the growth plate), which serves as a noncollapsible vein
  b. Needles used to obtain intraosseous access include: standard steel hypodermic, spinal, trephine, sternal, and standard bone marrow needles
4. Umbilical
  a. 3.5 to 5.0 French flexible rigid-walled radiopaque umbilical catheter inserted into an umbilical vessel upward toward the liver for 5 to 8 centimeters or until blood is noted
5. Selection determinants
  a. pH of solution
  b. Osmolality of solution
  c. Flow rate considerations and catheter capabilities
  d. Gauge needed to administer prescribed treatment and in accordance with vasculature size tolerance
  e. Duration of therapy (days, months, years/indefinite)
  f. Number of lumens needed to administer prescribed therapy (consider solution compatibilities, potential need for multiple therapies, blood products or blood sampling)
  g. Interval: frequency over 24-hour period for solutions or medications to be administered
  h. Available vasculature

6. Care and maintenance
   a. Dressing and cannula site change are essentially the same as with the adult
   b. Pediatric patients may require additional securing of the VAD as a safety measure

VI. VENIPUNCTURE

A. Site Selection

1. Peripheral: upper extremity
   a. Hand: dorsal venous network
      1) Most distal site of extremity
      2) Allows successive sites in a proximal location may be needed
      3) Stabilization by armboard/restraint necessary
      4) Possible difficult insertion secondary to excessive subcutaneous tissue in infants
      5) Increased pain may occur as a result of increased nerve endings in this area
      6) Digital veins: useful if unable to access other sites; however, infiltrates easily
      7) Metacarpal veins
   b. Forearm
      1) Bones act as natural splint
      2) Vessels in this area may be difficult to visualize and access in toddlers because of subcutaneous tissue
      3) Cephalic, basilic, and median anticubital found
   c. Antecubital fossa
      1) Accessory cephalic: may not be easily palpated on children
      2) Median basilic
      3) Median cephalic
      4) Median cubital: joins cephalic and basilic
   d. Upper arm (below axilla)
      1) Basilic: largest vein in upper arm with straightest pathway to thoracic vessels
      2) Cephalic: smaller than basilic; pathway in upper arm and thorax variable and unknown
      3) Brachial: adjacent to basilic; more frequently accessed by vascular surgeons to gain central access
      4) Axillary
2. Peripheral: lower extremity; used before walking age; large vessels usually easy to palpate
   a. Greater saphenous: located close to bifurcating veins connecting to deep veins of the leg
   b. Lesser (small) saphenous
   c. Foot (metatarsal veins)

1) Dorsal venous network
- May not be easily palpated secondary to age or disease-related changes
- Complications related to impaired circulation, difficulty stabilizing joint

2) Medial and lateral margins of foot
- May be large
- Usually easy to palpate and visualize

d. Popliteal

3. Scalp veins
   a. Use before 18 months
      1) Disadvantages
         - Cannot be used for chemotherapy or other vesicants
         - Hair must be clipped
         - Infiltrates easily
         - Difficult to secure
         - Increases family anxiety
   b. Superficial temporal: located at front of ear
   c. Occipital
   d. Metopic or frontal: located in middle of forehead
   e. Posterior auricular
   f. Supraorbital
   g. Posterior facial

4. Umbilical
   a. In newborns, provides temporary access in emergency situations or when conditions are compromised
   b. Insertion is a medical act
   c. A 3.5 to 5.0 French flexible, rigid-walled radiopaque umbilical catheter is inserted into the umbilical vessel upward toward the liver for 5 to 8 centimeters or until blood is noted
   d. Venous catheter tip resides in the IVC
   e. Arterial catheter tip resides above the level of aortic bifurcation
   f. Two umbilical arteries: used for blood sampling, arterial pressures, intravenous fluids, and most medications (no TPN or exchange transfusions)
   g. One umbilical vein: used for blood sampling, all intravenous fluids and medications, central venous pressure monitoring, exchange transfusions
   h. May access up to fourth day of life
   i. Remove within 1 week
   j. Daily dressing change
   k. Luer-Lok connection necessary
   l. Complications of umbilical catheterization
      1) Vascular compromise
      2) Hemorrhage
      3) Air embolism

4) Infection
5) Thrombosis
6) Vascular perforation
m. Nursing assessment
1) Frequent inspection of lower extremities and buttocks for blanching and cyanosis, which may indicate impaired circulation and thrombosis
2) Monitor umbilical site for bleeding, slipping of the catheter from designated insertion length, and infection
3) Monitor respiratory status, peripheral pulses, and check for edema, which may indicate emboli formation
5. Central
a. Access sites
1) Subclavian
2) Jugular (2 internal, 2 external)
   - External jugular more commonly accessed in infants
   - Increased complication secondary to motion of neck and difficulty stabilizing
3) Innominate (brachiocephalic)
4) Femoral
5) Median cephalic (PICC)
6) Median basilic (PICC)
b. Catheter tip located in SVC or IVC
c. Placed by physician
1) PICCs may be placed by registered nurses specially trained in the procedure
6. Intraosseous
a. Situations may occur in which rapid establishment of a systemic access is vital and in which venous access may be impaired by peripheral circulatory collapse, cardiopulmonary arrest, burns, or other conditions
b. Intraosseous site provides an emergency route for the rapid administration of intravenous fluids and medication
c. A large-bore intraosseous needle is inserted into the medullary cavity of a long bone (1 inch away from growth plate)
1) Method of infusion is used for children 3 years of age and younger
2) Preferred sites are the distal tibia, proximal tibia, and distal femur
3) Recommendation is to remove cannula within 24 hours following establishment of conventional intravenous access

B. Local Anesthesia (not routinely used, contraindicated in patients with known allergy or sensitivity to local anesthetics)

1. Injectable: lidocaine hydrochloride
2. Transdermal analgesic cream: EMLA (eutectic mixture of lidocaine-prilocaine anesthetic)

  a. May be considered before peripheral VAD insertion or port access
  b. Must be applied 60 minutes before accessing procedure
  3. Numby (Iomed)-iontophoresis is a drug delivery method that uses a small external current to deliver water-soluble, charged drugs (Iontocaine) into the skin to provide dermal anesthesia

C. Insertion Techniques

1. Actual method of venipuncture the same for children as for adults, but certain techniques enhance successful venipuncture
2. Have extra personnel to lend assistance during intravenous procedure
3. Pad tongue blades for use as arm boards
4. Use rubberbands or 3/8-inch penrose drains with a tape tab as tourniquets
5. Use stickers or drawings on the intravenous dressing as a reward
6. Stabilization is essential, particularly in the younger child whose level of comprehension concerning the importance of not manipulating the intravenous site is minimal
7. Fully explain venipuncture procedures to parents; obtain their consent before proceeding with a scalp vein access and offer to give them the clipped hair as a keepsake
8. During scalp vein insertions aim the catheter downward, toward the heart
9. Secure extremities with normal joint position maintained on padded boards; consider using a folded towel taped around the extremity or stretch netting
10. Use sandbags to secure the lower extremity in alignment
11. Perform toddler (and younger) intravenous procedures in a treatment room, thus preserving the child's room and bed as a "safe" place where invasive procedures are not performed
12. Use caution not to impair circulation with stabilization
13. Set up equipment and supplies before venipuncture
14. Perform site assessment (and documentation of observations) at least every 2 hours
15. Use warm wet towels, flashlights, warming lights, and fiberoptic vein lights to increase visibility and vasodilation; exercise caution not to burn the child's skin

D. Other Intravenous Therapies

1. Indications, complications, and interventions are the same as for adults

E. Complications and Risks

1. Similar to adult
2. Possible malposition of central catheter tip as a result of growth of the child; radiographic reconfirmation of catheter tip location with replacement as indicated

F. Nursing Interventions

1. Similar to adult

VII. PATIENT AND FAMILY EDUCATION

A. Underlying Principles

1. Include explanation, demonstration, return demonstration, and verbalization of understanding
2. Provide detail appropriate to child's growth and development and to caregiver's educational level

B. Introduction

1. Purpose and principle of therapy
2. Terminology

C. Aseptic Technique

1. Hand washing
2. Handling of sterile supplies
3. Establishment of work area/space

D. Catheter Care

1. Site inspection
2. Signs of infection
3. Signs of complications
4. Dressing change
5. Catheter cap change
6. Extension tubing change
7. Flushing the catheter

E. Preparing/Mixing the Solutions

1. Storing solutions
2. Inspection before and after
3. Appropriate dosage calculation
4. Preparation
5. Appropriate disposal of used supplies and equipment

F. Fluid Administration

1. Infusing of solution
2. Pump operation (include alarm features)
3. Lipid emulsion administration
4. Additives
5. Rate of administration
6. Gravity
7. Bolus
8. Changing solution containers/sets
9. Discontinuing infusions

G. Potential Complications Associated with Therapy

1. Physical signs and symptoms
2. Equipment failure
3. Action(s) to prevent/correct problems
4. Emergency actions

H. Self Monitoring

1. Urine
2. Serum glucose
3. Temperature
4. Other

I. Physical Limitations

1. Contact sports
2. Lifting
3. Other

REFERENCES

Barone MA, Johns Hopkins Hospital. Children's Medical and Surgical Center. The Harriet Lane Handbook: A Manual for Pediatric House Officers/The Harriet Lane Service. 14th ed. St. Louis, MO: Mosby, 1996.

Behrman RE, Keigman A (eds.) *Nelson's Textbook of Pediatrics,* 15th ed. Philadelphia, PA: Saunders, 1996.

Gahart BL, Nazzareno AR. *Intravenous Medications: A Handbook for Nurses and Other Allied Health Personnel,* 15th ed. St. Louis, MO: Mosby Year-Book, 1999.

Haekelman RA, Freidman SB, Nelson NM, Seidel HM, et al. (eds.) *Primary Pediatric Care,* 3rd ed. St. Louis, MO: Mosby Year-Book, 1997.

Intravenous Nurses Society. Position paper: Midline and midclavicular catheters. *Journal of Intravenous Nursing* 1997:20(4):175–178.

Intravenous Nurses Society. Position paper: Peripherally inserted central catheters. *Journal of Intravenous Nursing* 1997;20(4):172–174.

Intravenous Nurses Society. Intravenous Nursing Standards of Practice (revised 1998). *Journal of Intravenous Nursing* 1998;21(1):suppl: S1–S95.

Methany NM (ed.) *Fluid and Electrolyte Balance: Nursing Considerations,* 3rd ed. Philadelphia, PA: Lippincott-Raven, 1996.

Oncology Nursing Society. *Cancer Chemotherapy Guidelines and Recommendations for Practice.* Pittsburgh, PA: Oncology Nursing Press, 1996.

Phillips LD. *Manual of IV Therapeutics,* 2nd ed. Philadelphia, PA: FA Davis, 1996.

Tenenbaum L. *Cancer Chemotherapy and Biotherapy: A Reference Guide,* 2nd ed. Philadelphia, PA: Saunders, 1994.

Terhume LP. Intraosseous infusion: An emergency skill for the pediatrician. *Contemporary Pediatrics* 1992;9:48–60.

Terry J, Baranowski L, Lonsway RA, Hedrick D (eds.). *Intravenous Therapy: Clinical Principles and Practice.* Philadelphia, PA: Saunders, 1995.

Teusch and Ballard (eds.). *Avery's Diseases of the Newborn,* 7th ed. Philadelphia, PA: Saunders, 1998.

Trissel LA. *Handbook on Injectable Drugs,* 11th ed. Bethesda, MD: American Society of Health-System Pharmacists, 1998.

Weinstein SM. Math calculations for intravenous nurses. *Journal of Intravenous Nursing* 1990;13(4):231–236.

Weinstein SM (ed.). *Plumer's Principles and Practice of Infusion Therapy,* 6th ed. Philadelphia, PA: Lippincott-Raven, 1997.

Weir JA. Blood component therapy. In *Intravenous Therapy: Clinical Principles and Practice,* edited by Terry J, Baranowski L, Lonsway RA, and Hedrick C. Philadelphia, PA: Saunders, 1995:171–175.

Whaley LF, Wong DL. *Clinical Manual of Pediatric Nursing,* 4th ed. St. Louis, MO: CV Mosby, 1996.

Whaley LF, Wong DL. *Nursing Care of Infants and Children,* 5th ed. St. Louis, MO: CV Mosby, 1995.

Wheeler C, Frey AM. Intravenous therapy in children. In *Intravenous Therapy: Clinical Principles and Practice,* edited by Terry J, Baranowski L, Lonsway RA, and Hedrick C. Philadelphia, PA: Saunders, 1995:491–492.

CHAPTER **6**

Transfusion Therapy
....

Ann Corrigan, CRNI, BSN, MS
Gloria Pelletier, CRNI

I. IMMUNOHEMATOLOGY

A. Definition
....

1. Study of the immune system and immune response as it specifically relates to the antigens and antibodies found in the blood
   a. Antigens
      1) Found on surface of the red cell
      2) Are inherited
      3) Are glycoproteins or glycolipids
      4) Can invoke an immune system response
   b. Antibodies
      1) Also referred to as agglutinins
      2) Proteins found in plasma
      3) React to specific antigens found on red cells
      4) May naturally occur (inherited) or may result from immunization (acquired)
      5) Can cause agglutination in presence of red cells that exhibit corresponding antigen

B. ABO System
....

1. There are four identified blood groups: A, B, AB, and O
   a. Group A: contains antigen A on the red cell and antibody B in the plasma; thus may receive red cells from groups A and O
   b. Group B: contains antigen B on the red cells and antibody A in the plasma; thus may receive red cells from groups B and O
   c. Group AB: contains both antigen A and B on the red cells and does not have any corresponding antibodies
      1) As a result, group AB may receive red cells from blood groups A, B, AB, and O
      2) Group AB is considered a universal recipient for red cells
   d. Group O: contains no antigens on the red cells but has both antibodies A and B in the plasma

277

1) Must receive red cells from group O
2) In emergency situations, group O may be administered to any other blood group until ABO blood grouping has been established
   e. Rh factor: there are approximately 50 known Rh antigens; antigen D is the factor to be considered in transfusion therapy
   1) Rh positive: antigen D found on the red cell
   2) Rh negative: no antigen D found on the red cell
   3) Rh negative blood can be administered to Rh positive types
   4) Rh positive blood produces antibodies when administered to Rh negative types
   5) Rh compatibility extremely important in women of childbearing age to reduce potential for complications in pregnancy

TABLE 6-1 *Blood Group Antigens: ABO Systems*

ABO Group	Antigen	Antibody
A	A	B
B	B	A
AB	A and B	None
O	None	A and B

II. BLOOD AND BLOOD COMPONENTS

A. Whole Blood (use limited because of advances in the use of blood components)

1. Composition: contains red cells, white cells, platelets, and plasma
2. Volume: approximately 450 to 500 ml blood plus anticoagulant preservative in the collection unit
3. Indications
   a. To treat acute massive blood loss with signs and symptoms of hypotension, shortness of breath, tachycardia, pallor, and low hemoglobin/hematocrit (Hgb/Hct)
   b. Volume expansion required
   c. Patients who have a symptomatic deficit in oxygen-carrying capacity combined with hypovolemia of sufficient degree to be associated with shock
4. Administration of whole blood is contraindicated when blood loss can be managed with blood components and crystalloid and/or colloid solutions

5. Disadvantages
   a. Volume may lead to potential fluid volume excess
   b. Storage considerations
      1) Formation of microaggregates occurs
      2) Breakdown of cells resulting in increased potassium level
      3) Loss of coagulation factors
   c. Massive whole blood transfusion may cause calcium deficit in patients with severely damaged liver
6. Administration considerations
   a. Note patient's serum potassium before administration
   b. Number of units administered is determined by the clinical situation
   c. Administration of a single unit of whole blood is not appropriate
   d. Administer as rapidly as possible to stabilize hemodynamic status
   e. For pediatric patients, 20 ml/kg is administered initially, followed by the volume required for hemodynamic stabilization
7. Expected outcome
   a. Improved hemodynamic status and resolution of symptoms of hypovolemic shock
   b. Hct and Hgb may fluctuate because of rapid fluid shifts during active bleeding and result in erroneous laboratory values
8. Compatibility
   a. Must be ABO compatible

B. Red Blood Cells (prepared by separating the plasma from the cellular portion of whole blood)

1. Composition: contains red blood cells (RBCs) and has the same cell mass as whole blood
2. Volume: contains 250 to 350 ml/unit dependent on anticoagulant/preservative used
3. Indications
   a. Increase red cell mass when volume expansion is not required
   b. Restore or maintain oxygen-carrying capacity of the blood
   c. Symptomatic anemia unresponsive to other therapies
   d. Hypovolemic shock that can be managed with the administration of RBCs and crystalloid and/or colloid solutions
   e. Acute or chronic blood loss with tachycardia, shortness of breath, pallor, fatigue, and low Hgb/Hct
4. Administration considerations
   a. Number of units administered is determined by the clinical situation
   b. Each unit may be infused over 1 to 2 hours but must be infused within 4 hours
   c. Red cells with anticoagulant/preservative solution may be viscous and may require dilution with 0.9% sodium chloride

   d. For pediatric patients
      1) Administer 10 ml/kg
      2) Use of red cells stored with additives undesirable for massive transfusion settings and critically ill pediatric and neonatal patients
      3) Units may be divided into aliquots (smaller amounts) for administration
      4) Administer at rate of 2 to 5 ml/kg/hr
   5. Expected outcome
      a. Resolution of symptoms of anemia
      b. Increased Hct of 3% and increased Hgb of 1 g/dL per unit
   6. Compatibility
      a. Should be ABO compatible
      b. Recipients whose ABO group is unknown may receive group O red cells until ABO typing is complete
   7. Variations
      a. Leukocyte-reduced
         1) A unit of leukocyte-reduced RBCs contains fewer than 5×10^8 leukocytes
         2) Indications
            • In cases of known febrile, nonhemolytic transfusion reactions caused by donor white cell antigens reacting with recipient white cell antibodies
            • To reduce incidence of urticarial and anaphylactic reactions
            • To prevent transmission of cytomegalovirus (CMV) or alloimmunization to human leukocyte antigens
            • Immunosuppressed patients
         3) Reduction methods: may be performed before or during transfusion
            • Filtration: may be done during processing or at bedside; removes up to 99% of leukocytes
            • Washed RBCs: done before transfusion; may reduce number of red cells by 20%; must be used within 24 hours of preparation; more expensive and time-consuming method

C. Fresh Frozen Plasma (prepared by separating plasma from the cells)

   1. Composition: contains albumin, globulins, antibodies, and clotting factors
   2. Volume: 200 to 250 ml/unit
   3. Indications
      a. Increase level of clotting factors in patients with a demonstrative deficiency
      b. Counteract the effects of warfarin (Coumadin) therapy
   4. Should not be used for volume expansion or as a protein supplement for nutrition

5. Administration considerations
    a. Number of units administered is determined by the clinical situation and underlying disease
    b. Administer at 200 ml/hr or more slowly if there is potential for circulatory overload
    c. For pediatric patients, the usual dose is 10 to 15 ml/kg at a rate of 1 to 2 ml/min
    d. Transfuse within 24 hours of thawing to avoid loss of clotting factors V and VIII
6. Expected outcome: improved coagulation function
7. Compatibility: must be ABO compatible

D. Platelets (a component of plasma obtained by separation)

1. Indications: thrombocytopenia or abnormal platelet function
2. Administration considerations
    a. Number of units administered is determined by the clinical situation
        1) Random donor: usually 6 to 10 units obtained from various donors
        2) Plateletpheresis: obtained from a single donor with content similar to that of 6 to 8 units random donor
    b. Infusion rate determined by volume tolerance
        1) May be infused as rapidly as 30 minutes but must be infused within 4 hours
    c. For pediatric patients, the usual dose is 1 unit (50 to 70 ml) per 7 to 10 kg of body weight
3. Expected outcome
    a. Prevention or resolution of bleeding
    b. Increased platelet count
4. Compatibility
    a. ABO compatibility not required
    b. ABO grouping recommended to reduce potential for refractoriness to platelets
5. Special considerations
    a. Store with gentle agitation at room temperature up to 5 days
    b. Random donor units may be pooled into a single bag before release from blood bank
    c. Plateletpheresis units may reduce the risk of transfusion-transmitted diseases and human leukocyte antigen (HLA) antibody formation
6. Variations
    a. HLA-matched
        1) Collected by pheresis from donor who is HLA-compatible with recipient
        2) Decreases premature destruction of transferred platelets by HLA antibodies
        3) Frequently used in patients being prepared for tissue/organ transplantation

4) Generally more suitable matching obtained from immediate family; less perfect match from nonrelated donor may be sufficient

b. Leukocyte-reduced

1) Reduction achieved by filtration with approximately 99% of leukocytes being removed

2) Used to decrease incidence of febrile reaction; helps prevent HLA alloimmunization in patients who require long-term platelet support or may require transplantation

E. Cryoprecipitate (a component derived from a unit of fresh frozen plasma)

1. Composition: factor VIII (antihemophilia factor), von Willebrand's factor, and factor XIII
2. Volume: 10 to 20 ml/unit
3. Indications
   a. Treatment of deficiencies of factor XIII and fibrinogen
   b. May be used in the treatment of von Willebrand's disease if factor XIII concentrate is not available
4. Administration considerations
   a. Number of units is dependent on the clinical situation
      1) Dose may need to be repeated every 8 to 12 hours
      2) Laboratory evaluation required to assess effectiveness of treatment
   b. Rate of infusion is 1 to 2 ml/min for both the adult and pediatric patient
   c. Single units must be infused within 6 hours of thawing; pooled units infused within 4 hours of being pooled
   d. 0.9% sodium chloride may be added to facilitate infusion
5. Expected outcome
   a. Correction of deficiencies
   b. Cessation of bleeding episode
6. Compatibility: ABO and Rh match preferred whenever possible; plasma compatibility also preferred but not required

F. Factor VIII Concentrate (commercially prepared from large pools of donor plasma)

1. Contains large quantities of factor VIII
2. Indications: factor VIII deficiency (hemophilia A)
3. Administration considerations
   a. Amount to be administered depends on prophylactic use or as treatment for active bleeding based on a factor VIII calculation formula
   b. Dilution is required for reconstitution and should be administered within 3 hours of reconstitution

    c. Some of the newer preparations can be used in von Willebrand's disease

    d. Factor assays should be performed at appropriate intervals to assess response

  4. Expected outcome: hemostasis is caused by increased levels of factor VIII and/or von Willebrand's factor activity

  5. Compatibility: not required

G. Factor IX Concentrate (commercially prepared from quantities of donor plasma; may also contain trace amounts of factor II, VII, and X)

  1. Indications: factor IX deficiency (hemophilia B), also known as Christmas disease

  2. Administration considerations

    a. Amount to be administered depends on the clinical situation and can be calculated using the formula for factor VIII dosage

    b. Units to be given should be doubled because half of the infused factor IX disappears immediately following infusion

    c. Recommended dose and treatment schedule varies with the severity and type of bleeding

    d. Diluent provided with factor for reconstitution

    e. Factor assays should be performed at intervals to assess response

  3. Expected outcome: hemostasis because of increased level of factor IX activity

  4. Compatibility: not required

H. Colloid Solutions

  1. Albumin: commercially extracted from plasma; eliminates risk of transfusion transmitted viruses; contains no clotting factors

    a. Indicators

      1) Volume expansion when crystalloid solutions not adequate

      2) Treatment of hypoproteinemia

      3) May be used as plasma substitute in treatment of hypovolemic shock and massive hemorrhage

    b. Administration considerations

      1) Amount administered dependent on clinical situation

        • 5% solution: an isotonic solution oncotically equivalent to plasma; available in 250 ml

        • 25% solution: contains 25 grams albumin per 100 ml; available in 50 or 100 ml

      2) Rate of administration varies dependent on indication, present blood volume, and patient response; circulatory overload may occur if albumin infused too rapidly

    c. Expected outcome

      1) Expansion of blood volume

      2) Prevention of marked hemoconcentration

3) Decreased edema

4) Increased serum protein levels

2. Protein plasma fraction: commercially extracted from plasma; contains a high degree of plasma products and no clotting factors

  a. Indications

    1) Plasma volume expansion in treatment of shock or in conditions in which circulatory volume deficit is present

    2) Not as preferable as albumin as it is more likely to cause hypotensive reactions

  b. Administration considerations

    1) Rate and dose dependent on patient's condition and response to therapy; however, administration should not exceed 10 ml/min to reduce potential for hypotensive episode

    2) Available as a 5% solution

  c. Expected outcome

    1) Expansion of plasma volume

    2) Prevention of marked hemoconcentration

    3) Decreased edema

    4) May increase serum protein levels

III. ADVERSE REACTIONS

A. Acute (occurs within minutes or hours of administration)

1. Hemolytic

  a. Intravascular: due to donor red cells being incompatible with recipient's plasma, potential fatality may occur with the administration of as little as 10 to 15 ml of incompatible blood

    1) Causes: misidentification or improper labeling resulting in the wrong unit of blood

    2) Signs and symptoms

      • Fever with or without chills

      • Hypotension

      • Lumbar pain

      • Hemoglobinemia

      • Hemoglobinuria

      • Dyspnea

      • Shock

      • Oliguria and/or anuria

      • Abnormal bleeding

    3) Interventions

      • Stop transfusion

      • Change administration set and administer 0.9% sodium chloride at a rate to maintain a patent intravenous line

      • Notify physician and blood bank immediately

      • Institute transfusion reaction protocol

      • Initiate treatment to reverse effects of reaction

4) Preventions
- Proper patient identification
- Proper labeling of blood sample
- Verification of ABO/Rh compatibility between donor and recipient before administration

b. Extravascular: results from incompatibility between recipient red cells and donor plasma
1) Causes: improperly identified blood sample, blood unit, or patient
2) Signs and symptoms
- Chills
- Fever, usually several hours after transfusion
- Positive direct antiglobulin test
3) Interventions
- Stop transfusion
- Change administration set and administer 0.9% sodium chloride at a rate to maintain a patent intravenous line
- Notify physician and blood bank immediately
- Institute transfusion reaction protocol
- Initiate treatment to relieve symptoms
4) Preventions
- Proper patient identification
- Proper labeling of blood sample

2. Febrile nonhemolytic
a. Causes: white blood cell antigen-antibody reaction
b. Signs and symptoms
1) Increase in temperature of 1°C or 2°F or more without any other clinical reason; may begin early in transfusion or up to several hours after completion
2) Chills
3) Rigors
4) General malaise
c. Interventions
1) Stop transfusion
2) Change administration set and administer 0.9% sodium chloride at a rate to maintain a patent intravenous line
3) Notify physician and blood bank
4) Institute transfusion reaction protocol
5) Administer antipyretics to treat fever
d. Preventions
1) Obtain transfusion history
2) Premedicate, as ordered
3) Use of leukocyte-reduced products

3. Allergic
a. Causes: sensitivity reaction to foreign plasma protein in transfused product

b. Signs and symptoms
1) Urticaria
2) Hives
3) Local erythema
c. Interventions: based on severity of reaction
1) Severe
- Stop transfusion
- Notify physician
- Initiate treatment to relieve symptoms
2) Mild
- Interrupt transfusion
- Administer antihistamines, as ordered
- Following resolution of symptoms, proceed with transfusion
d. Preventions
1) Obtain transfusion history
2) Pretreatment with an antihistamine may be ordered
4. Anaphylaxis: may occur after infusion of only a few milliliters of blood or plasma
a. Causes: generally unknown but thought to be associated with sensitization to a foreign protein
b. Signs and symptoms
1) Respiratory distress
2) Bronchospasm
3) Abdominal cramps
4) Nausea, vomiting, and/or diarrhea
5) Shock
6) Loss of consciousness
7) Death
c. Interventions
1) Stop transfusion
2) Maintain patent intravenous line
3) Initiate treatment to relieve symptoms
d. Preventions
1) Obtain transfusion history
2) Use of deglycerolized red cells or autologous blood for future transfusions
5. Circulatory overload
a. Causes: rapid infusion to patients with compromised cardiac or pulmonary status
b. Signs and symptoms
1) Pulmonary edema
2) Dyspnea
3) Cyanosis
4) Severe headache
5) Hypertension
6) Congestive heart failure

c. Interventions
1) Stop transfusion
2) Place patient in sitting position
3) Administer diuretics and oxygen, as ordered
d. Preventions: infuse blood and blood components at a rate appropriate for patient's condition, age, and tolerance to treatment
6. Bacterial contamination
a. Causes: introduction of bacteria at the time of donation or component preparation; gram-negative organisms are most commonly involved; occurs rarely
b. Signs and symptoms
1) High fever
2) Hypotension
3) Flushing of the skin
4) Shock
5) Renal failure
6) Disseminated intravascular coagulation
c. Interventions
1) Stop transfusion
2) Change administration set and administer 0.9% sodium chloride at a rate to maintain a patent intravenous line
3) Initiate measures to prevent shock
4) Notify physician and blood bank
5) Culture patient's blood, suspected component, administration set, filter, and 0.9% sodium chloride
d. Preventions: use of aseptic technique and sterile equipment in the collection processing and administration of blood components
7. Hypothermia
a. Causes: rapid infusion of refrigerated blood or blood components
b. Signs and symptoms
1) Shaking chills
2) Hypotension
3) Cardiac arrhythmias
c. Interventions
1) Initiate measures to warm blood
2) Initiate treatment to relieve symptoms
d. Preventions: warm blood using a fluid/blood warmer device
8. Citrate toxicity
a. Causes: large volume transfusion to patients with liver impairment; liver is unable to metabolize the citrate
b. Signs and symptoms
1) Hypocalcemia
2) Circumoral tingling
3) Hypotension
4) Nausea and vomiting
5) Hypokalemia
6) Cardiac arrhythmias

    c. Interventions
      1) Slow or discontinue transfusion
      2) Monitor serum calcium and potassium levels
    d. Preventions: ascertain history of liver impairment

B. Delayed (onset within days to years)

  1. Primary alloimmunization
    a. Causes: sensitization to foreign red blood cell antigens not found in the ABO system; examples include Rh, Kell, Duffy, Kidd antigens
    b. Signs and symptoms
      1) Fever of unknown origin
      2) Continued anemia
      3) Declined Hgb
      4) Mild jaundice
      5) Hemoglobinuria
    c. Interventions: monitor renal function
  2. Secondary alloimmunization
    a. Causes: re-exposure to some antigen increasing antibody production
    b. Signs and symptoms
      1) Fever
      2) Unexpected drop in Hgb
      3) Mild jaundice
      4) Hemoglobinuria
    c. Interventions: monitor renal function
    d. Preventions: administer future transfusions that do not contain corresponding antigen
  3. Iron overload
    a. Causes: progressive and continued accumulation of iron as a result of chronic transfusions, especially in those patients with hemoglobinopathies; each unit of red cells contains approximately 200 mg of iron
    b. Signs and symptoms
      1) Hepatic failure
      2) Cardiac toxicity
    c. Interventions
      1) Removal of iron without reducing circulating Hgb
      2) Administration of deferoxamine mesylate (Desferal mesylate)
  4. Graft versus host disease
    a. Causes: infusion of immunocompetent lymphocytes into a severely immunosuppressed recipient
    b. Signs and symptoms
      1) Fever
      2) Skin rash
      3) Hepatitis
      4) Diarrhea

   5) Bone marrow suppression

   6) Overwhelming infection that may progress to fatal outcome

  c. Interventions: initiate treatment of symptoms; condition fatal in 75 to 90% of cases

  d. Preventions: pretransfusion irradiation of all blood components containing lymphocytes

 5. Hepatitis: hepatitis viruses associated post-transfusion are hepatitis B and hepatitis C

  a. Causes: transmission of hepatitis virus from donor to recipient

  b. Signs and symptoms: can occur from 2 weeks to 6 months after transfusion

   1) Abnormal liver function test

   2) Elevated liver enzymes

   3) Fatigue

   4) Nausea

   5) Jaundice

 6. Human T-cell lymphotropic virus (HTLV)

  a. Causes: transmission of HTLV from donor to recipient

   1) Four types of HTLV are identified

   2) HTLV-III is the type that causes acquired immunodeficiency syndrome (AIDS)

  b. Signs and symptoms

   1) Fever

   2) Night sweats

   3) Weight loss

   4) Skin lesions

   5) Adenopathy

   6) Opportunistic infections

 7. Cytomegalovirus (CMV): immunocompromised patients are at greater risk of CMV transmission because of the higher risk for significant morbidity and mortality as a result

  a. Causes: member of the herpes virus family; known to be one of the infectious agents most frequently transmitted by transfusion

  b. Signs and symptoms

   1) Most CMV infections are asymptomatic

   2) May have mononucleosis-like syndrome

IV. PATIENT ASSESSMENT

A. History

 1. Pertinent medical history: includes current and chronic conditions and medications

 2. Transfusion history: includes history of any reactions or adverse effects during previous transfusions

 3. Social history: includes religious and cultural beliefs

B. Clinical

1. Review of laboratory values for appropriateness of therapy
   a. Hct
   b. Hgb
   c. Platelets
   d. Electrolytes, especially calcium and potassium
   e. Liver function tests
   f. Albumin
   g. Clotting factor assays
   h. Serum iron binding
2. Vital signs: abnormal findings before the start of a transfusion may delay recognition of a transfusion reaction
3. Renal status: determine function
4. Venous status: to determine whether appropriate access is available
5. Mental status: ability to comprehend and/or cooperate before and during transfusion

V. ADMINISTRATION

A. Physician's Order

1. Type of component and number of units to be administered
2. Premedication orders, as appropriate
3. Special considerations such as leukocyte-reduced components, blood warmer

B. Informed Consent

1. Must be signed before administration of blood, blood components
2. Physician is responsible for informing the patient of benefits, risks, alternative treatments, and prognosis

C. ABO, Rh Determination

1. Type and cross match must be done, as appropriate

D. Patient Education

1. Reaffirm purpose of transfusion, benefits, and risks involved

E. Identification Verification

1. Obtain component from blood bank/transfusion services
   a. Verification of patient identification and results of ABO, Rh compatibility are essential before removing from blood bank/transfusion services
2. Verify patient identification
   a. The nurse, before initiating the transfusion, must verify the following information at the bedside:

1) Patient name
2) Identification number
3) Name of component
4) Donor and recipient ABO and Rh type
5) Expiration date of unit
6) Compatibility results
7) Blood component number

F. Equipment

1. Cannula
   a. Generally recommended that blood/blood components be transfused through an 18 to 20 gauge cannula
   b. Pediatric and adult patients in whom large veins are inaccessible may require use of a smaller-gauge cannula; use of external pressure to administer a transfusion through a small-gauge cannula may result in damage to the red cells
2. Filter
   a. Designed to retain clots and other debris from blood/blood components
   b. Available in various micron sizes
      1) Standard: 170 to 260 microns
      2) Microaggregate: 20 to 40 microns; recommended for administration of whole blood and/or packed cells that have been stored for 5 or more days; may impede flow rates when rapid transfusion required
      3) Leukocyte-reduction: specifically designed for red cells or platelets; removes at least 99% of leukocytes from the component
   c. To maximize effectiveness, it is important that the whole surface area of the filter be used
   d. May be an integral part of the blood administration set or be added to a nonvented administration set
3. Blood administration sets
   a. Straight: designed to administer a single unit; not recommended for use when multiple units are to be administered
   b. Y-type: designed for the administration of multiple units; one arm of the Y is designated for the administration of 0.9% sodium chloride, the other arm is designated for the blood
   c. Component recipient sets: designed for the administration of platelets and cryoprecipitate; generally of a shorter length and has a smaller filter surface area to reduce lysis of component to the filter and wall of the administration set
   d. Component infusion set: designed to allow for administration of components by direct intravenous push
4. Electronic infusion device
   a. Follow manufacturer's recommendation for use with blood/blood components

    b. Consideration must be given to the configuration of the pumping mechanism and to the PSI rating to minimize risk of damage to the cells

  5. External pressure cuff

    a. Designed to assist in the delivery of blood by exerting even pressure to the bag

    b. Cuff must have a gauge to monitor pressure; pressure should not exceed 300 mm Hg

    c. Not used routinely; may be used in situations where rapid administration is required

  6. Blood/fluid warmer

    a. Device that increases the temperature of blood

    b. Indications

      1) Rapid massive infusion of refrigerated blood

      2) Exchange transfusion in newborns

      3) In patients with known potent cold agglutinins

    c. Types

      1) Warm water bath: blood passes through coiled plastic tubing and is placed in a monitored water bath

      2) Electric heated plates: blood passes through a plastic bag that has been placed between the electronically heated plates

    d. All blood warmers must have a temperature gauge; temperature should not exceed 42°C; hemolysis may occur if temperature exceeds 42°C

    e. Warmer must be equipped with an audible alarm system

    f. Use of warmer may decrease flow rate and may increase amounts of priming fluid required

G. Special Considerations

  1. 0.9% sodium chloride is the recommended solution for use with blood administration; other solutions may potentiate agglutination and/or hemolysis if used with blood

  2. A nonvented blood administration set must be used to reduce the potential for air contamination

  3. Blood must be stored in blood bank-approved, temperature-controlled refrigeration units

  4. Blood must be returned to the blood bank within 30 minutes if unable to initiate transfusion

  5. When required, blood is warmed only using a specifically designed blood warmer

  6. Blood should be administered within 4 hours; units may be split into aliquots if longer hang time is required because of patient's condition and/or age

  7. No medications should be added to blood

  8. Blood must be filtered

  9. Blood should not be piggybacked into a main intravenous line that has been used for any solution other than 0.9% sodium chloride

VI. DOCUMENTATION

A. The administration of blood must be documented and should include name of component; date and time started and completed; vital signs pre-, during, and post-infusion; and patient responses and nursing interventions initiated

REFERENCES

American Association of Blood Banks. *Technical Manual,* 12th ed., Vengelen-Tyler (ed.). Bethesda, MD: AABB, 1996.

American Hospital Formulary Service, AHFS Drug Information 98. Bethesda, MD: American Society of Health-System Pharmacists.

Dailey JF. *Blood.* Arlington, MA: Medical Consulting Group, 1998.

Gahart BL, Nazareno AR. *Intravenous Medications: A Handbook for Nurses and other Allied Health Personnel,* 14th ed. St. Louis, MO: Mosby Year-Book, 1998.

Intravenous Nurses Society. Intravenous Nursing Standards of Practice (revised 1998). *Journal of Intravenous Nursing* 1998;21(1):suppl.

Terry J, Baranowski L, Lonsway RA, Hedrick C (eds.). *Intravenous Therapy: Clinical Principles and Practice.* Philadelphia, PA: Saunders, 1995:165–187.

CHAPTER **7**

Antineoplastic Therapy

Michaelle M. Wetteland, CRNI, BA

I. THE CELL CYCLE

A. Overview

1. Knowledge of the cell cycle is necessary to understand antineoplastic therapy[1]
2. The cell cycle is a series of phases in normal and cancer cell growth
3. Knowledge of cell growth and division helps to understand the functions and side effects of antineoplastic therapy[1]

B. Cell Cycle of Normal Cells

1. The cell cycle is called the cell generation time
2. Normal cells re-enter the cell cycle and reproduce only when necessary
3. A controlled mechanism prevents cell replication unless a cell needs to be replaced as a result of damage or death
4. The cell cycle consists of five stages or phases
   a. G_0, resting stage (most normal cells are in this phase)
   b. G_1, stage of ribonucleic acid (RNA) and protein synthesis
   c. S, stage of deoxyribonucleic acid (DNA) synthesis
   d. G_2, premitotic stage (manufactures mitotic spindle)
   e. M, mitosis stage (actual cell division)

C. Cancer Cell Development

1. Cancer cells possess characteristics that allow faster proliferation and uncontrolled cell division, resulting in cell mass[1]
   a. Cancer cells continue to divide regardless of the need
   b. They quickly push into surrounding spaces and structures
2. Cancer cells move quickly through the cell cycle without entering the resting phase
   a. However, large solid tumors may have cells in the resting phase
   b. Normal cells will reproduce 10% of existing cells during the reproduction phase; cancer cells reproduce 50% of existing cells
   c. The distribution of dividing cancer cells is called "growth fraction"; Figure 7-1 demonstrates normal cell division compared to uncontrolled cell division of the cancer cell[1,3]

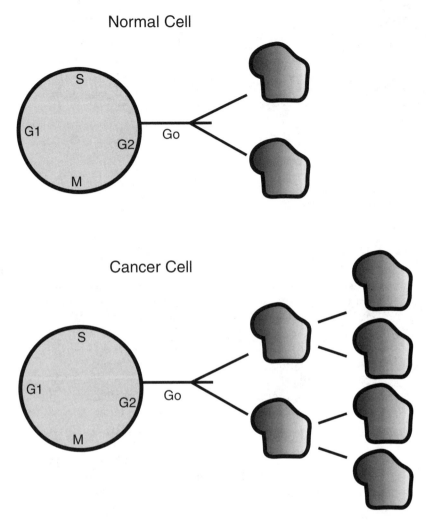

FIGURE 7-1 Cell Division: Controlled and uncontrolled.

II. DRUG SPECIFICITY

A. Overview

1. Antineoplastic agents are generally effective in the cell cycle's active phase
   a. Normal cells are equally susceptible to antineoplastic therapy during the same phase of development
      1) Normal cells that continuously replace dying cells or "actively proliferate" are the blood, epithelial, gastrointestinal, and germ cells
   b. Side effects such as myelosuppression, alopecia, nausea, vomiting,

stomatitis, and altered reproductive systems are results of destruction of normal cells

2. Goal of cancer cell-kill is to determine a dose that is effective and destroys a consistent fraction of cancer cells
   a. Ideally, the antineoplastic agent kills cancer cells while allowing enough normal cells to recover adequately
   b. To eradicate cancer cells most effectively, the therapy should be started when the cancer cell population is small or when the patient can tolerate the maximum medication dose
   c. Cancer cell type often determines how responsive the cancer will be to the antineoplastic therapy
      1) Hodgkin's disease is highly responsive to treatment because the number of dividing cells is high
      2) Malignant melanoma has a poor response to treatment because of the large number of cells in the G_0 phase

3. Primary action of antineoplastic therapy is to disrupt cancer cell division
   a. Treatment during the highest rate of cell replication is desirable
   b. Some antineoplastic agents will be effective regardless of the cell phase; such agents are called cell cycle-specific and cell cycle-nonspecific[1,3]

B. Cell Cycle-specific Agents

1. Act on the cells at various phases of the cell cycle
   a. Inhibit mitosis (vinca alkaloids)
   b. Interfere with DNA synthesis, preventing cell reproduction; also called cell cycle-dependent (antimetabolites)
   c. Most effective when a large number of cells are dividing
2. Agents affecting G_1 phase
   a. Asparaginase (Elspar)
3. Agents affecting G_2 phase
   a. Bleomycin sulfate (Blenoxane)
   b. Etoposide (VePesid)
4. Agents affecting S phase
   a. Cytarabine (Cytosar-U)
   b. Fluorouracil (5-FU)
   c. Gemcitabine hydrochloride (Gemzar)
   d. Irinotecan hydrochloride (Camptosar)
   e. Methotrexate sodium (Mexate)
5. Agents affecting M phase
   a. Vinblastine sulfate (Velban)
   b. Vincristine sulfate (Oncovin)[1,3]

C. Cell Cycle-nonspecific Agents

1. Act on the cells that are not going through the division phase
   a. Prevent cell division by causing chromosome breakage and formation of new cellular DNA (alkylating agents)

    b. Interfere with cell division, destroying completed DNA and inhibiting transcription of RNA (antitumor antibiotics)

    c. Act nonselectively on cancer cells (nitrosourea)

2. Dose-intensity curve measures the significant relationship between the number of cells and the amount of drug administered (miscellaneous antineoplastics agents)[1,3]

3. Agents

    a. Carboplatin (Paraplatin)

    b. Carmustine (BiCNU)

    c. Cisplatin (Platinol)

    d. Cladribine (Leustatin)

    e. Cyclophosphamide (Cytoxan)

    f. Dacarbazine (DTIC-Dome)

    g. Dactinomycin (Cosmegen)

    h. Daunorubicin hydrochloride (Cerubidine)

    i. Doxorubicin hydrochloride (Adriamycin)

    j. Ifosfamide (Ifex)

    k. Mechlorethamine hydrochloride (Mustargen)

    l. Mitomycin (Mutamycin)

    m. Paclitaxel (Taxol)

    n. Plicamycin (Mithracin)

    o. Streptozocin (Zanosar)

    p. Thiotepa (Thioplex)

III. PHARMACOLOGICAL CATEGORIES

A. Alkylating Agents

1. Drug specificity: cell cycle-nonspecific
2. Action: interfere with DNA replication
3. Toxicity: hematologic, gastrointestinal, reproductive; also carcinogenic (however, the benefits far exceed the risks)
4. Agents

    a. Carboplatin (Paraplatin)

    b. Cisplatin (Platinol)

    c. Cyclophosphamide (Cytoxan)

    d. Dacarbazine (DTIC-Dome)

    e. Ifosfamide (Ifex)

    f. Mechlorethamine hydrochloride (Mustargen)

    g. Thiotepa (Thioplex)

B. Antitumor Antibiotics

1. Drug specificity: cell cycle-nonspecific
2. Action: interfere with RNA synthesis, inhibit DNA synthesis by binding or reacting to DNA (some anti-infective action)
3. Toxicity: hematologic, gastrointestinal, reproductive

4. Agents
   a. Bleomycin sulfate (Blenoxane)
   b. Dactinomycin (Cosmegen)
   c. Daunorubicin hydrochloride (Cerubidine)
   d. Doxorubicin hydrochloride (Adriamycin)
   e. Mitomycin (Mutamycin)
   f. Mitoxantrone hydrochloride (Novantrone)
   g. Plicamycin (Mithracin)

C. Antimetabolites

1. Drug specificity: cell cycle-specific
2. Action: interfere with DNA synthesis, prevent cell division
3. Toxicity: hematologic, gastrointestinal
4. Agents
   a. Cladribine (Leustatin)
   b. Cytarabine (Cytosar-U)
   c. Floxuridine (FUDR)
   d. Fluorouracil (5-FU)
   e. Gemcitabine hydrochloride (Gemzar)
   f. Methotrexate sodium (Mexate)

D. Nitrosoureas

1. Drug specificity: cell cycle-nonspecific
2. Action: inhibit DNA repair
3. Toxicity: hematologic, gastrointestinal
4. Agents
   a. Carmustine (BiCNU)
   b. Streptozocin (Zanosar)

E. Vinca Alkaloids

1. Drug specificity: cell cycle-specific
2. Action: metaphase arrest results from the mitotic spindle crystallization
3. Toxicity: neurologic
4. Agents
   a. Etoposide (VePesid)
   b. Vinblastine sulfate (Velban)
   c. Vincristine sulfate (Oncovin)

F. Miscellaneous

1. Drug specificity: action and toxicity vary
2. Agents
   a. Asparaginase (Elspar)
   b. Irinotecan hydrochloride (Camptosar)
   c. Paclitaxel (Taxol)

G. Biological Response Modifiers

1. Drug specificity: antitumor activity, colony-stimulating
2. Action: augment and/or restore the immune system and interfere with tumor cell metastasis
3. Toxicity: pulmonary
4. Agents
   a. Filgrastim (G-CSF)
   b. Interferon alpha
   c. Levamisole hydrochloride (Ergamisol)
   d. Sargramostim (GM-CSF)

IV. PROPERTIES OF ANTINEOPLASTIC AGENTS

A. Overview

1. Placed into three groups, determined by the amount of irritation or potential damage caused to the subcutaneous tissue
2. Include vesicants, irritants, and nonvesicants[1,3]

B. Vesicants

1. Toxic to soft tissue, inducing tissue necrosis if extravasation occurs
2. Examples
   a. Dacarbazine (DTIC-Dome)
   b. Dactinomycin (Cosmegen)
   c. Daunorubicin hydrochloride (Cerubidine)
   d. Doxorubicin hydrochloride (Adriamycin)
   e. Irinotecan hydrochloride (Camptosar)
   f. Mechlorethamine hydrochloride (Mustargen)
   g. Mitomycin (Mutamycin)
   h. Mitoxantrone hydrochloride (Novantrone)
   i. Plicamycin (Mithracin)
   j. Vinblastine sulfate (Velban)
   k. Vincristine sulfate (Oncovin)

C. Irritants

1. Burning or inflammation without soft tissue necrosis
2. Examples
   a. Carmustine (BCNU)
   b. Paclitaxel (Taxol)
   c. Streptozocin (Zanosar)

D. Nonvesicants

1. No significant damage to soft tissue if infiltrated

2. Examples
   a. Asparaginase (Elspar)
   b. Bleomycin sulfate (Blenoxane)
   c. Carboplatin (Paraplatin)
   d. Cisplatin (Platinol)
   e. Cyclophosphamide (Cytoxan)
   f. Cytarabine (Cytosar-U)
   g. Etoposide (VePesid)
   h. Floxuridine (FUDR)
   i. Fluorouracil (5-FU)
   j. Gemcitabine hydrochloride (Gemzar)
   k. Ifosfamide (Ifex)
   l. Methotrexate sodium (Mexate)
   m. Mitoxantrone hydrochloride (Novantrone)
   n. Thiotepa (Thioplex)

V. ANTINEOPLASTIC AGENTS

A. Asparaginase (Elspar)

1. Classification
   a. Pharmacological category: miscellaneous
   b. Drug specificity: cell cycle-specific
   c. Group: nonvesicant
2. Indications
   a. Lymphosarcoma, acute lymphocytic leukemia, acute myeloid leukemia
3. Dose: used as a single agent or in combination with other agents; individualized, based upon tolerance of and response to agent and in accordance with published protocol
4. Method of administration
   a. Intramuscular (IM), IV push, continuous infusion, intrathecal
5. Complications
   a. Common: nausea, vomiting, hypersensitivity reactions including anaphylaxis, slight immunosuppression, hepatic dysfunction, hyperglycemia, hyperlipidemia, onset of pancreatitis in children
   b. System-specific: neurologic (lethargy and somnolence)
   c. Dose-limiting effects: none
6. Considerations
   a. Perform intradermal skin testing and desensitization as recommended
   b. Have emergency supportive care available in the event of an anaphylactoid response

B. Bleomycin Sulfate (Blenoxane)

1. Classification
   a. Pharmacological category: antitumor antibiotic

b. Drug specificity: cell cycle-nonspecific

c. Group: vesicant

2. Indications

a. Hodgkin's disease; non-Hodgkin's lymphoma; squamous cell carcinoma of the skin, vulva, head and neck, penis, esophagus, cervix and testes; mycosis fungoides

3. Dose

a. 0.25 to 0.5 U/kg weekly or twice a week

4. Method of administration

a. IV push, subcutaneous injection, IM, intrapleural, intraperitoneal

5. Complications

a. Common: fever, chills, stomatitis, nausea, vomiting, hyperpigmentation, alopecia, hypersensitivity reactions, erythema, rash, photosensitivity

b. System-specific: pulmonary (dry cough and dyspnea)

c. Dose-limiting effects: pulmonary fibrosis and pneumonitis

6. Considerations

a. Administer test dose as recommended

b. Prepare for possible anaphylactic reaction

c. Lifetime cumulative dose should not exceed 400 mg

C. Carboplatin (Paraplatin)

1. Classification

a. Pharmacological category: alkylating agent

b. Drug specificity: cell cycle-nonspecific

c. Group: nonvesicant

2. Indications

a. Ovarian cancer

3. Dose: used as a single agent or in combination with other agents; individualized, based upon tolerance of and response to agent and in accordance with published protocol

4. Method of administration

a. Continuous infusion

5. Complications

a. Common: anemia, mild nausea and vomiting, paresthesias

b. System-specific: none

c. Dose-limiting effects: bone marrow suppression

6. Considerations

a. Be alert for renal toxicity; increases when aminoglycosides are given concomitantly

b. Monitor patient's urine creatinine and hematologic studies, especially platelets

D. Carmustine (BiCNU)

1. Classification

a. Pharmacological category: nitrosourea

b. Drug specificity: cell cycle-nonspecific
c. Group: irritant
2. Indications
   a. Acute lymphocytic leukemia with central nervous system involvement; Hodgkin's disease; melanoma; myeloma; cancer of gastrointestinal tract
3. Dose: used as a single agent or in combination with other agents; individualized, based upon tolerance of and response to agent and in accordance with published protocol
4. Method of administration
   a. Continuous infusion
5. Complications
   a. Common: delayed bone marrow suppression, nausea, vomiting
   b. System-specific: pulmonary (dry cough and dyspnea)
   c. Dose-limiting effects: delayed leukopenia and thrombocytopenia
6. Considerations
   a. Monitor blood urea nitrogen (BUN), SGOT, SGPT, LDH, creatinine, CBC and platelet count, and notify physician if studies fall outside normal parameters
   b. Rapid intravenous infusion may cause eyes to burn and skin to flush

E. Cisplatin (Platinol)

1. Classification
   a. Pharmacological category: alkylating agent
   b. Drug specificity: cell cycle-nonspecific
   c. Group: nonvesicant
2. Indications
   a. Metastatic testicular tumors; neuroblastoma; cancer of the bladder, head, neck, ovary, and prostate
3. Dose: used as a single agent or in combination with other agents; individualized, based upon tolerance of and response to agent and in accordance with published protocol
4. Method of administration
   a. Continuous infusion
5. Complications
   a. Common: bone marrow suppression, severe nausea and vomiting, hyperuricemia
   b. System-specific: neurological (high-frequency hearing loss, tinnitus, tendon twitching, tetany, and positive Chvostek's sign); nephrotoxic (usually reversible)
   c. Dose-limiting effects: hematuria, frequent or burning urination
6. Considerations
   a. Ensure adequate hydration before and after administration of the medication to minimize impaired renal function
   b. Monitor BUN and creatinine closely; notify physician if studies fall outside normal parameters

   c. Obtain orders for premedication with antiemetics to reduce or
      eliminate nausea and vomiting

F. Cladribine (Leustatin)

   1. Classification
      a. Pharmacological category: antitumor antineoplastic
      b. Drug specificity: cell cycle-nonspecific
      c. Group: nonvesicant
   2. Indications
      a. Hairy cell leukemia
   3. Dose
      a. .09 mg/kg/day (4 mg/m²/day) as a single course
   4. Method of administration
      a. Continuous infusion
   5. Complications
      a. Common: bone marrow suppression, anemia, thrombocytopenia,
         fever, gastroenteritis
      b. System-specific: renal (with high doses)
      c. Dose-limiting effects: bone marrow suppression
   6. Considerations
      a. Monitor CBC, platelet count, uric acid level

G. Cyclophosphamide (Cytoxan)

   1. Classification
      a. Pharmacological category: alkylating agent
      b. Drug specificity: cell cycle-nonspecific
      c. Group: nonvesicant
   2. Indications
      a. Ewing's sarcoma; Burkitt's tumor; Hodgkin's disease; non-
         Hodgkin's lymphoma; mycosis fungoides; lymphocytic leukemia;
         chronic lymphocytic leukemia; myeloma; neuroblastoma; Wilms
         tumor; cancer of the breast, lung, and ovary
   3. Dose: used as a single agent or in combination with other agents;
      individualized, based upon tolerance of and response to agent and in
      accordance with published protocol
   4. Method of administration
      a. IV push, continuous infusion
   5. Complications
      a. Common: bone marrow suppression, nausea, vomiting, alopecia,
         sterility, dermatitis, hemorrhagic cystitis
      b. System-specific: pulmonary (dry cough and dyspnea), renal
         (frequent or burning urination, hematuria)
      c. Dose-limiting effects: bone marrow suppression
   6. Considerations
      a. Hydration essential to reduce potential for hemorrhagic cystitis
      b. Monitor renal status

H. Cytarabine (Cytosar-U)

1. Classification
   a. Pharmacological category: antimetabolite
   b. Drug specificity: cell cycle-specific
   c. Group: nonvesicant
2. Indications
   a. Acute myeloid leukemia, acute lymphocytic leukemia, chronic myeloid leukemia in blast crisis, Burkitt's tumor
3. Dose: used as a single agent or in combination with other agents; individualized, based upon tolerance of and response to agent and in accordance with published protocol
4. Method of administration
   a. IV push, intermittent, continuous infusion, intrathecal
5. Complications
   a. Common: nausea, vomiting, stomatitis, diarrhea, bone marrow suppression, fever, malaise, myalgia
   b. System-specific: none
   c. Dose-limiting effects: bone marrow suppression
6. Considerations
   a. Warn patients receiving radiation therapy during cytarabine administration that skin peeling may occur
   b. Monitor for common symptoms occurring 6 to 12 hours post-infusion
      1) Fever
      2) Myalgia
      3) Bone pain
      4) Malaise
      5) Maculopapular rash
      6) Conjunctivitis
   c. Monitor CBC

I. Dacarbazine (DTIC-Dome)

1. Classification
   a. Pharmacological category: alkylating agent
   b. Drug specificity: cell cycle-nonspecific
   c. Group: vesicant
2. Indications
   a. Melanoma; soft tissue sarcomas; Hodgkin's disease
3. Dose: used as a single agent or in combination with other agents; individualized, based upon tolerance of and response to agent and in accordance with published protocol
4. Method of administration
   a. IV push, continuous infusion
5. Complications
   a. Common: nausea, vomiting, bone marrow suppression, fever, malaise, myalgia

b. System-specific: none

c. Dose-limiting effects: bone marrow suppression

6. Considerations

a. Severe tissue damage may occur if medication extravasates

b. Instruct patients to avoid sun exposure or to use protection in sunlight while receiving this drug

c. Change in the color of the solution from ivory to pink indicates decomposition

d. Monitor CBC

J. Dactinomycin (Cosmegen)

1. Classification

a. Pharmacological category: antitumor antibiotic

b. Drug specificity: cell cycle-nonspecific

c. Group: vesicant

2. Indications

a. Wilms tumor; choriocarcinoma; testicular tumors; neuroblastoma; Ewing's sarcoma; soft tissue sarcomas; rhabdomyosarcoma; carcinoid tumor; melanoma

3. Dose: used as a single agent or in combination with other agents; individualized, based upon tolerance of and response to agent and in accordance with published protocol

4. Method of administration

a. IV push, continuous infusion, regional perfusion

5. Complications

a. Common: nausea, vomiting, fever, alopecia, bone marrow suppression, erythema, hyperpigmentation, acneiform skin manifestations, radiation recall

b. System-specific: none

c. Dose-limiting effects: mucositis, bone marrow suppression, concurrent radiation therapy

6. Considerations

a. Severe tissue damage may occur if the medication extravasates; administer suggested antidote, 10% sodium thiosulfate and ascorbic acid injection[6] as treatment

b. Monitor CBC

c. Instruct patient to report discomfort from oral irritation

K. Daunorubicin Hydrochloride (Cerubidine)

1. Classification

a. Pharmacological category: antitumor antibiotic

b. Drug specificity: cell cycle-nonspecific

c. Group: vesicant

2. Indications

a. Acute myelogenous monocytic or erythroid leukemia, solid tumors in children, non-Hodgkin's lymphoma

3. Dose
   a. Adult: 60 mg/m^2/day for 3 days, repeat in 3 to 4 weeks; reduced when used in combination chemotherapy in acute myelogenous leukemia for remission or induction
   b. Children: 25 mg/m^2 on day one of each week for acute lymphocytic leukemia in conjunction with vincristine sulfate and prednisone
   c. Consult published protocols for additional dosing regimens
4. Method of administration
   a. IV push
5. Complications
   a. Common: bone marrow suppression, nausea, vomiting, alopecia, radiation recall
   b. System-specific: cardiac (ECG changes and cardiomyopathy)
   c. Dose-limiting effects: bone marrow suppression and cardiotoxicity
6. Considerations
   a. Instruct patients to expect reddish-colored urine after receiving this medication
   b. Total cumulative dose should not exceed 600 mg/m^2
   c. Extravasation may result in severe tissue damage
   d. Monitor laboratory values

L. Doxorubicin Hydrochloride (Adriamycin)

1. Classification
   a. Pharmacological category: antitumor antibiotic
   b. Drug specificity: cell cycle-nonspecific
   c. Group: vesicant
2. Indications
   a. Acute myeloid leukemia; acute lymphocytic leukemia; Hodgkin's disease; non-Hodgkin's lymphoma; Wilms tumor; osteogenic sarcoma; soft tissue sarcoma; neuroblastoma; Ewing's sarcoma; cancer of the bladder, breast, lung, thyroid
3. Dose: used as a single agent or in combination with other agents; individualized, based upon tolerance of and response to agent and in accordance with published protocol
4. Method of administration
   a. IV push, continuous infusion
5. Complications
   a. Common: bone marrow suppression, alopecia, stomatitis, nausea, vomiting, fever, hyperpigmentation of nailbed
   b. System-specific: cardiac (flattening of T waves and ST depression noted on ECG)
   c. Dose-limiting effects: bone marrow suppression and cardiac toxicity
6. Considerations
   a. Instruct patients to expect reddish-colored urine after the first few voidings

b. Total cumulative lifetime dose should not exceed 550 mg/m^2

c. Extravasation may result in severe tissue damage

d. Assess patient for quality and rhythm of heart rate

M. Etoposide (VePesid)

1. Classification
   a. Pharmacological category: vinca alkaloid
   b. Drug specificity: cell cycle-specific
   c. Group: irritant
2. Indications
   a. Small cell carcinoma of the lung, Hodgkin's disease, carcinoma of the breast, refractory testicular tumors, non-Hodgkin's lymphoma
3. Dose: used as a single agent or in combination with other agents; individualized, based upon tolerance of and response to agent and in accordance with published protocol
4. Method of administration
   a. Continuous infusion
5. Complications
   a. Common: bone marrow suppression, nausea, vomiting, alopecia, stomatitis, diarrhea, orthostatic hypotension with rapid intravenous administration, paresthesias
   b. System-specific: none
   c. Dose-limiting effects: bone marrow suppression
6. Considerations
   a. Although anaphylaxis is rare, have emergency medications and oxygen readily available
   b. Monitor CBC

N. Fluorouracil (5-FU)

1. Classification
   a. Pharmacological category: antimetabolite
   b. Drug specificity: cell cycle-specific
   c. Group: nonvesicant
2. Indications
   a. Cancer of the breast, ovary, skin, gastrointestinal tract, and hepatoma
3. Dose: used as a single agent or in combination with other agents; individualized, based upon tolerance of and response to agent and in accordance with published protocol
4. Method of administration
   a. IV push, continuous infusion
5. Complications
   a. Common: nausea, vomiting, diarrhea, bone marrow suppression,

alopecia, glossitis, cerebellar ataxia, skin manifestations, teratogenic effects

    b. System-specific: none

    c. Dose-limiting effects: stomatitis, gastrointestinal ulcers, bone marrow suppression

  6. Considerations

    a. Instruct patient to avoid sun exposure and to use sun protection when in sunlight

    b. Instruct patient to report discomfort due to oral irritation

    c. Monitor CBC, electrolytes

O. Gemcitabine Hydrochloride (Gemzar)

  1. Classification

    a. Pharmacological category: antimetabolite

    b. Drug specificity: cell cycle-specific

    c. Group: nonvesicant

  2. Indications: locally advanced or metastatic adenocarcinoma of the pancreas

  3. Dose

    a. 800 to 1250 mg/m^2 weekly for three consecutive weeks

    b. Consult published protocols

  4. Method of administration: continuous infusion

  5. Complications

    a. Common: nausea, vomiting, fever, rash, water retention, flu-like symptoms, thrombocytopenia, bone marrow suppression

    b. System-specific: hematologic (bone marrow suppression)

    c. Dose-limiting effects: bone marrow suppression

  6. Considerations

    a. Monitor CBC and platelet count

P. Ifosfamide (Ifex)

  1. Classification

    a. Pharmacological category: alkylating agent

    b. Drug specificity: cell cycle-specific

    c. Group: nonvesicant

  2. Indications

    a. Testicular, ovary, and breast sarcoma; lymphoma

  3. Dose: individualized, based upon tolerance of and response to agent and in accordance with published protocol

  4. Method of administration

    a. Continuous infusion

  5. Complications

    a. Common: thrombocytopenia, nausea, vomiting, alopecia, fatigue, hemorrhagic cystitis

b. System-specific: hematuria, frequent or burning urination
c. Dose-limiting effects: bone marrow suppression and hemorrhagic cystitis
6. Considerations
  a. Ensure patient receives at least 2 liters of fluid, intravenously or orally, to prevent bladder toxicity
  b. Always give mesna (Mesnex) in conjunction with ifosfamide as a uroprotective agent

Q. Irinotecan Hydrochloride (Camptosar)

1. Classification
  a. Pharmacological category: miscellaneous
  b. Drug specificity: cell cycle-specific
  c. Group: vesicant
2. Indications
  a. Metastatic carcinoma of the colon and rectum whose disease has recurred or progressed following fluorouracil base therapy
3. Dose: individualized, based upon tolerance of and response to agent and in accordance with published protocol
4. Method of administration: continuous infusion
5. Complications
  a. Common: diarrhea, nausea, vomiting, malaise, alopecia, anemia, bone marrow suppression
  b. System-specific: hematologic (anemia and neutropenia); gastrointestinal (diarrhea)
  c. Dose-limiting effects: neutropenia, diarrhea
6. Considerations
  a. Obtain orders for an antiemetic to reduce or eliminate nausea and vomiting
  b. Monitor CBC
  c. Obtain orders for antidiarrheal medications as needed
  d. Severe tissue damage may occur if medication extravasates

R. Mechlorethamine Hydrochloride (Mustargen)

1. Classification
  a. Pharmacological category: alkylating agent
  b. Drug specificity: cell cycle-nonspecific
  c. Group: vesicant
2. Indications
  a. Hodgkin's disease; non-Hodgkin's lymphoma; cancer of the lung; mycosis fungoides; lymphosarcoma
3. Dose
  a. Intravenous: single dose: 0.4 mg/kg, may divide into two to four doses and give daily for 2 to 4 days; repeat 3 to 6 weeks
  b. Intracavitary: 0.2 to 0.4 mg/kg
  c. Consult published protocols for additional dosing regimens

4. Method of administration
   a. IV push, intracavitary
5. Complications
   a. Common: severe nausea and vomiting, bone marrow suppression, metallic taste in mouth, local cellulitis
   b. System-specific: none
   c. Dose-limiting effects: bone marrow suppression
6. Considerations
   a. Has a short period of stability
   b. Mix immediately before administration
   c. Severe tissue damage may occur if medication extravasates
   d. Medical personnel must take precautions to avoid skin or eye contact

S. Methotrexate Sodium (Mexate)

1. Classification
   a. Pharmacological category: antimetabolite
   b. Drug specificity: cell cycle-specific
   c. Group: nonvesicant
2. Indications
   a. Acute myeloid leukemia; acute lymphocytic leukemia; Burkitt's lymphoma; choriocarcinoma; solid tumors; cancer of the breast, cervix, head and neck, lung, testes; osteogenic sarcoma
3. Dose: used as single agent or in combination with other agents; individualized, based upon tolerance of and response to agent and in accordance with published protocol
4. Method of administration
   a. IV push, intrathecal
5. Complications
   a. Common: bone marrow suppression, nausea, vomiting, stomatitis (severe with high doses)
   b. System-specific: hepatic and renal (with high doses)
   c. Dose-limiting effects: oral and gastrointestinal ulcerations, bone marrow suppression, pulmonary infiltrates and fibrosis
6. Considerations
   a. Check CBC, SGOT, LDH, bilirubin, liver function studies, creatinine, and notify physician if results are abnormal
   b. With high-dose methotrexate sodium (Mexate), ensure adequate hydration before and after administration
   c. Within 24 hours following high-dose administration, give citrovorum factor (Leucovorin)

T. Mitomycin (Mutamycin)

1. Classification
   a. Pharmacological category: antitumor antibiotic
   b. Drug specificity: cell cycle-nonspecific
   c. Group: vesicant

2. Indications
  a. Cancer of the breast, cervix, head and neck, lung; melanoma; disseminated adenocarcinoma of the stomach and pancreas
3. Dose: used as a single agent or in combination with other agents; individualized, based upon tolerance of and response to agent and in accordance with published protocol
4. Method of administration
  a. IV push, continuous infusion
5. Complications
  a. Common: bone marrow suppression (particularly thrombocytopenia), vomiting, diarrhea, alopecia
  b. System-specific: pulmonary (dyspnea and nonproductive cough); renal (diminished urinary output)
  c. Dose-limiting effects: bone marrow suppression
6. Considerations
  a. Monitor BUN, urine output, and creatinine clearance
  b. Severe tissue damage may occur if medication extravasates
  c. Potential for nephrotoxicity increases when dose exceeds 50 mg/m^2

U. Paclitaxel (Taxol)

1. Classification
  a. Pharmacological category: miscellaneous
  b. Drug specificity: cell cycle-nonspecific
  c. Group: irritant
2. Indications
  a. Metastatic ovarian, breast, non-small cell lung cancer
3. Dose: used as a single agent or in combination with other agents; individualized, based upon tolerance of and response to agent and in accordance with published protocol
4. Method of administration
  a. Continuous infusion
5. Complications
  a. Common: nausea, vomiting, alopecia, anemia, bone marrow suppression
  b. System-specific: neurologic
  c. Dose-limiting effects: bone marrow suppression and peripheral neuropathy
6. Considerations
  a. Do not administer if patient has a history of hypersensitivity to cyclophosphamide
  b. Do not use polyvinylchloride infusion bags or administration sets
  c. Use a 0.22 micron filter
  d. Premedicate to reduce incidence of hypersensitivity reactions

V. Plicamycin (Mithracin)

1. Classification
  a. Pharmacological category: antitumor antibiotic

     b. Drug specificity: cell cycle-nonspecific
     c. Group: vesicant
  2. Indications
     a. Carcinoma of the testes and hypercalcemia in malignant disease
  3. Dose
     a. Testicular cancer: 25–30 µg/kg/day for 8 to 10 days
     b. Hypercalcemia: 25 µg/kg/day for 3 to 4 days; repeat every week as needed
     c. Consult published protocol
  4. Method of administration
     a. Continuous infusion
  5. Complications
     a. Common: fever, vomiting, diarrhea, bone marrow suppression, (specifically thrombocytopenia), anorexia
     b. System-specific: none
     c. Dose-limiting effects: bone marrow suppression
  6. Considerations
     a. Assess for hypocalcemia: muscle cramps, weakness and/or tingling in extremities
     b. Monitor CBC, electrolytes, prothrombin time, liver and renal function

W. Streptozocin (Zanosar)

  1. Classification
     a. Pharmacological category: nitrosourea
     b. Drug specificity: cell cycle-nonspecific
     c. Group: irritant
  2. Indications
     a. Metastatic islet cell carcinoma of the pancreas
  3. Dose: individualized, based upon tolerance of and response to agent and in accordance with published protocol
  4. Method of administration
     a. IV push, continuous infusion
  5. Complications
     a. Common: bone marrow suppression, nausea, vomiting, diarrhea
     b. System-specific: renal
     c. Dose-limiting effects: nephrotoxicity
  6. Considerations
     a. Monitor BUN, creatinine, SGOT, LDH, and CBC closely, and notify physician if results are abnormal
     b. Pretreat with antiemetics to reduce incidence of nausea and vomiting
     c. Ensure adequate hydration

X. Thiotepa (Thioplex)

  1. Classification
     a. Pharmacological category: alkylating agent

         b. Drug specificity: cell cycle-nonspecific

         c. Group: nonvesicant

     2. Indications

         a. Cancer of the breast, ovary, bladder

     3. Dose: individualized, based upon tolerance of and response to agent and in accordance with published protocol

     4. Method of administration

         a. IV push, continuous infusion

     5. Complications

         a. Common: bone marrow suppression, mild nausea and vomiting, hyperkeratosis, pigmentation

         b. System-specific: none

         c. Dose-limiting effects: bone marrow suppression

     6. Considerations

         a. Monitor CBC

Y. Vinblastine Sulfate (Velban)

     1. Classification

         a. Pharmacological category: vinca alkaloid

         b. Drug specificity: cell cycle-specific

         c. Group: vesicant

     2. Indications

         a. Hodgkin's disease; lymphocytic and histiocytic leukemias; Kaposi's sarcoma; mycosis fungoides; cancer of the breast and testes (teratocarcinoma); choriocarcinoma (resistant to the other therapies)

     3. Dose: used as a single agent or in combination with other agents; individualized, based upon tolerance of and response to agent and in accordance with published protocol

     4. Method of administration

         a. IV push

     5. Complications

         a. Common: bone marrow suppression, constipation, alopecia, jaw pain, paresthesia

         b. System-specific: neurologic

         c. Dose-limiting effects: bone marrow suppression, numbness and/or tingling fingers and/or toes, loss of deep tendon reflexes

     6. Considerations

         a. Severe tissue damage may occur if medication extravasates

         b. Assess neurological status prior to administration

Z. Vincristine Sulfate (Oncovin)

     1. Classification

         a. Pharmacological category: vinca alkaloid

         b. Drug specificity: cell cycle-specific

         c. Group: vesicant

2. Indications
   a. Acute lymphocytic and myeloid leukemia; chronic myeloid leukemia in blasts crisis; Ewing's sarcoma; Hodgkin's disease; non-Hodgkin's lymphoma; rhabdomyosarcoma; melanoma; soft tissue sarcoma; Wilms tumor; cancer of the brain, breast, cervix, ovary, testes
3. Dose: used as a single agent or in combination with other agents; individualized, based upon tolerance of and response to agent and in accordance with published protocol
4. Method of administration
   a. IV push
5. Complications
   a. Common: alopecia, constipation, nausea, and vomiting
   b. System-specific: neurologic
   c. Dose-limiting effects: peripheral neuropathy, numbness and/or tingling fingers and/or toes, loss of deep tendon reflexes
6. Considerations
   a. Severe tissue damage may occur if medication extravasates
   b. Assess neurological status prior to administration
   c. Monitor bowel function

VI. BIOLOGICAL RESPONSE MODIFIERS

A. Overview

1. Biotherapy is a form of treatment that uses the body's immune response
2. This method will change the way the body's immune response functions and the direct action on the tumor and cancer cell cycle
3. Because this treatment modality is new, many of the biological response modifiers are still in clinical studies[10,11]

B. Filgrastim (G-CSF)

1. Classification
   a. Pharmacological category: cytokine
   b. Action: stimulates proliferation of neutrophils in the bone marrow
2. Indications
   a. Decreases incidence of infection in neutropenic patients
3. Dose
   a. 5 μg/kg/day
4. Method of administration
   a. IV push over 1 minute, continuous infusion
5. Complications
   a. Rash, flu-like symptoms, redness, swelling at injection site, hypersensitivity reaction, transient bone pain
6. Considerations
   a. Monitor CBC and determine absolute neutrophil count
   b. Use only 5% dextrose in water for dilution

C. Interferon Alpha

1. Classification
   a. Pharmacological category: cytokine
   b. Action: to reduce the proliferation of malignant cells and inhibit tumor growth
2. Indications
   a. Hairy cell leukemia
3. Dose: consult published protocols
4. Method of administration
   a. Intermittent, continuous infusion
5. Complications
   a. Flu-like symptoms, chills, and nausea
6. Considerations
   a. Monitor fluid intake

D. Sargramostim (GM-CMF)

1. Classification
   a. Pharmacological category: cytokine
   b. Action: stimulates hematopoietic system to increase monocytes and macrophages
2. Indications
   a. To increase bone marrow recovery, especially after a bone marrow transplant
3. Dose: consult published protocols
4. Method of administration
   a. Continuous infusion over 2 hours
5. Complications
   a. Diarrhea, malaise, rash, peripheral edema, bone pain, hypersensitivity reaction, including anaphylaxis, headache, dyspnea, supraventricular arrhythmias
6. Considerations
   a. Monitor WBC[11]

VII. INVESTIGATIONAL AGENTS AND PROTOCOLS

A. Overview

1. Clinical investigation of new antineoplastic agents is accomplished in three phases
2. The agent becomes commercially available after successful completion of phase III[9]

B. Phase I

1. Purpose: to define dose-limiting toxicities and determine the maximum tolerated dose
2. Analysis: descriptive, no comparison

3. Nursing intervention: observe and record toxicities according to severity scale[10]

C. Phase II

1. Purpose: to further define toxicities and determine the antitumor activity at specific doses and schedules
2. Analysis: the ability of the agent to decrease the size or slow the growth rate of the cancer
3. Nursing intervention: observe and record the response to treatment in addition to monitoring toxicities[9]

D. Phase III

1. Purpose: to determine usefulness in comparison with other drug regimens
2. Analysis: documentation of response criteria
3. Nursing intervention: to collect accurate and complete data[9]

E. Protocols (describe the clinical investigation)

1. Background information about the study
2. Objectives
3. Patient selection criteria
4. Diagram schema (schematics)
5. Toxicity information
6. Required laboratory and diagnostic procedures
7. Evaluation parameters
8. Consent form
9. References
10. Resource person and contact information

F. Institutional Review Boards (IRBs)

1. All investigational agents, studies, and protocols must be approved by an IRB
2. The objective of the IRB is to protect participants and to determine the validity of a study
3. Membership and actions of the IRB are determined and monitored by federal regulations[10]

G. Consent Forms

1. Any patient participating in a protocol or receiving an investigational agent must sign a consent form[2,9]

H. Policies and Procedures

1. Institutional policies and procedures must be followed
2. National standards are references for the development of procedures

VIII. PREADMINISTRATION CONSIDERATIONS

A. Patient Assessment, Patient History, and Relevant Information Regarding the Diagnosis

1. Diagnosis and whether the disease is local or disseminated
2. Food and drug allergies
3. Current medications
4. Prior chemotherapy, including resultant toxicities and side effects
5. Prior radiation therapy
6. History of cardiac, liver, or pulmonary disease

B. Systems Clinical Assessment (done prior to, during, and after prescribed treatment)

1. Emphasis placed on system most affected by the specific medication
2. Cardiovascular
   a. Baseline parameters; ECG, MUGA scan as indicated
   b. Blood pressure
   c. Pulse
3. Gastrointestinal
   a. Constipation
   b. Diarrhea
   c. Esophagitis
   d. Jaundice
   e. Nausea
   f. Stomatitis
   g. Taste alterations
   h. Vomiting
   i. Weight loss
4. Genitourinary
   a. Renal function
   b. Urine color, amount, and frequency
5. Integumentary
   a. Alopecia
   b. Cellulitis
   c. Desquamation
   d. Erythema
   e. Facial flushing
   f. Hyperpigmentation
   g. Nail ridges
   h. Pain
   i. Phlebitis
   j. Pruritus
   k. Radiosensitization
6. Neurologic
   a. Alterations in sensorium

     b. Ataxia

     c. Paresthesia

     d. Hearing loss

  7. Pulmonary

     a. Baseline parameters; pulmonary function studies as indicated

     b. Breath sounds

     c. Edema

     d. Respirations

  8. Hepatic

     a. Baseline parameters; liver function studies as indicated

     b. Jaundice

     c. Ascites

C. Evaluation of Current Laboratory Values and Diagnostic Tests Significant to the Treatment Plan

  1. Complete blood count with platelet count and differential

  2. BUN and creatinine

  3. Liver function studies

  4. ECG or MUGA scan

  5. Pulmonary function study

D. Calculations

  1. Body surface area (BSA)

     a. Patient's weight and height are used as a basis

     b. Nomogram chart is used by drawing a line from the patient's weight to height (Fig. 7-2(A))

     c. Note that there are different nomogram charts (Fig. 7-2(B)) for children and adults[1,2]

  2. Treatment dose

     a. Determined using BSA

     b. Formula: $BSA \times mg/m^2 =$ treatment dose

  3. Lifetime cumulative dose

     a. Formula: $BSA \times$ recommended limit $=$ lifetime dose

  4. Absolute granulocyte count (AGC)

     a. Basis for knowing a patient's risk for infection

     b. Granulocytopenia usually has an AGC of less than 2,000 cells/mm^3

     c. Normal granulocyte count ranges from 3,000 to 7,000 cells/mm^3

     d. Formula: $WBC \times \%$ of granulocytes $= AGC$

       1) AGC less than 1500 considered guarded

       2) AGC less that 1000 considered severe[1,2,9]

     e. Treatment may be held when AGC low

E. Compounding

  1. Limit to qualified personnel

HEIGHT   BODY SURFACE AREA   WEIGHT

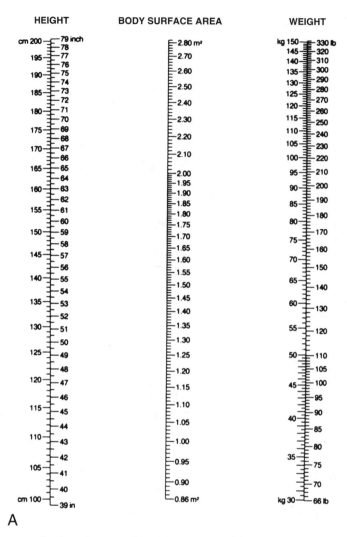

A

FIGURE 7-2(A) Nomogram of body surface area for adults. *Directions:* (1) Find height. (2) Find weight. (3) Draw a straight line connecting the height and weight. (4) Where the line intersects on the BSA column is the body surface area (m²). (Reprinted with permission from Kee/Hayes: *Pharmacology: A Nursing Process,* 2E. W.B. Saunders (1997) pg 59-fig. 4B-2.)

2. Provide protection for personnel
   a. Barrier gowns with closed front and fitted cuffs
   b. Disposable, powder-free latex gloves
   c. Goggles
3. Specific equipment
   a. Class II biological vertical laminar airflow safety cabinet
   b. Syringes with Luer-Lok connections
   c. Vented vials[8]

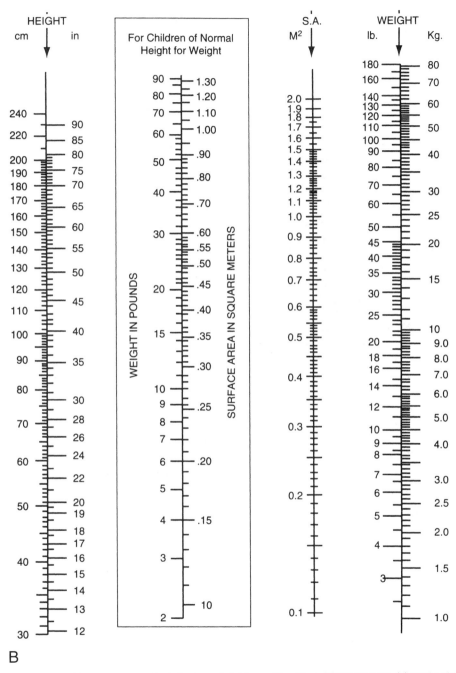

FIGURE 7-2(B) West nomogram for infants and children. Di*rections:* (1) Find height. (2) Find weight. (3) Draw a straight line connecting the height and weight. (4) Where the line intersects on the SA column is the body surface area (m²). (Reprinted with permission from Kee/Hayes: *Pharmacology: A Nursing Process,* 2E. W.B. Saunders (1997) pg 58-fig. 4B-2.)

IX. PATIENT INFORMATION

A. Treatment Goal

1. Cure: disease-free
2. Control: increased survival and/or prevention of metastatic disease
   a. Complete remission (CR): no apparent evidence of disease
   b. Partial remission (PR): reduced tumor mass by greater than 50% that lasts longer than 1 month
3. Palliation: reduced severity and/or alleviation of symptoms without cure[1,2,9]

B. Medications

1. Drug name
2. Route
3. Action
4. Side effects
   a. Related complications and toxicities
   b. Methods to minimize or prevent occurrence
5. Special instructions while receiving the medication
   a. Infection and bleeding precautions
   b. Mouth care
   c. Avoid exposure to sun
   d. Avoid aspirin and aspirin-containing products
   e. Adequate fluid intake
   f. Rest
   g. Good nutrition
6. Chemotherapy regimens
   a. Single-agent chemotherapy: one medication used to combat the disease process
   b. Combination chemotherapy: more than one agent used to increase response actions, provides multiple modes of actions with synergistic activity, and may circumvent drug resistance[1,2,3,9]
7. Plan and schedule of treatment
   a. Approximate number of cycles, number of days of treatment, and the number of weeks between treatments
   b. Adjuvant treatment: from 3 months to 1 year
   c. Active disease: from 6 months to 1 year after remission
   d. Possibility of treatment delay because of toxicities
8. Monitoring
   a. Routine laboratory tests before treatments
   b. Laboratory tests, radiological studies, and other tests required to determine response to treatment or to restage disease
9. Patient rights: treatment refusal

C. Side Effects

1. Immediate
   a. Allergic

   b. Extravasation
   c. Gastrointestinal
   d. Phlebitis
   e. Psychosocial
2. Delayed
   a. Alopecia
   b. Bone marrow suppression
   c. Genetic
   d. Oncogenetic
   e. Psychosocial
   f. Reproductive
3. Potential risks
   a. Kidney toxicity
   b. Liver toxicity
   c. Lung toxicity
   d. Heart toxicity

X. ADMINISTRATION

A. Vein Selection

1. Avoid areas of impaired circulation
2. Avoid veins distal to previous venipunctures
3. Avoid joints and hands
   a. Use of the antecubital fossa is controversial
   b. Use is based on institutional policies or recognized standards of practice
4. Avoid side of mastectomy
5. Avoid areas of bruising, inflammation, or phlebitis
6. Alternate arms if possible[8,11]

B. Venipuncture

1. Individual with expertise in venipuncture to initiate and administer the chemotherapy
2. Helps alleviate patient anxiety and preserve venous access[4,5,8]

C. Alternative Vascular Access

1. Peripheral
   a. Used for administration of nonvesicant medications
   b. May be used for IV push administration of vesicant medications
2. Short-term catheters
   a. Short-term therapy, usually 30 to 60 days
   b. Subclavian or jugular catheter: catheter tip is located in the superior vena cava (SVC)
   c. Peripherally inserted central catheter (PICC): catheter placed via the basilic or cephalic vein at the antecubital fossa with the tip located in the SVC[8,11]

3. Long-term catheters
   a. Used when extended therapy is expected
   b. Designed to provide protection against infection and to promote catheter security
   c. Tunneled catheter: percutaneously placed with tip in SVC
      1) Subcutaneous tunnel is made and catheter exits on lower chest wall
      2) Dacron cuff aids in prevention of infection and helps to secure catheter in the tunnel
      3) Available as a single, double, or triple lumen
      4) Patients with limited venous access, anticipated long-term treatment, and receiving vesicants or irritating chemotherapy benefit from this catheter[1,8]
   d. Implanted catheter: percutaneously placed with tip in SVC
      1) Has an attached reservoir, which has a resealing septum
      2) A pocket is made in subcutaneous tissue to house reservoir and is sutured closed
      3) The septum is accessed through the skin with a noncoring needle
      4) Single and double lumen systems are available
      5) Patients with limited venous access, anticipated long-term treatment, and unable to care for external catheters are good candidates for this type of catheter[1,8]
      6) Due to potential dislodgement of the needle accessing the reservoir, these devices should be used with caution in the administration of vesicants

D. Methods

1. IV push
   a. Direct: administering medication by manual pressure
   b. Side-arm free-flow: administering medication by manual pressure through the port of an administration set
2. Intermittent: administering medication at prescribed intervals
3. Continuous: administering medication over a prescribed period of time
4. Other
   a. Antineoplastic agents are most often considered either oral or intravenous medications
   b. Other methods have been employed to achieve higher concentrations of the medication at the tumor site
      1) Intra-arterial
         • Administered via intra-arterial catheter or implanted pump with a catheter into hepatic artery
         • Used commonly to treat metastatic liver disease
      2) Intrathecal (intraventricular)
         • Administered by way of cerebrospinal fluid reservoir or lumbar puncture by the physician

- Surgically implanted cerebrospinal fluid reservoirs with catheter placed into ventricle; accessed through the scalp
- Limited lumbar puncture procedures if reservoir used

E. Specific Considerations for Administration

1. Physician orders
   a. Verify medication dose, route, and patient identification
   b. Double check orders and medication with another registered nurse
2. Recommendations when administering antineoplastic agents
   a. Employ safe and protective techniques to minimize potential risk
   b. Follow the Occupational Safety and Health Administration (OSHA) guidelines for handling antineoplastics
      1) Wear disposable, powder-free surgical latex gloves
      2) Change gloves at regular intervals and when integrity is compromised
      3) Wear closed-front gowns with long sleeves and fitted cuffs; fabric of low permeability material
3. Maintain sterile technique
4. Assure patency of intravenous site
   a. Administer 0.9% sodium chloride before antineoplastic given and observe for signs of infiltration
   b. Instruct patient to report any burning or pain during infusion
   c. Assess patency by periodic check of blood return[8,11]

F. Termination

1. Assess intravenous site
2. Remove catheter
3. Apply sterile dressing over venipuncture site
4. Assess patient
   a. Assure that patient or significant other can identify potential problems
   b. Instruct to contact nurse or physician should problems occur
5. Document during administration and on completion of the chemotherapy administration
   a. Intravenous site
   b. Catheter size and type
   c. 0.9% sodium chloride flush before, between, and/or post-administration
   d. Appearance of intravenous site after treatment
   e. Any adverse reaction or symptom during or after treatment
   f. Patient's response during and after treatment
   g. Premedications given to alleviate reactions

XI. COMPLICATIONS

A. Leukopenia (hematologic)

1. Decreased WBC predisposing patient to risk of infection

2. Interventions
   a. Assess patient for fever, chills, sore throat, cough, dyspnea, frequency and/or urgency with voiding, edema, or purulent drainage of skin
   b. Monitor WBC and AGC
   c. Notify physician of WBC less than 3000/mm^3 or AGC less than 2500/mm^3
   d. Obtain cultures and administer antibiotics as ordered

B. Thrombocytopenia (hematologic)

1. Decreased platelet count
2. Interventions
   a. Assess patient for bleeding in gums and nose, presence of blood in urine, stools, and easy bruising of skin
   b. Monitor platelet count and notify physician if less than 50,000/mm^3
   c. Instruct patient on bleeding precautions, including use of electric razors and soft toothbrush, avoiding nose blowing
   d. Caution against activities that may cause abrasions, cuts, or trauma
   e. Apply pressure to sites of bleeding and notify physician if bleeding persists

C. Anemia (hematologic)

1. Reduced number of red blood cells with a decrease in the blood's oxygen-carrying capacity
2. Interventions
   a. Assess patient for fatigue, dyspnea, pallor, tinnitus, tachycardia, and fainting
   b. Monitor hemoglobin and hematocrit and notify physician of abnormal results
   c. Administer red blood cells and/or oxygen as ordered
   d. Instruct patient on need for rest

D. Nausea and Vomiting (gastrointestinal)

1. Increased risk of dehydration and compromised nutritional status
2. Interventions
   a. Monitor oral intake
   b. Provide adequate antiemetic therapy and information on nutrition and nutritional supplements
   c. Administer antiemetics
      1) Dexamethasone sodium (Decadron)
         • Administer 20 mg single-dose over 1 minute IV push, before chemotherapy
         • Give in combination with other medications

  2) Lorazepam (Ativan)
- Administer 1.5 mg/m^2 by intravenous push or through the tubing of an intravenous line over 1 minute
- Dilute with equal volume of sterile water, 5% dextrose, or 0.9% sodium chloride
- Give in combination with other medications

  3) Metoclopramide hydrochloride (Reglan)
- Administer 2 mg/kg intravenously over 2 minutes or by infusion over at least 15 minutes before chemotherapy
- Give in combination with other medications

  4) Ondansetron hydrochloride (Zofran)
- Administer a single dose of 0.15 mg/kg doses by intravenous infusion 30 minutes before chemotherapy[4]
- Subsequent doses of 0.15 mg/kg may be administered 4 and 8 hours after the first dose

  5) Granisetron hydrochloride (Kytril)
- Administer 10 mg/kg intravenously over 5 minutes, 30 minutes before chemotherapy
- Dilute with 0.9% sodium chloride or 5% dextrose to a total volume of 25 to 50 ml
- May be administered by intravenous push, undiluted, over 30 seconds

E. Anorexia (gastrointestinal)

1. Increased risk of compromised nutritional status
2. Interventions
   a. Monitor patient's weight
   b. Monitor laboratory values (serum albumin, nitrogen balance, glucose, transferrin, electrolytes)
   c. Instruct patient to eat foods high in protein and calories, use nutritional supplements, and try eating smaller but more frequent meals
   d. Teach good oral care and methods to stimulate taste buds and appetite

F. Constipation (gastrointestinal)

1. Decreased bowel elimination
2. Interventions
   a. Assess patient for dry skin and mucous membranes and for poor skin turgor and bowel sounds
   b. Instruct patient on eating high-fiber foods and those with high bulk, and use of laxatives, stool softeners, or enemas as indicated

G. Diarrhea (gastrointestinal)

1. Increased risk of fluid and electrolyte disturbance and dehydration

2. Interventions
   a. Assess the frequency and character of stools
   b. Monitor patient's weight
   c. Monitor serum electrolytes
   d. Notify physician and administer antidiarrheal agents as ordered
   e. Instruct patient on low residue, high-protein diet; to eat small meals with high fluid intake at frequent intervals
   f. Advise avoiding caffeine and tobacco

H. Alopecia (integumentary)

1. Increased risk of depression from poor self-image
2. Interventions
   a. Instruct patient on the use of wigs or turbans
   b. Provide psychological reassurance and encourage expression of feelings
   c. For mild to moderate hair loss, instruct on the use of mild shampoo, gentle brushing, and avoiding hair dryers, curling irons, and curlers

I. Stomatitis (integumentary)

1. Increased risk of compromised nutritional status, sepsis, and pain
2. Interventions
   a. Assess oral mucosa for bleeding, erythema, ulceration, and white or yellow film
   b. Instruct patient on good oral care with saline mouth rinse, after-meals teeth cleaning with soft toothbrush or soft swab
   c. Avoid commercial mouthwashes, elective dental work, alcohol, and tobacco
   d. Encourage soft, bland, and even-temperature foods and fluids
   e. Notify physician and instruct patient on the use of topical anesthetics and swish-and-swallow medications
   f. For severe stomatitis, provide adequate analgesics for pain

J. Hyperuricemia (renal)

1. Increased risk of impaired renal function
2. Interventions
   a. Assess intake and output, skin turgor, pain, frequency or urgency on urination
   b. Monitor BUN, serum creatinine, creatinine clearance, urinalysis, and electrolytes
   c. Notify physician if patient is unable to maintain adequate fluid intake, and arrange for the administration of hydration fluids and diuretics as ordered

K. Cardiotoxicities (cardiac)

1. Risk of myocardial damage, decreased cardiac output, and tissue perfusion leading to congestive heart failure, cardiac arrhythmias, or cardiomyopathy
2. Interventions
   a. Assess patient for ankle edema, cough, cyanosis, dyspnea, decreased peripheral pulses, jugular vein distention, rales, tachycardia
   b. Monitor ECG, cardiac enzymes and electrolytes, vital signs with apical pulse
   c. Notify physician of irregularities and administer medication as ordered

L. Neurotoxicity (neurologic)

1. May be central or peripheral
2. Interventions
   a. Assess patient for paresthesias, deep tendon reflexes, jaw pain, bowel sounds, numbness in extremities, inability to walk on heels, confusion, or slurred speech
   b. Instruct patient to take adequate fluids and use stool softeners
   c. Contact physical therapy, if needed, to assist with mobility, exercise, and physical aids

M. Ototoxicity (neurologic)

1. Risk of decreased or lost hearing
2. Interventions
   a. Assess patient for changes in hearing, sense of coordination, and tinnitus
   b. Hearing loss is more commonly seen in the pediatric patient
   c. Implement strategies to provide communication in the event of any hearing loss

N. Nephrotoxicity (renal)

1. Risk of impaired renal function
2. Interventions
   a. Adequate hydration by pre- and post-intravenous fluids, encourage oral fluid intake
   b. Assess for any difficulty, frequency, or urgency with voiding
   c. Monitor BUN, serum creatinine, creatinine clearance, urinalysis, and uric acid
   d. Notify physician of any abnormal results
   e. Encourage patient to empty bladder every 4 hours, especially at night
   f. Monitor urine pH if on high dose of methotrexate sodium

O. Hepatic (liver)

1. Risk of liver damage
2. Interventions
   a. Assess patient for previous or current radiation therapy, active hepatitis, or current medications (especially those that may be hepatotoxic)
   b. Monitor SGOT, SGPT, LDH, bilirubin, and liver function studies
   c. Notify physician of any abnormalities

P. Pulmonary (lungs)

1. Risk of decreased pulmonary function
2. Interventions
   a. Assess breath sounds; observe for dry, hacking cough and signs of dyspnea
   b. Notify physician of abnormal findings and administer oxygen, as ordered

REFERENCES

1. Tennenbaum L. *Cancer Chemotherapy and Biotherapy: A Reference Guide.* Philadelphia, PA: Saunders, 1994:3–262.
2. Gahart BL. *Intravenous Medications,* 15th ed. St. Louis, MO: Mosby, 1997.
3. Skeel RT, Lachant NA. *Handbook of Cancer Chemotherapy,* 5th ed. Boston, MA: Little, Brown & Company, 1999:573.
4. Phillips LD, Kuhn MA. *Manual of IV Medications,* 2nd ed. Philadelphia, PA: Lippincott-Raven, 1998.
5. Intravenous Nurses Society. Intravenous Nursing Standards of Practice (revised 1998). *Journal of Intravenous Nursing* 1998;21(1):suppl.
6. Coleman C. Overview of biotherapy and nursing considerations. *Journal of Intravenous Nursing* 1998;6(21):367–373.
7. San Angel F. Current controversies in chemotherapy administration. *Journal of Intravenous Nursing* 1995;1(18):16–23.
8. Weinstein SM. *Plumer's Principles and Practices of Intravenous Therapy,* 6th ed. Philadelphia, PA: Lippincott-Raven, 1997.
9. Fischer DS, Knobf MT. *The Cancer Chemotherapy Handbook,* 5th ed. 1997.
10. Terry J. *Clinical Intravenous Therapy: Clinical Principles and Practice.* Philadelphia, PA: Saunders, 1995.
11. Ott S, Larocco T. *Mosby's Pocket Guide: Intravenous Therapy,* 3rd ed. St. Louis, MO: Mosby, 1997.

CHAPTER 8

Parenteral Nutrition

Leslie Baranowski, CRNI, BSN

I. OVERVIEW

A. Definition

1. The provision of partial or total nutrient requirements through the venous system

B. Goals[1,3]

1. To provide all essential nutrients in adequate amounts to sustain nutritional balance during periods when oral or enteral routes of feedings are not possible or are insufficient to meet the patient's caloric needs
2. To preserve or restore the body's protein metabolism and prevent the development of protein and/or caloric malnutrition
3. To diminish the rate of weight loss, maintain or increase body weight
4. To promote wound healing
5. To replace nutritional deficits

C. Types

1. Peripheral parenteral nutrition (PPN)
    a. A partial nutritional solution that involves the infusion of low osmolarity dextrose, amino acids, fat, electrolytes, vitamins, and trace elements using the peripheral intravenous route
    b. This form of nutritional therapy only meets partial nutritional requirements and is therefore used for short-term or supplemental nutritional support
2. Total parenteral nutrition (TPN)
    a. The infusion of high concentrations of dextrose, amino acid, fat, electrolytes, vitamins, and trace elements via a central vein
    b. This form of nutritional therapy provides sufficient nutrients to satisfy total nutritional requirements

D. Considerations (evaluation for parenteral nutrition is based on multiple objective parameters)

1. Patients who are candidates for parenteral nutrition support cannot, should not, or will not eat adequately to maintain their nutrient

331

stores; these patients are already or have the potential of becoming malnourished[5]

2. Any patient unable to ingest sufficient nutrients via the gastrointestinal (GI) tract is a potential candidate for parenteral nutrition

3. The least invasive, least expensive means of supporting a patient's nutritional status must be considered

4. The GI route should always be used if appropriate
   a. Serious adverse effects can be associated with a totally resting GI tract
   b. Enteral nutrition preserves intestinal mass and structures, as well as hormonal, enzymatic, and immunological function better than does intravenous nutrition

5. Nutritional risk or deficit must be defined when evaluating a patient for parenteral nutrition

6. Generally, nourished patients unable to eat for as long as 7 to 10 days do not require parenteral nutrition; however, the general rule is that parenteral nutrition should be considered whenever 5 to 7 days pass with insufficient enteral intake[2]

7. The indications and disease states for which parenteral nutrition is clearly beneficial are continually being established and reassessed

II. INDICATIONS

A. TPN Versus PPN

1. The decision to use PPN versus TPN is determined by the extent of nutritional depletion, duration of illness, and clinical course before initiation of parenteral nutrition

B. PPN

1. Indications[4,8]
   a. Used to provide partial or total nutritional support for up to 2 weeks in patients who cannot ingest or absorb oral or enteral tube-delivered nutrients, or when central vein parenteral nutrition is not feasible
   b. Patients with mild to moderate deficits in adipose and protein stores
   c. Patients who cannot be fed by the oral or enteral route, requiring nutritional support by the parenteral route for anticipated therapy of 7 to 10 days
   d. Supplemental nutritional support to oral or enteral nutrition or as a transition to enteral nutrition
   e. A transitional support until TPN can be initiated or resumed
   f. Patients in whom central venous access is either impossible or contraindicated

2. Specific pediatric indications[5,9,10]
   a. Indications are similar to those for the adult
      1) PPN is suggested for nonstressed infants for brief courses of maintenance therapy when full growth and development are not the primary goal
      2) TPN is a more logical choice for supporting normal growth and maintaining body composition
   b. Generally used for nutrition support for a short time (up to 2 weeks) because of limited access to peripheral veins
      1) In older infants, children, and adults, nutrition repletion or aggressive nutrition support may be possible by this route, except in patients requiring fluid restriction
3. Contraindications
   a. Long-term support is needed
   b. Poor or inaccessible peripheral venous access
   c. Severe malnourished state
   d. Large volumes of fluid cannot be tolerated
   e. Nutrient needs are greater than what can be safely met with PPN
   f. Functional GI tract

C. TPN

1. Indications[5,8]
   a. Necessary when parenteral feeding is indicated for longer than 2 weeks, peripheral venous access is limited, nutrient needs are large, or fluid restriction is required and the benefits of TPN support outweigh the risks
   b. Used for patients requiring intravenous nutrition as primary or supportive therapy
      1) TPN frequently indicated for patients with disease states that result in impaired ability to ingest nutrients by the oral route in quantities sufficient to satisfy nutritional requirements and when unable to absorb enough nutrients from GI tract
   c. Disease states in which the use of TPN may be indicated as a primary therapy[11]
      1) Short gut syndrome
      2) Enterocutaneous fistula
      3) Renal failure caused by acute tubular necrosis
      4) Hepatic failure (acute decompensation in the face of cirrhosis)
      5) Burns
   d. There are other disease states in which TPN may be indicated as supportive therapy or conditions in which the efficacy of parenteral nutrition has not been clearly demonstrated (e.g., inflammatory bowel disease, anorexia nervosa)
   e. The use of TPN for cancer support, sepsis, trauma, and general perioperative support may be appropriate in selected situations
2. Specific pediatric indications[3,9,10]

    a. Disease states that affect the pediatric populations as outlined for adult

    b. Extremely premature infant

    c. Disorders of the respiratory system

    d. Disorders of the GI tract

        1) Congenital anomalies

        2) Surgical conditions

        3) Intractable diarrhea of infancy

        4) Inflammatory conditions

        5) Neuromuscular disorders

    e. Hypercatabolic states

3. Contraindications

    a. Functional GI tract

    b. Sole dependence on TPN is clearly less than 5 days

    c. Inability to obtain central venous access

    d. Prognosis does not warrant aggressive nutritional support

    e. Patient or legal guardian refuses TPN

    f. Risks of TPN outweigh its benefits

    g. Minimal stress and trauma or immediate postoperative or poststress period in a well-nourished patient when it is anticipated that convalescence will be short and the GI tract can be used within 7 to 10 days

    h. Malnutrition caused by a rapidly progressive disease not amenable to curative or palliative therapy; disease is proven or suspected of being untreatable

    i. *Candida* septicemia (with hypertonic dextrose regimen)

III. NUTRIENT BALANCE AND MALNUTRITION

A. Nutrient Balance

1. Nutrients

    a. Constituents in food that supply the body with its necessary elements; certain nutrients (carbohydrates, fats, proteins, and alcohol) provide energy and other nutrients (water, electrolytes, minerals, and vitamins) are essential to the metabolic process

2. Nutritional status[11,12]

    a. The condition of the body resulting from the utilization of the essential nutrients available to the body

    b. Nutritional status depends on the quality and quantity of nutrients consumed, on the relative need for nutrients, and on the ability of the body to utilize nutrients

3. Nutritional deficiency

    a. Occurs when adequate amounts of essential nutrients required for proper functioning are not provided to the body tissues; may be primary or secondary[12]

   b. Primary deficiency occurs when the diet is deficient in a particular nutrient or nutrients
   c. Secondary deficiency results from impairment in normal digestion, absorption, and utilization of essential nutrients resulting in nutrient deficiency and may occur despite adequate ingestion, or metabolic stress

B. Malnutrition

   1. Classification
      a. Patients should be considered malnourished or at risk of developing malnutrition if they have inadequate nutrient intake for $\geq$ 7 days or if they have weight loss $\geq$ 10% of their pre-illness body weight[5]
      b. Protein and/or calorie deficiency are the most common causes of malnutrition
      c. Three types of protein-calorie malnutrition have been identified: marasmus, kwashiorkor, and marasmus-kwashiorkor; it is important to determine the nature and severity of protein-calorie depletion so that appropriate nutritional support can be given
   2. Marasmus
      a. Characteristics
         1) A gradual wasting of adipose and somatic muscle with preservation of visceral proteins; patient is cachectic
         2) Chronic condition in which basal metabolic rate (BMR) is reduced; fat is the major energy substrate and visceral proteins are preserved
         3) Presents with weight loss, adipose and skeletal muscle atrophy, decreased anthropometric measurements, and development of immune incompetence, which is accompanied by decreased total lymphocyte counts and skin test energy
      b. Causes
         1) Occurs when there is an acceptable ratio of protein-caloric intake but inadequate total dietary intake
         2) Seen with prolonged starvation, anorexia, chronic illness, old age
      c. Goal of therapy: to restore fat and protein stores over prolonged period
   3. Kwashiorkor (Hypoalbuminemia)
      a. Characteristics
         1) Presents with increase in extracellular water spaces, pitting edema, salt retention, occasionally ascites, and anasarca
         2) Visceral protein stores are depleted with depressed concentrations of serum albumin, transferrin, thyroxin-binding prealbumin, and retinol-binding protein
         3) Immunocompetence is impaired and patient is susceptible to infection
      b. Causes

1) Caloric intake is adequate or excessive but diet consists of almost all carbohydrates with little or no protein

2) Seen during periods of decreased protein intake accompanied by increased carbohydrate intake (e.g., liquid diets, fat diets, long-term use of intravenous fluids containing dextrose)

   c. Goal of therapy: to preserve remaining protein stores

4. Marasmus-Kwashiorkor

   a. Characteristics

1) Presents with skeletal muscle and visceral protein wasting, depleted fat stores, immune incompetence; individuals appear cachetic and are usually undergoing acute catabolic stress; can also present with vitamin and mineral deficiencies

2) Associated with the highest risk of morbidity and mortality

   b. Causes

1) Individuals share some aspect of both marasmus and kwashiorkor

2) Two phases of abnormal dietary intake occur: initial reduced protein intake with subsequent decreased total intake or vice versa

3) May occur in hospitalized patient with pre-existing marasmus complicated by hospital-induced kwashiorkor resulting from administration of intravenous dextrose solutions

IV. NUTRITIONAL REQUIREMENTS

A. Determination of Nutrient Requirements[12]

1. The requirement for a nutrient is the minimum intake that will maintain normal function and health

2. The United States standard for determining nutrient intake and planning and evaluating diet is the Recommended Dietary Allowance (RDA)

   a. RDAs are recommendations established for a healthy population and do not address therapeutic nutritional needs

   b. RDAs have not been established for all nutrients

3. Changes in physical activity, climate, aging, drug therapy, and/or illness may require adjustment of the RDA

B. Energy Balance[12]

1. Positive balance exists when food intake exceeds expenditure; excess energy is stored primarily as fat, and weight gain results

2. Negative balance exists when energy expenditure exceeds food intake; weight loss results as the body uses its own energy stores to meet requirements

3. Equilibrium exists when energy in food equals energy expended; body weight remains constant

C. Energy Requirements[13,14]

1. Energy requirements are dependent on a number of factors, which include the body surface area (derived from height and weight), age, and sex; they are usually estimated from tables or from simple formulas
2. Energy expenditure
   a. Total daily energy (TDE) expenditure has three components:
      1) Basal energy expenditure (BEE) or BMR
      2) Energy expenditure related to activity
      3) Specific dynamic action of food
   b. Determination of energy needs can be determined from the BEE or resting metabolic expenditure (RME); BEE is the amount of energy produced per unit of time under "basal" conditions; RME is the amount of energy expended at any time other than during basal conditions but with the patient at thermal neutrality
      1) Terms BEE and RME are frequently used interchangeably; however, RME is usually approximately 10% higher than BEE in normal persons
      2) BEE accounts for 65 to 75% of energy expenditure and may be measured or estimated
      3) Traditional method used to estimate BEE is the Harris-Benedict equation, which takes into consideration influence of patient's weight in kilograms, height in centimeters, age, and sex
         • For men: BEE (kcal/day) = 66.5 + (13.7 × Weight) + (5.0 × Height) − (6.8 × Age)
         • For women: BEE (kcal/day) = 65.5 + (9.6 × Weight) + (1.7 × Height) − (4.7 × Age)
      4) May be modified for activity factors (AF) and injury factors (IF)
         • TDE = (BEE) (AF) (IF)
         • AF: Confined to bed = 1.2, Out of bed = 1.3
         • IF: Surgery = 1.1 to 1.2; Infection = 1.2 to 1.6, Trauma = 1.35 to 1.6; Burns = 1.5 to 1.9
      5) A simpler, widely accepted method used to estimate daily adult caloric requirements is to use 30 to 35 calories/kg
      6) Two methods are available to measure the BMR: direct or indirect calorimetry; the term calorimetry derives from heat metabolism
         • Direct calorimetry methods directly measure heat produced by the body; this technique is cumbersome, expensive, and difficult to apply to acutely ill or injured patients
         • Indirect calorimetry indirectly measures heat production of the body through measurement of oxygen consumption and carbon dioxide production; is the most accurate method of determining caloric requirements
   c. Energy expenditure of activity: second largest component of daily energy expenditure

1) Energy requirement can vary from 1.1 to 10.3 kcal/kg/hr depending on the type of activity
   d. Specific dynamic action (SDA) of food: the increased heat production that occurs with food ingestion or infusion of parenteral nutrients
      1) Add 10% to the sum of BMR plus energy expenditure of activity to account for SDA

D. Protein

1. Classifications
   a. Amino acids are the basic units of protein; there are essential and nonessential amino acids
      1) Essential amino acids cannot be synthesized in the body and must be received in the diet
      2) Conditionally, essential amino acids are nonessential under normal circumstances but are required in the diet during certain disease states because utilization exceeds synthesis
   b. The amino acids are classified as aromatic amino acids (AAA) or branched-chain amino acids (BCAA)
      1) BCAAs are oxidized principally by skeletal muscle
      2) Rate of oxidation of BCAAs in muscle is stimulated by stress, fasting conditions associated with muscle protein wasting, and negative nitrogen balance
   c. Essential amino acids: isoleucine (BCAA), leucine (BCAA), lysine (AAA), methionine (AAA), phenylalanine (AAA), threonine (AAA), tryptophan (AAA), valine (BCAA)
   d. Conditionally essential amino acids: histidine, cysteine, tyrosin
   e. Nonessential amino acids: alanine, arginine, aspartic acid, asparagine, glutamic acid, glutamine, glycine, proline, serine
2. Function
   a. The major function of protein is contributing to tissue growth, repair, and replacement of all body cells
   b. Proteins are components of the body's defense mechanism and are found in antibodies, scar tissue, and clots; the body's functional molecules (enzymes, hormones, and carrier substances) require protein for development
   c. Although protein can contribute to energy needs (approximately 4 kcal/g), this is not its major purpose
3. Metabolism
   a. Body protein is constantly being turned over by the process of synthesis and catabolism, with approximately 40% of the body's resting energy expenditure used for these processes
      1) During periods of inadequate nutrient intake, mobilization and catabolism (breakdown) of the body's protein compartment occur to supply energy substrate as glucose
      2) Positive balance of calories and nitrogen is needed to promote anabolism (build-up)

b. There is no storage form of amino acids other than the body muscle mass

c. The amino acids released as a result of skeletal muscle catabolism are the main sources of nitrogen, which is released in the urine as urea

d. Factors regulating rate of metabolism, extreme environmental stress, infection, fever, trauma, and surgical procedures can result in substantial urinary loss of nitrogen

    1) In illness or trauma that has led to severe protein depletion, protein requirements for repletion of wasted tissues is increased; this is similar to the process that occurs in infants and children who are in a state of rapid growth

    2) The degree of stress, possible hypercatabolic state, and special clinical conditions such as renal failure and hepatic insufficiency affects protein need and tolerance

4. Protein compartments: the body's protein resides in two compartments

a. Somatic compartment: includes skeletal muscle, skeleton, and skin-supporting structure

b. Visceral compartment: includes solid viscera and secretory proteins

5. Requirements

a. Protein needs are determined according to the results of nitrogen balance studies

    1) Predicted protein requirements are equated with the lowest quantity of protein needed to maintain health and nitrogen equilibrium

    2) An important objective is to maintain a positive nitrogen balance

b. Requirement is dependent on a number of metabolic factors such as the previous nutritional status, degree of nutritional depletion, provision of nonprotein energy, and the rate of desired repletion

    1) Requirements increase in certain states (athletic training, growth, pregnancy) or in catabolic states (stress, trauma)

c. The more calories given, the better the nitrogen retention; retention also depends on the calorie-to-nitrogen ratio

    1) The optimal calorie-to-nitrogen ratio in the patient requiring nutritional support remains individualized

    2) The currently used calorie-to-nitrogen ratio ranges from 100 and 200 to 1 (nonprotein calories/1g of nitrogen provided in amino acid solution)

d. 1 g nitrogen is equal to 6.25 g of protein

e. Effective nitrogen supplementation during TPN in patients with limited activity, based on the level of stress, is as follows[7]:

    1) No stress: 0.5 to 0.8 g/kg/day

    2) Mild stress: 0.8 to 1.0 g/kg/day

3) Moderate stress: 1.0 to 1.5 g/kg/day
4) Severe stress: 1.5 to 2.0 g/kg/day
5) Up to 2.5 g/kg/day may be required (burn patients)[16]
 • Watch for adverse reactions associated with protein supplementation (i.e., renal solute load, increased respiratory drive, altered medicinal kinetics)
 f. Pediatrics
  1) Child > 12 months: 1.5 to 2 g/kg/day
  2) Neonate: 2.5 to 3 g/kg/day

E. Carbohydrates[16]

1. Types
  a. Dextrose (glucose)
   1) Primary source of carbohydrate calories in parenteral nutrition solutions
   2) Is a physiological substrate, easily purified for intravenous administration, inexpensive, and can be provided in high concentrations
   3) 1 gram of dextrose provides approximately 3.4 calories
  b. Fructose
   1) Naturally occurring monosaccharide that offers an alternative to dextrose as a source of carbohydrate calories
   2) Fructose does not require insulin for conversion to glucose; however, most adult tissues cannot use fructose directly and require its conversion to glucose in the liver
   3) Hyperglycemia and glycosuria occur less frequently with fructose than with corresponding amounts of glucose
   4) Rapid infusion of fructose has been associated with lactic acidosis, hypophosphatemia, elevated serum bilirubin and uric acid levels, and depletion of hepatic adenine nucleotides
   5) Its use has not gained popularity in the United States[17]
  c. Sorbitol and xylitol
   1) Alcohol sugars that are only partially insulin-independent
   2) Both require conversion to glucose in the liver and are associated with numerous toxic effects, including lactic acidosis, hepatic failure, hyperuricemia
  d. Glycerol
   1) Naturally occurring sugar alcohol that provides 4.3 calories/g
   2) The use of glycerol as an exclusive energy source is relatively recent and requires further clinical investigation[17]
2. Functions
  a. Major function is as an energy providing nutrient
  b. Carbohydrate is protein-sparing; when the body does not receive sufficient energy calories it will turn to protein and fat stores for energy
3. Metabolism

a. When glucose is supplied as a nutrient, the quantity not immediately used for energy calories is stored in the liver and muscle as glycogen
  1) Glycogen is the storage form of glucose
  2) When glycogen storage capacity is exhausted, excess carbohydrate is stored as fat
b. Carbohydrate metabolism, like all forms of metabolism, has a constructive phase called catabolism and a destructive phase called anabolism
  1) The three major processes involved in carbohydrate catabolism are glycolysis (initial process in which sugar is broken down into simpler compounds), the Kreb's cycle (completed carbohydrate catabolism), and glycogenolysis (conversion of glycogen stores into glucose)
  2) The two major processes involved in carbohydrate anabolism include glycogenesis (glucose converted to glycogen) and gluconeogenesis (transformation of fats and proteins into glucose or glycogen for use by cells for fuel)
c. Rate of glucose metabolism varies between 0.4 to 1.4 g/kg/hr; maximum glucose utilization rate is approximately 5 mg/kg/min
  1) Overfeeding by supplying glucose in excess of this rate does not further accentuate nitrogen retention and produces adverse effects such as fatty liver and increased carbon dioxide production, which may aggravate pre-existing respiratory distress

4. Requirements
  a. There is no specific requirement for carbohydrates; individual requirements are determined by estimating or measuring energy requirements
    1) It can be synthesized from amino acids and glycerol by gluconeogenesis, although it is preferable to ingest carbohydrates
  b. Carbohydrates are generally used to provide at least 50% of total calories

F. Fat

1. Types
  a. Essential fatty acids
    1) Linoleic acid is the primary essential fatty acid required for growth
    2) Linolenic acid may not be essential for adults, but it may be essential for proper visual and neural development and in certain disease states
  b. Major lipid substances within the body include triglycerides, phospholipids, cholesterol, and fatty acids
2. Functions
  a. Responsible for a wide range of metabolic and structural functions

b. Essential for structural integrity of cell membranes and is necessary for absorption of fat-soluble vitamins

c. In parenteral nutrition, lipids are a major source of metabolic fuel and a source of essential fatty acids

3. Metabolism

a. The most concentrated source of heat and energy, providing more than twice as many energy calories per gram (9 kcal/g) as either protein or carbohydrates; fat stores are a reserve of body energy that is mobilized when necessary

b. Lipids are isotonic and can be infused in peripheral veins

c. Allows a decrease in the concomitant intake of glucose and a reduction in the complications associated with large glucose loads in critically ill patients

d. Fat deposition in the liver is markedly reduced by lipid-containing (versus glucose-based) parenteral nutrition preparations

e. There are lower levels of circulating insulin in lipid-containing parenteral nutrition preparations[18]

4. Requirements

a. The main purpose of intravenous fat is to prevent the onset of essential fatty acid deficiency (EFAD), manifested as dermatitis, hemolytic anemia, thrombocytopenia, impaired wound healing, and hepatic dysfunction secondary to fatty metamorphosis

b. There is no recommended dietary allowance for fat as a nutrient in the diet; EFAD can occur in as little as 5 days without fat supplementation

c. The minimum human requirement needed to prevent EFAD should represent 2 to 4% of the total caloric intake

d. The optimum dose of lipid for the provision of calories is not known

1) Most patients receive 10 to 40% of the daily caloric intake, 2.5 g/kg for adults or 4 g/kg for pediatric patients

2) The maximum safe dose is no more than 60%[1,17]

G. Fluid

1. Requirements

a. Maintenance: 30 to 35 ml/kg/day or 1500 ml for first 20 kg plus 20 ml/kg for actual weight beyond 20 kg[2]

b. Factors increasing requirements: extraordinary exogenous losses (e.g., fistulas, diarrhea, nasogastric tube drainage)

2. Fluid changes induced by starvation

a. Extracellular fluid (ECF)

1) Most of early water loss in starvation originates from ECF

2) If fasting continues, loss of ECF is markedly reduced

3) Water and sodium are conserved, and catabolism of body cell mass results in a proportionally high extracellular water content[19]

      b. Intracellular fluid
        1) Oxidation of cell substrates results in net production of free water
        2) Water normally bound to macromolecules such as glycogen and protein is free to diffuse to the ECF[19]
  3. Fluid changes induced by acute injury
      a. Acute injury is followed by characteristic fluid and electrolyte distortions that tend to maintain plasma volume and tissue perfusion
      b. Sodium and water retention occurs along with the formation of third spaces in injured areas or in the GI tract[19]
  4. Fluid changes induced by parenteral nutrition
      a. Fluid overload can occur if parenteral nutrition is administered with a predetermined number of calories without regard for the volume infused
      b. To prevent fluid overload, concentration of glucose calories needs to be increased, or fat needs to be added as a caloric source

H. Essential Macronutrients (Electrolytes)

  1. Considerations
      a. The following three factors should be considered when determining the electrolyte requirements for a patient receiving parenteral nutrition
        1) Pre-existing electrolyte deficits
        2) Excessive fluid and electrolyte losses
        3) Daily electrolyte needs
      b. With protein-calorie malnutrition there is loss of the intracellular ions potassium, magnesium, and phosphorus, together with a gain in sodium and water
      c. It is necessary to give potassium, magnesium, phosphorus, and zinc to ensure optimum nitrogen retention
  2. Sodium
      a. Recommendations/requirements
        1) Daily needs range from 100 to 150 mEq[20]
        2) Supplement to cover abnormal losses
      b. Considerations related to parenteral nutrition
        1) Abnormalities of sodium commonly linked to fluid administration
        2) Initially, sodium balance may become markedly positive and cause edema during refeeding
        3) Less sodium should be given to patients with renal or cardiovascular disease
  3. Potassium
      a. Recommendations/requirements
        1) Daily needs range from 80 to 100 mEq; an anabolic patient may require 150 to 200 mEq/day[20]

b. Considerations related to parenteral nutrition
    1) Glucose infusions will increase the need for potassium; approximately 3 mEq are retained with each gram of nitrogen

4. Chloride
  a. Recommendations/requirements
    1) Add quantity similar to total sodium content[20]
  b. Considerations related to parenteral nutrition
    1) To prevent hyperchloremic metabolic acidosis, crystalline amino acid formulations are acetate-balanced, with acetate substituted as an anion, and chloride is maintained in a 1:1 ratio with sodium
    2) Hypochloremic metabolic acidosis remains a risk in patients undergoing sustained gastric decompression

5. Phosphorus
  a. Recommendations/requirements
    1) 15 to 45 mmol/day[20]
    2) Increases when glucose alone is given as a source of energy; this is partly because lipid emulsions have phospholipids that act as an additional source of phosphorus, and high insulin levels associated with the glucose system increase cellular uptake of phosphorus
  b. Considerations related to parenteral nutrition
    1) Hypophosphatemia is commonly found during the initial phase of nutritional support in previously debilitated, malnourished patients
    2) With refeeding there is a redistribution of phosphate into muscle, which can induce hypophosphatemia.
      • Signs and symptoms include tremors, paresthesias, ataxia, decreased platelet and erythrocyte survival, impaired leukocyte function, and weakness

6. Calcium
  a. Recommendations/requirements
    1) 5 to 15 mEq/day[20]
  b. Considerations related to parenteral nutrition
    1) Administration of large amounts of phosphate salts can contribute to a lowering of serum calcium levels
    2) In contrast, administration of intravenous phosphate and acetate-balanced solutions has been shown to decrease hypercalciuria and may be beneficial in maintaining calcium stores in patients receiving long-term TPN
    3) In malnourished patients, serum calcium levels may be low as a result of decreased levels of albumin to which half of calcium is bound, while ionized calcium levels remain normal[21]

7. Magnesium
  a. Recommendations/requirements
    1) 8 to 30 mEq/day

  2) Additional amounts may be required to cover losses from GI secretions[20]

 b. Considerations related to parenteral nutrition

  1) Inadequate replacement aggravated by high losses can lead to clinical syndrome of hypomagnesemia

  2) Renal potassium and phosphate losses are increased by hypomagnesemia[21]

I. Essential Micronutrients (Trace Elements)

 1. Definition

  a. Trace elements are found in the body in minute amounts; dosage parameters to meet basic requirements are usually very small (in milligrams)

  b. Each trace element is a single chemical and has an associated deficiency state; functions of trace elements are many and often their actions are synergistic

  c. The American Medical Association (AMA) Department of Food and Nutrition established guidelines for essential trace elements for parenteral use; these recommendations are used for determining base requirements[22]

 2. Iron

  a. Uses/function

   1) Predominant function is oxygen transport

   2) Lowered serum iron observed in malnourished patients may be secondary to defects in iron mobilization rather than lowered whole body stores

   3) The body has a large capacity to store iron in usable nutritional reserves and has limited potential to excrete excesses

   4) There are potential problems associated with compatibility, bioavailability, and administration with parenteral nutrition solutions[20]

  b. Signs/symptoms of deficiency

   1) Pallor, fatigue, exertional dyspnea, tachycardia, headache, listlessness, paresthesias, glossitis, stomatitis, altered attention span, abnormal skin and nail formation, microcytic anemia

  c. Recommendations/requirements

   1) Iron dextran is not routinely added to parenteral solutions; however, when required, it is added as 1 mg/ml daily

 3. Iodine

  a. Uses/function

   1) Thyroid hormone synthesis

  b. Signs/symptoms of deficiency

   1) Goiter, hypothyroidism

  c. Recommendations/requirements

   1) 0.07 to 0.5 mg/day intravenous

4. Zinc
   a. Uses/function
      1) Most abundant of all the trace elements; an integral part of many enzymes and enzyme cofactors; is necessary for RNA, DNA, and protein synthesis
   b. Signs/symptoms of deficiency
      1) Alopecia, scaling, pustular rash, periorbital and nasolabial dermatitis, diarrhea, mental depression/apathy, glucose intolerance, night blindness, and impaired taste sensation, wound healing, T-lymphocyte function, and cutaneous energy
   c. Recommendations/requirements
      1) 2.5 to 4.0 mg/day intravenous; additional 2 mg for acute catabolic state, additional 12 mg/L for small bowel fluid loss, additional 17.1 mg/kg for stool or ileostomy output[20,22]
5. Copper
   a. Uses/function
      1) Essential with iron for normal erythropoiesis
      2) Constituent of many oxidative enzymes such as ceruloplasmin, cytochrome oxidase, monoamine oxidase, and tyrosinase
         • Ceruloplasmin aids the oxidation of ferrous iron in tissue stores to the ferric form to enable it to be transported by transferrin
         • Copper deficiency results in anemia with an iron deficiency picture
   b. Signs/symptoms of deficiency
      1) Microcytic anemia, leukopenia, neutropenia, skin and hair depigmentation, skeletal demineralization, hypothermia
   c. Recommendations/requirements
      1) 0.5 to 1.5 mg/day intravenous
         • Withhold in jaundiced patients or in those with liver dysfunction
6. Chromium
   a. Uses/function
      1) Potentiates insulin reaction with tissue receptors; in its absence, insulin-resistant diabetes and neurological changes have been noted during TPN
   b. Signs/symptoms of deficiency
      1) Insulin-resistant glucose intolerance, neurological changes (neuropathy), elevated serum lipids
   c. Recommendations/requirements
      1) 10 to 15 µg/day intravenous
      2) 20 µg/day intravenous in the presence of intestinal losses
7. Manganese
   a. Uses/function
      1) Antioxidant protection and energy metabolism
      2) Formation of connective tissue

3) Soluble cofactor in a number of enzymatic reactions

4) Affects carbohydrate synthesis from pyruvate

b. Signs/symptoms of deficiency

1) Extrapyramidal symptoms, bony abnormalities, central nervous system dysfunction, weight loss, transient dermatitis, occasional nausea and vomiting, changes in hair color

c. Recommendations/requirements

1) 0.15 to 0.80 mg/day intravenous

8. Selenium

a. Uses/function

1) Catalyst for the enzyme glutathione peroxidase, an important antioxidant pathway

b. Signs/symptoms of deficiency

1) Muscle dysfunction (including cardiac muscle changes), myalgias

c. Recommendations/requirements

1) 100 to 200 μg/day intravenous

9. Molybdenum

a. Uses/function

1) Cofactor for sulfite oxidase and xanthine oxidase

b. Signs/symptoms of deficiency

1) Headache, night blindness, irritability, lethargy, coma

c. Recommendations/requirements

1) 150 to 500 μg/day intravenous

J. Vitamins

1. Definition

a. Vitamins are organic compounds necessary for normal growth and maintenance of the body but are required only in minute quantities; they cannot be synthesized by the body in sufficient amounts and thus must be provided in the diet

2. Properties/requirements

a. Act as cofactors for the operation of certain enzyme systems

b. The exact vitamin requirements for patients receiving parenteral nutrition are not known

c. Recommendations are typically based on estimations derived from the requirements of normal adults and adjusted for patients who have increased requirements as a result of illness, nutritional depletion, or stress[16]

d. The composition of parenteral multivitamin preparations is based on recommendations established by the AMA Department of Food and Nutrition[23]

3. Classifications

a. Fat soluble: vitamins A, D, E, and K

b. Water soluble: ascorbic acid, thiamin, riboflavin, niacin, B_6, pantothenic acid, folacin, B_{12}, and biotin

4. Factors that alter status[24]
   a. Malnutrition, specific disease states, and drug therapy may predispose some patients to vitamin deficiencies
   b. Continuous parenteral infusion of a multivitamin preparation is physiologically different than oral administration; the gut and liver play important roles in modifying and storing orally ingested vitamins
5. Vitamin A
   a. Uses/function
      1) Essential for the integrity of epithelial surfaces, synthesis of retinal pigments, and protection against infection
      2) Fat-soluble and stored in the liver
   b. Signs/symptoms of deficiency
      1) Night blindness, xerophthalmia, mucosal keratinization
   c. Recommendations/requirements
      1) 3300 IU daily intravenous
6. Vitamin D
   a. Uses/function
      1) Promotes intestinal calcium and phosphate absorption
      2) Mediates the mobilization of calcium from bone
   b. Signs/symptoms of deficiency
      1) Bone pain and tenderness, proximal muscle weakness, skeletal deformity, low serum calcium and serum phosphotate, elevated alkaline phosphate, tetany caused by hypocalcemia
   c. Recommendations/requirements
      1) 200 IU daily intravenous
7. Vitamin E
   a. Uses/function
      1) Acts as an antioxidant at the tissue level
   b. Signs/symptoms of deficiency
      1) Edema, reticulocytosis, decreased erythrocyte survival time, excessive creatinuria, skeletal muscle lesions, increased platelet aggregation
   c. Recommendations/requirements
      1) 10 IU daily intravenous
      2) A portion may come from lipid emulsions and part from added vitamin
8. Vitamin K
   a. Uses/function
      1) Required for synthesis of clotting factors II, VII, IX, X
   b. Signs/symptoms of deficiency
      1) Bleeding, prolonged prothrombin time, hematuria
   c. Recommendations/requirements
      1) 2 to 4 mg intravenous once weekly (in absence of anticoagulant therapy)
9. Thiamine (B_1)

a. Uses/function
  1) An integral part of the cocarboxylase enzyme complex, which is necessary for the metabolism of alpha-keto acids such as pyruvate
  2) Cells, such as neurons, that depend exclusively on carbohydrates as an energy substrate need thiamine
b. Signs/symptoms of deficiency
  1) Beriberi, peripheral neuropathy, decreased or absent deep tendon reflex, muscle tenderness, muscle atrophy, fatigue, decreased attention span
c. Recommendations/requirements
  1) 3 mg/day intravenous
10. Riboflavin (B_2)
  a. Uses/function
    1) Coenzyme or active prosthetic group of flavoproteins involved with tissue oxidation and respiration
  b. Signs/symptoms of deficiency
    1) Cheilosis, lip inflammation, oral fissures, seborrhea dermatitis, corneal vascularization, ocular disturbances
  c. Recommendations/requirements
    1) 3.6 mg/day intravenous
11. Niacin
  a. Uses/function
    1) Component of coenzymes NAD and NAD phosphate (NADP), which are essential for glycolysis, fat synthesis, and energy production
  b. Signs/symptoms of deficiency
    1) Weakness, pellagra, diarrhea, tongue fissures, mental disorders, anorexia, oral inflammation, irritability
  c. Recommendations/requirements
    1) 40 mg/day intravenous
12. Pantothenic acid
  a. Uses/function
    1) As part of coenzyme A, involved in the release of energy from carbohydrate synthesis of sterols, fatty acids, and steroid hormones
  b. Signs/symptoms of deficiency
    1) Abdominal pain and cramps, headache, nausea/vomiting, lethargy
  c. Recommendations/requirements
    1) 15 mg/day intravenous
13. Pyridoxine (B_6)
  a. Uses/function
    1) Cofactor for many amino acid-metabolizing systems
    2) Affects many neurotransmitters
    3) Required for synthesis of heme proteins

     b. Signs/symptoms of deficiency
        1) Central nervous system disorders, nasolabial seborrhea, glossitis, hypochromic microcytic anemia
     c. Recommendations/requirements
        1) 4 mg/day intravenous

14. Biotin (B_7)
     a. Uses/function
        1) Essential cofactor for several enzymes
        2) Has direct and indirect effects on fatty acid synthesis, carbohydrate metabolism, and protein and nucleic acid synthesis
     b. Signs/symptoms of deficiency
        1) Skin rash, alopecia, lethargy, depression, paresthesias, anemia, anorexia, nausea, muscle pain
     c. Recommendations/requirements
        1) 60 μg/day intravenous
        2) 300 μg/day intravenous for repletion

15. Folacin (folic acid)
     a. Uses/function
        1) Transfer single carbon units as tetrahydrofolate
     b. Signs/symptoms of deficiency
        1) Macrocytic anemia, diarrhea, stomatitis, glossitis, malabsorption
     c. Recommendations/requirements
        1) 0.4 to 1.0 mg/day intravenous

16. Vitamin B_{12}
     a. Uses/function
        1) Affects nucleic acid formation
     b. Signs/symptoms of deficiency
        1) Megaloblastic anemia, glossitis, stomatitis, constipation, neuropathy
     c. Recommendations/requirements
        1) 5 μg/day intravenous

17. Ascorbic acid (vitamin C)
     a. Uses/function
        1) Affects growth of fibroblasts, osteoblasts, and odontoblasts
        2) Plays a role in hydroxylation of proline and lysine
        3) Enhances absorption of iron and inhibits absorption of copper from the GI tract
        4) Aids formation of active compounds from tetrahydrofolates
     b. Signs/symptoms of deficiency
        1) Delayed wound healing, scurvy, hemorrhagic petechiae, gingivitis, delayed wound healing
     c. Recommendations/requirements
        1) 100 mg/day intravenous
        2) 500 mg/day intravenous with catabolic stress

V. DISEASE STATES THAT AFFECT NUTRITIONAL STATUS

A. Diseases of the Esophagus and Stomach

1. Gastric dysfunction: dysfunction of the stomach may cause nausea, vomiting, or an inability to ingest food orally or to pass on to the small intestine
2. Disorders of the stomach affecting nutrition
   a. Delayed gastric emptying related to mechanical obstruction, diabetic gastroparesis, or following vagotomy and gastric surgery
   b. Rapid gastric emptying (dumping syndrome) may result from gastric resection or vagotomy
   c. Peptic ulcer disease
   d. Gastric cancer

B. Diseases of the Intestine

1. Short bowel syndrome[25]: virtually any nutrient, electrolyte, mineral, vitamin, or trace element deficiency can occur; nutritional alterations depend on site and length of resection, degree of adaptation, and existing disease
   a. Short bowel syndrome has three postoperative phases, and nutritional support needs change as time allows adaptation of the bowel to proceed
      1) First phase is characterized by fluid and electrolyte loss caused by massive diarrhea
      2) Second phase is marked by eventual stabilization of the diarrhea and fluid and electrolyte requirements; in this period, adaptation occurs in the remaining bowel, although absorption deficiencies in fat, calcium, magnesium, and vitamins may persist
      3) Final phase is full adaptation, which may not be achieved by all patients; usually requires 3 to 12 months, diarrhea is controlled, and patients have improved tolerance of feedings
2. Inflammatory bowel disease[1]
   a. Inflammatory bowel disease describes two inflammatory intestinal conditions that affect nutrient intake and absorption: Crohn's disease and ulcerative colitis
   b. Malnutrition is caused by several factors
      1) Decreased oral intake results from nausea and vomiting associated with the disease process; pain and cramping, which often increases with oral intake; and side effects of the medications used to treat the disease
      2) Excessive protein losses occur during acute diarrhea
      3) Malabsorption of vitamins and minerals almost always accompanies the disease process
   c. Severe diarrhea can lead to varying degrees of dehydration and losses of sodium, potassium, chloride, and protein

    d. Iron-deficiency anemia is common

  3. Pancreatitis[1]

    a. Almost all patients exhibit impaired carbohydrate metabolism, fluid and electrolyte imbalance, and hypoalbuminemia

    b. Malabsorption causes weight loss, diarrhea, steatorrhea

    c. Pain, often severe and associated with anorexia and nausea associated with hyperbilirubinemia, results in significant voluntary reduction in oral intake

C. Cardiac Failure[26]

  1. Malnutrition may precede or follow severe cardiac failure

  2. Cardiac failure patients frequently decrease their dietary intake because of anorexia, dietary restrictions, intestinal malabsorption, angina, GI hypomotility, or digitalis intoxication

  3. Patients have an elevated BMR

  4. Malabsorption of neutral fats occurs with severe congestive heart failure

  5. Sodium retention and potassium loss from diuretics may occur; sodium and fluids may be restricted by methyldopa

D. Liver and Gallbladder Disease[1,27]

  1. Liver failure

    a. Primary diseases of the liver include hepatitis and cirrhosis

    b. Liver has a supportive role in efficient digestion by modulating the physical characteristics of nutrients, making them accessible for digestion

    c. Metabolic changes include glucose intolerance, alteration in fat metabolism, protein intolerance, and an increase in nitrogen demand as a result of hepatocellular destruction

    d. Impaired dietary intake from nausea, vomiting, anorexia, depression, lethargy, weakness, alcohol intake

    e. Increased losses from vomiting, diarrhea, ascites, steatorrhea

    f. Decreased vitamin and mineral storage, decreased glycogenesis, glyconeolysis, gluconeogenesis, and decreased protein synthesis

  2. Cholecystitis

    a. Poor intake secondary to nausea, vomiting, pain, anorexia, fat intolerance; increased losses from vomiting and diarrhea

    b. Increased requirements for calories and protein secondary to possible fever and postoperative stress

  3. Biliary tract obstruction

    a. Poor intake dependent on obstruction and GI symptoms

    b. Steatorrhea: malabsorption of fat as a result of a decrease in bile salts; decreased absorption of fat-soluble vitamins secondary to fat malabsorption

    c. Increased requirements for calories and protein secondary to possible fever and infection, postoperative stress

E. Renal Disease[28]

1. Acute renal failure
    a. Poor intake as a result of anorexia, nausea, stomatitis, dry mucous membranes, alterations in taste perceptions, lethargy, possible impending coma
    b. Increased losses secondary to vomiting, diarrhea; protein losses may occur during dialysis
    c. Severe endogenous protein catabolism with accumulation of toxic protein metabolites and electrolyte imbalance
    d. Increased nutritional substrates required to repair injured tissues, eliminate infections and maintain hemodynamic, respiratory, and metabolic balances
    e. Consider potassium and sodium content of medications
2. Chronic renal failure
    a. Poor intake secondary to anorexia, nausea, stomatitis, gum ulceration with bleeding, esophagitis, gastritis, alterations in taste perception
    b. Increased losses from vomiting, GI bleeding; protein losses may occur during dialysis
    c. Wasting of lean body tissue and muscle mass with concurrent fluid retention that may mask cachexia; increased nutrient substrates are required to repair injured tissues, eliminate infections, and maintain hemodynamic, respiratory, and metabolic balance

F. Diabetes Mellitus[29]

1. Markedly elevated plasma glucose levels lead to glucosuria, which causes osmotic diuresis and urinary loss of calories, electrolytes, and water; prolonged periods of elevated blood sugars induce a hyperosmolar state and osmotic diuresis
2. Decreased peripheral glucose uptake, increased endogenous glucose productions, reduced suppression of glucose production with glucose infusion, diminished capacity to oxidize infused glucose
3. Increased lipolysis, increased fat oxidation, increased glycerol turnover
4. Increased protein breakdown, decreased protein synthesis, net body protein catabolism, decreased uptake of BCAAs by skeletal muscle, increased amino acid efflux from skeletal muscle

G. Respiratory Diseases[30]

1. Acute respiratory distress syndrome
    a. Prone to develop hypophosphatemia, which causes reduced oxygen transport
    b. Drug nutrient reactions from bronchodilators, adrenergic agonists, antibiotics, and corticosteroids
2. Chronic obstructive pulmonary disease

a. Weight loss (24 to 26%) and malnutrition are common
1) Degree of nutritional risk is estimated to be high when a patient with chronic obstructive pulmonary disease weighs less than 90% of ideal weight or has lost more than 15% of usual weight
b. Malnutrition is most likely related to an elevated energy expenditure secondary to increased work of breathing and deterioration of peripheral substrate metabolism during oxygen deficiency

H. Cancer[31]

1. Severe malnutrition that occurs with cancer is called cancer cachexia
2. Severe malnutrition with cancer is common; anorexia is common and may be secondary to the tumor, depression, and cancer-related treatments
3. Depletion of host muscle and protein stores is common; abnormalities in protein metabolism include abnormal elevations in levels of whole body protein turnover and synthesis, elevated levels of whole body protein catabolism, and elevated levels of liver protein synthesis
4. Lipid abnormalities include elevated serum levels of lipids and marked depletion of host lipid reserves
5. Insulin resistance is a common finding in patients with cancer

I. Acquired Immune Deficiency Syndrome (AIDS)[32,33]

1. Malnutrition occurs commonly
2. Food intake may be diminished because of a variety of reasons; nutrient malabsorption as a result of intestinal injury may occur
3. Patients with chronic infections with fevers experience hypermetabolism or other metabolic derangements

J. Stress/Trauma/Burns[34]

1. Stress
a. The metabolic response is a complex process mediated by the interaction of neurohormonal signals and increased production of cytokines, which creates severe nutritional–metabolic deficits in critically ill patients
b. Alteration in glucose metabolism includes hyperglycemia, which increases with increased glucose loads and is resistant to insulin administration; increases resting energy expenditure
c. Protein needs increase
d. Lipolysis is increased during sepsis, and patients are more dependent on lipids for oxidation
2. Trauma[35]
a. Trauma results in profound metabolic alterations, beginning at the time of injury and persisting until wound healing and recovery are complete

       b. Hypermetabolism, marked protein catabolism with increased nitrogen loss and muscle wasting occurs

       c. Hyperglycemia, glucosuria, and impaired glucose tolerance occurs

   3. Burns[36]

       a. Marked hypermetabolism and increased nitrogen loss

          1) Nitrogen loss parallels energy expenditure; as a result, energy requirements are determined by the severity of the injury

       b. GI tract is a major target organ of altered pathophysiology response following burn injury

          1) Patients with burns covering more than 30% of the body surface area commonly develop ileus immediately following injury

K. Eating Disorders

   1. Metabolic and endocrine abnormalities occur related to the degree of starvation

       a. Marked muscle and fat wasting presents a classic form of malnutrition similar to marasmus

       b. On average, normal visceral protein status is present; vitamin deficiencies are rarely reported

VI. NUTRITIONAL ASSESSMENT

A. Definition

   1. Nutritional assessment incorporates a review of systems combined with physical, anthropometric, and biochemical measurements that provide the data necessary to make a statement of nutritional health

       a. Repeat assessments may be used as a monitoring tool to follow the patient's progress during nutritional support or starvation

B. Medical History

   1. Identify presence of disease states that affect nutritional status

   2. Past surgeries

   3. Recent acute illness

C. Fluid and Electrolyte Status

   1. Increased losses as a result of diarrhea, vomiting, draining wounds, fistulas, abscesses, and effusions

D. Vital Signs

E. Medications

   1. Use of medications on a chronic basis

   2. Use of over-the-counter medications such as antacids and laxatives may lead to depletion of vitamins and minerals

F. Psychosocial Assessment/Social History

1. Social factors that may affect nutrient intake are income, education, ethnic background, religion, environment during mealtimes, and the individual who purchases and prepares meals
2. Psychological and stress-related factors that may affect nutrient intake are weakness, lethargy, malaise, depression, altered body image, decreased libido

G. Dietary History

1. Past dietary intake and appetite
   a. Number of meals usually eaten
   b. Types of food consumed
   c. 24-hour dietary intake report of what patient recalls eating during the previous 24 hours
2. Recent changes in dietary patterns
3. Foods allergies and intolerances
4. Factors affecting dietary intake
   a. Dietary modifications secondary to chronic disease, e.g., sodium restriction for cardiac disease, and protein and electrolyte restrictions for liver or renal disease
   b. Poor dentition or ill-fitting dentures
   c. Chewing and/or swallowing difficulties
   d. Alteration in smell/taste
   e. Frequent NPO orders for tests, x-rays, bowel preparation
   f. Inability to feed self
   g. Food preference or idiosyncrasies

H. Physical Assessment

1. General physical examination provides several indicators of a patient's nutritional status
   a. Changes in body systems may represent nutritional deficiencies
   b. Signs of nutritional deficiencies are observed most commonly in the skin, hair, eyes, and mouth; less commonly affected are the glands and nervous system
2. General appearance and condition
   a. Normal weight for height, age, and sex
   b. Good muscle tone and posture
3. Hair
   a. Changes associated with malnutrition include dull, sparse, thinning hair; changes in pigmentation; easy to pull out; alopecia
4. Skin
   a. Consider general characteristics of skin; dryness, flakiness may be associated with vitamin A and essential fatty acid deficiencies
   b. Follicular hyperkeratosis is associated with vitamin A and essential fatty acid deficiencies; looks like gooseflesh

c. Petechiae is associated with vitamin C and K deficiencies; may occur with liver disease or anticoagulation

d. Pellagrous dermatosis (hyperpigmentation on body parts exposed to the sun) is associated with niacin deficiency

5. Nails

a. Iron deficiency causes thin, concave, spoon-shaped nails

6. Mouth

a. Tongue may change color: magenta (purplish red); glossitis (beefy red)

b. May be painful and hypersensitive with fissures; most changes are associated with deficiencies of one or more B vitamins

c. Taste buds may be atrophied, may appear smooth, pale

d. Teeth enamel may be mottled with white or brownish patches, associated with fluorine excess

e. Spongy, bleeding gums indicate Vitamin C deficiency

I. Anthropometric Measurements[37,38]

1. Definition

a. Anthropometrics is the physical measurement of subcutaneous fat and of muscle mass (somatic protein) stores; muscle mass represents the largest concentration of body protein stores

2. Reliability: anthropometrics can be unreliable indicators of an individual's nutritional gains

a. Peripheral edema can inflate measurements

b. Repeated measurements can be highly variable as a result of differences in technique used by those collecting data

c. Benefits from nutritional repletion primarily affect cellular function and cannot be readily detected through increases in somatic mass

3. Height: should be accurately measured

4. Evaluation of weight

a. Evaluate weight loss history

1) Usual weight should be determined for comparison to current weight

2) Serial weight determinations over a long period provide the most reliable and clinically relevant information for nutritional assessment

b. Present weight can be compared with ideal values

1) Ideal body weight may not be a clinically reliable determination of weight loss and malnutrition

c. Current weight as a percentage of usual weight may be a more accurate indication if a reliable usual weight cannot be determined

1) Mild malnutrition: 85 to 95%

2) Moderate malnutrition: 75 to 84%

3) Severe malnutrition: < 75%

d. Consider recent percentage of weight change

        1) Losses greater than 10% over any period of time may be clinically significant

  5. Midarm muscle circumference measurements

    a. Estimates somatic muscle mass and skeletal muscle reserves; protein-calorie malnutrition results in muscle wasting and a reduction in subcutaneous fat deposits

    b. Midarm muscle circumference is determined by measuring, in millimeters, the circumference of the arm halfway between the acromial process of the scapula and the olecranon process of the ulna

    c. For best overall impression, results should be interpreted in relation to weight percentiles

  6. Skinfold thickness

    a. Used to determine/assess body fat stores; estimates fat content of subcutaneous tissue, which can be reduced and eventually disappear in malnutrition

    b. Can be measured at several sites (biceps, subscapula, suprailiac), but the triceps is the most common and easiest to measure

    c. Triceps skin fold measurement is taken at the midpoint of the upper arm by pinching a fold of skin with calipers as the arm hangs freely at the side; multiple measurements are taken and averaged to improve accuracy

    d. Averaging several skin fold measurements at various body sites may improve accuracy of determination of body fat stores

    e. Anthropometric measurements may be observed every 14 to 21 days

  7. Creatinine-height index (CHI)

    a. Used to assess somatic protein stores via a 24-hour urine specimen

        1) Creatinine is derived from the breakdown of creatine

        2) An assay of creatinine excretion in a 24-hour urine collection directly reflects level of total body creatinine and thus indicates total body muscle mass

        3) The quantity of creatinine excreted from the body is directly proportional to skeletal muscle mass in the case of rapid loss of skeletal muscle, which occurs in association with severe sepsis or trauma

    b. Urine is collected for 24 hours and assayed for creatinine

        1) Total amount of creatinine excreted is compared with the expected creatinine excretion for nutritionally normal persons of the same height at ideal body weight

        2) CHI is tabulated as a percent of the expected standard

          • CHI: measured creatinine divided by ideal creatinine $\times$ 100

          • Ideal creatinine: 23 mg/kg/day for males and 18 mg/kg/day for females

    c. An index of:

        1) Normal muscle mass: 100%

2) Moderate somatic muscle repletion: 60 to 80%

3) Severe muscle repletion: < 60%

d. Not clinically reliable because small errors in urine collection can greatly affect results

e. Reliability is also affected by dietary intake of creatinine, variability in creatinine excretion, and renal disease

J. Laboratory Data Measurements[2,13,37]

1. Routine laboratory tests may be helpful in detecting malnutrition from a biochemical standpoint; several laboratory tests reveal certain aspects of nutritional deficiencies

   a. Note: all visceral protein measurements should be interpreted in the context of the patient's clinical condition because they are also affected by changing fluid balance, sepsis, medications, and any stressful insult

2. Serum albumin

   a. Measures visceral protein; maintains plasma oncotic pressure and functions as a carrier protein

   1) Represents 50 to 65% of total protein

   2) Approximately 40% of the protein mass is in circulation

   b. Popular indicator of malnutrition because protein synthesis is depressed and existing protein is consumed to maintain bodily functions when nitrogen intake is inadequate

   c. Although albumin levels may have prognostic or diagnostic values, they have been found to be poor indicators of nutritional support adequacy

   1) Low levels may reflect decreased liver function rather than nutritional deficiency as it is a liver-synthesized protein

   2) Plasma levels may also be decreased from fluid changes secondary to increased vascular permeability, increased catabolism, or losses from GI tract or burn wounds

   d. Half-life is 18 days; therefore, changes in synthesis are reflected slowly and acute changes in nutrition will not be reflected at all

   1) Normal levels: > 3.5 gm/dL

   2) Mild depletion: 2.8 to 3.2 gm/dL

   3) Moderate depletion: 2.1 to 2.7 gm/dL

   4) Severe depletion: < 2.1 gm/dL

3. Serum transferrin

   a. Measures visceral protein; carrier protein for iron and plays important role in iron metabolism

   1) Assayed directly or can be estimated from the total iron-binding capacity

   2) Levels measured directly are consistently lower than those measured indirectly

   b. Half-life is 8 days and thus is a more sensitive indicator to acute nutritional changes

1) Normal (measured directly): > 200 mg/dL
2) Mild depletion: 150 to 200 mg/dL
3) Moderate depletion: 100 to 150 mg/dL
4) Severe depletion: < 100 mg/dL
5) Note: normal levels can range from 160 to 356 mg/dL with a mean of 258 (49 mg/dL); this wide range of normal values is the main drawback in using this test

  c. Studies vary regarding the correlation between transferrin and nitrogen balance in TPN support[38,39]

4. Prealbumin
  a. Measures visceral protein; carrier protein for retinol-binding protein
  b. Half-life is 24 to 48 hours and sensitive to acute changes in protein status
    1) Because of extreme sensitivity to sudden demands on protein synthesis, it may not always be clinically useful
      • Normal level: 20 mg/dL
      • Mild depletion: 10 to 20 mg/dL
      • Moderate depletion: 5 to 10 mg/dL
      • Severe depletion: < 5 mg/dL

5. Retinol-binding protein
  a. Carrier protein for retinol in plasma
  b. Half-life is 10 to 18 hours, reflecting acute changes in protein status and therefore is extremely sensitive to sudden changes in protein synthesis
    1) May not be clinically useful because of the short half-life
      • Normal values: 3 to 5 mEq/dL

K. Immunocompetence Testing[40]

1. Nutritional state is among the many factors influencing the immune response of the body
2. Immunocompetence can be adversely affected by malnutrition, stress, and disease
3. Immunological testing is designed to assess nutritional deficiencies; it may be assessed by the total lymphocyte count or by delayed cutaneous hypersensitivity, also known as anergy testing
  a. Total lymphocyte count
    1) Derived from routine blood count with differential
      • Total lymphocyte count: % lymphocytes × WBC divided by 100
      • Mild depletion: 1200 to 2000/mm³
      • Moderate depletion: 800 to 1199/mm³
      • Severe depletion: < 800/mm³
  b. Levels below 1200/mm³ are often taken as a sign of malnutrition
    1) Must be interpreted with caution because many other non-nutritional factors may contribute to decreased lymphocyte counts

4. Delayed cutaneous hypersensitivity testing
    a. Uses a battery of four or more common skin test antigens that are injected intradermally to elicit an inflammatory reaction
        1) The skin test antigens chosen are those to which normal persons in a given geographical area commonly would have had prior exposure and would be expected to develop an immunological response on re-exposure
        2) Most commonly used antigens include purified protein derivative, *Candida*, mumps, *Trichophyton*, streptokinase-streptodornase
    b. A positive skin test occurs within 48 to 72 hours if T lymphocytes are functioning properly
        1) Normal: with a panel of 5 to 7 antigens, response to 2 is positive; response to 1 is partial anergy
        2) Anergy: no reaction observed; anergy is the failure to mount an acceptable response to any antigen, and its presence may indicate severe malnutrition
    c. Its value as a test of nutritional state or therapy is unclear
        1) Affected by variation in concentrations of antigens used and measurement and interpretation of responses and by potential booster effect or repeated antigen administration
        2) May not be clinically useful because factors other than malnutrition, such as trauma, burns, hemorrhage, and general anesthesia, may affect reactivity[41]

L. Serum Glucose

1. Hyperglycemia: signs and symptoms include glucose excretion in urine, polyuria, dehydration and thirst, fatigue, visual disturbances, and weight loss
2. Hypoglycemia: signs and symptoms include tachycardia, anxiety, trembling, hunger, sweating, and piloerection

M. Nitrogen Balance

1. The difference between the amount of nitrogen intake and output
    a. The clinical measurement of nitrogen balance allows for determination of the daily net of protein balance; it is useful for assessment of baseline nutritional status and as a method for monitoring the progress of nutritional support
        1) Anabolism: positive nitrogen balance
        2) Catabolism: negative nitrogen balance
2. Measurement
    a. Nitrogen intake is compared with the amount of nitrogen excreted
        1) Nitrogen balance equals nitrogen intake minus total urinary nitrogen minus insensible losses minus GI losses
    b. Urinary losses are obtained from a 24-hour urine collection
        1) 90% of the nitrogenous breakdown products of protein

metabolism are easily measured in the urine as urine urea
nitrogen

2) Other nitrogen losses are estimated as follows: insensible:
5 mg/kg; GI: 12 mg/kg

c. Nitrogen intake is determined from caloric counts by dividing
protein intake by 6.25

d. Baseline measurement should be taken

1) As soon as the predicted daily nutritional requirements are
determined, a nitrogen balance should be calculated

2) If patient has not achieved the desired positive nitrogen
balance, the amount of nutrient should be increased and the
nitrogen balance should be repeated 1 or 2 days later; repeat
until desired balance is achieved

3) Thereafter, the nitrogen balance should be performed once
each week or whenever the patient undergoes a major change
in disease process

N. Hemoglobin/Hematocrit

1. Anemia usually accompanies protein deficiency

O. Other Laboratory Values to Monitor

1. Serum electrolytes
2. Serum vitamin levels
3. Serum trace element levels
4. Serum liver enzymes
5. Coagulation studies
6. Serum lipids
7. Urinary protein, glucose, and acetone

VII. PARENTERAL SOLUTION COMPOSITION

A. Carbohydrates, Fats, and Proteins

1. The three essential nutrients included in parenteral nutritional
solutions and required for protein anabolism and tissue synthesis

B. Protein Solutions

1. Composition
   a. Protein is parenteral nutrition in the form of crystalline amino acids
2. Concentrations/caloric value
   a. Amino acids provide 4.0 calories/g but are not always included in
   the calculated intake; all amino acids should be used to create
   endogenous proteins, not oxidized to produce energy
   b. Final TPN amino acid concentrations of > 60 g/L are difficult to
   formulate if they are to contain adequate calories; 3 L/day places
   an upper limit on amino acids of approximately 180 g/day

3. Formulations[16]
   a. Protein solutions are available in concentrations from 3 to 15% and come with or without electrolytes; these products are produced by several companies that manufacture similar amino acid mixtures
   b. Special branched-chain formulas are sometimes used for highly stressed and septic patients, hepatic insufficiency accompanied by hepatic encephalopathy, and in patients with acute renal failure; the need for disease-specific formulations has been controversial

C. Carbohydrate Solutions

1. Many carbohydrate sources are capable of being used for energy, but only a few can be physically absorbed and infused parenterally
   a. Dextrose is the most common and least expensive source used for parenteral nutrition and is the carbohydrate of choice in parenteral nutrition
2. Dextrose (glucose)
   a. Concentrations
      1) Primarily supplied in water in varied concentrations
         • Available commercially in concentrations varying from 5 to 70%
         • Can be given in high concentrations and in large amounts that are well tolerated by most patients after a period of adaptation
         • Infusion of concentrations greater than 10% require central venous access
      2) Individual formulas are chosen according to the patient's estimated energy requirements and his or her cardiac, renal, and volume status
   b. Caloric value
      1) Provides 3.4 calories/g
         • Note: it is possible to meet daily caloric needs with carbohydrate solutions alone
      2) May be used as the exclusive nonprotein caloric source or may be administered in varying proportions with lipids
         • When used with lipids, at least 100 to 150 g of glucose should be supplied to achieve maximum impact on nitrogen balance and to utilize it for certain key tissues, notably the central nervous system, peripheral nerves, red blood cells, white blood cells, active fibroblasts, and certain phagocytes that normally require glucose as the sole or major energy source
   c. Considerations
      1) Administration rates are dependent on the concentration as well as the patient's needs
      2) For the dextrose to be used effectively, concentrated solutions must be administered slowly; when administered rapidly, these

solutions act as an osmotic diuretic and pull interstitial fluid into the plasma

3) With glucose infusions of more than 4 to 5 mg/kg/min, progressive hyperglycemia may occur because tissues that traditionally utilize the glucose become insulin-resistant and do not extract it from the bloodstream

4) Excessive glucose intake should be avoided because it may precipitate an increase in the synthesis and storage of fat, hepatic dysfunction, and excessive production of carbon dioxide causing respiratory failure in some patients

5) The pancreas secretes extra insulin to metabolize infused glucose; if a hypertonic solution is discontinued suddenly, a temporary excess of insulin in the body may cause nervousness, sweating, and weakness

3. Fructose
   a. Used in 5 and 10% solutions combined with glucose and xylitol in Europe; its use is not popular in the United States

4. Glycerol
   a. Commercially available source that contains 3% amino acids and 3% glycerin and is intended for use with PPN
   b. Provides a protein-sparing effect similar to that of an intravenous fat emulsion
   c. The use of glycerol as an exclusive energy source is relatively recent and requires further clinical investigation

D. Lipid Emulsions

1. Used as a caloric source and to correct or prevent EFAD
2. Composition
   a. Lipids are provided by administration of commercially available fat emulsions that are aqueous dispersions composed of a neutral triglyceride such as soybean or safflower oil
      1) Egg yolk phospholipid is added as an emulsifying agent
      2) Glycerin is added to achieve isotonicity with plasma
   b. Fat emulsions contain only long-chain fatty acids and are a rich source of essential fatty acid, linoleic acid
      1) Medium-chain triglycerides are only used clinically in enteral nutrition; their use intravenously is investigational
   c. Safflower oil emulsions contain 77% linoleic acid and 4% linolenic acid
   d. Soybean oil emulsions contain 49 to 60% linoleic acid and 6 to 9% linolenic acid

3. Available preparations
   a. Of the four brands currently marketed in the United States, three use soybean oil and one uses safflower oil; both soybean and safflower oil emulsions are effective as energy sources and in reversing EFADs
   b. Available in 10 and 20% concentrations

4. Osmolality
   a. Lipid emulsions range in osmolality from 280 to 340 mOsm/L, depending on the concentration of the emulsion; because of their isotonic nature, they can be administered peripherally as well as centrally
5. Caloric value
   a. 10%: 1.1 calories/ml
   b. 20%: 2.0 calories/ml
6. Dosage
   a. At least 2 to 4% of calories from linoleic acid should be provided to prevent EFAD; 500 ml of 10% fat emulsion twice a week should provide adequate amounts of essential fatty acid
   b. Optimal fat intake is unknown; general recommendations are to provide 20 to 50% of calories from fat, not to exceed 60% of nonprotein calories
      1) Higher percentages of fat are useful with patients with hyperglycemia, carbon dioxide retention, and hypermetabolism
7. Adverse reactions include anaphylaxis, back pain, chest pain, cyanosis, dizziness, dyspnea, elevated temperature, headache, nausea, and vomiting
8. Monitoring patient tolerance
   a. Review liver function tests, blood coagulation studies, and cholesterol
   b. Be alert for complications such as transient increases in liver enzymes, blood dyscrasia, and hyperlipidemia
9. Contraindications
   a. Presence of pancreatitis and significant hypertriglyceridemia

E. Electrolyte Preparations

1. Commercially available as single salts or mixture for injection
2. Multiple-component electrolyte injections contain sodium, potassium, calcium, magnesium, chloride, and acetate salts
   a. It is important to consider that most amino acid formulations are available with and without electrolytes
3. Individual needs are highly variable in patients receiving TPN
   a. The choice of preparation depends on acid-base balance, renal and cardiac function, disease-specific needs, and abnormal losses requiring replacement
   b. Suggested doses per 1000 calories or 1 liter may be based on the following:
      1) Sodium: 40 to 50 mEq
      2) Potassium: 40 mEq
      3) Chloride: 40 mEq
      4) Magnesium: 8 to 12 mEq
      5) Calcium: 2 to 5 mEq
      6) Phosphate: 15 to 25 mmol
4. Acetate or lactate salts may be substituted for chloride salts if the

patient receives excessive amounts of chloride and develops a hyperchloremic acidosis

a. The use of acetate or lactate salts will reduce the chloride load, and the acetate or lactate may serve as a precursor for bicarbonate synthesis

F. Vitamin Preparations

1. The daily intravenous vitamin requirements established by the AMA Department of Food and Nutrition are provided by several commercial formulas in a 10 ml volume
2. Vitamin K is not included in adult multivitamin formulations and must be provided separately; it must be supplemented weekly either by adding 5 mg to the parenteral nutrition solution or administering 5 mg intramuscularly

G. Trace Elements

1. Commercial preparations of trace elements are available to meet basal requirements; individual dosage should be adjusted according to any identified deficiencies or increased losses

H. Insulin

1. Only regular insulin is appropriate for intravenous administration; addition of regular insulin is unlikely to cause hypoglycemia after tapering because of its short half-life
2. Insulin is considered chemically stable in parenteral nutrition solutions; a certain degree of absorptive loss of insulin to the solution container, tubing, and filter has been demonstrated
   a. It has been demonstrated that availability of insulin can range from 50 to 95% with the use of regular human insulin[42]
   b. Absorptive losses of insulin can be overcome by increasing the dose with subsequent solution admixtures until the desired effect is reached
3. Indications
   a. Many patients receiving concentrated glucose solutions require insulin to maintain normal blood glucose levels and to achieve maximum utilization
   b. Acute hyperglycemic episodes are managed by intravenous or subcutaneous insulin administration
   c. Maintenance with insulin is best provided through the administration of subcutaneous injections; the appropriate amount of insulin may also be added to the nutritional solution at the time of solution preparation

I. Heparin

1. Heparin in low doses (1000 to 3000 U/L) is sometimes added to parenteral nutrition solutions to decrease potential formation of a

fibrin sleeve, which may lead to venous thrombosis; concerns related to the possibility of heparin-induced thrombocytopenia have decreased this practice

    a. Another pharmacological effect of heparin is improving the clearance of intravenous fat emulsion from the bloodstream through activation of the lipoprotein lipase system

2. Physically compatible in parenteral nutrition solutions in concentrations up to 20,000 U/L

J. Albumin

1. Albumin is not used for nutritional purposes

    a. The essential amino acid content of albumin is poor and its half-life of 18 days too long for it to be an immediate or efficient source of usable protein

2. May be administered to increase or maintain colloid osmotic pressure so that concomitantly administered amino acids will be readily available for tissue protein synthesis rather than being diverted to albumin synthesis

3. Physically compatible

K. Histamine Antagonists (ranitidine/cimetidine)

1. Rationale for use[1]

    a. Histamine antagonists inhibit gastric acid secretion and are used by some as a prophylactic measure to prevent stress ulceration

2. Stability

    a. Both are considered visually and chemically stable

    b. May not be compatible with other additives such as aminophylline, iron, or antibiotics

L. Total Nutrient Admixture (three-in-one)

1. Description

    a. A nutritional solution composed of amino acids, dextrose, lipids, electrolytes, and trace metals in one container; the addition of lipids is the unique part of this type of admixture versus the traditional method of providing the lipids as a separate infusion

2. Considerations[43,44]

    a. May be clinically useful in patients with diabetes and in patients with compromised respiratory function by decreasing the amount of calories provided from glucose

    b. Has been reported as safe, efficacious, and cost-effective for infants less than 1 year of age

    c. May reduce the potential risk of microbial contamination because of fewer manipulations of the administration set

    d. Provides ease of administration and can be more cost-effective than standard solutions

e. Modified solutions have been successfully used peripherally
f. Since three-in-one solutions cannot be filtered through a 0.2-micron bacterial-retentive filter, the growth of microorganisms could prove detrimental
   1) *Staphylococcus epidermidis, Candida albicans,* and *Escherichia coli* are able to survive in three-in-one solutions
   2) A 1.2-micron filter may be used and will remove *Candida;* however, it will not remove *Staphylococcus* or *Escherichia coli*[45]
g. Stability of various amino acids, lipid solutions, and electrolyte and mineral additives is variable and must be considered during preparation
   1) There are possibilities of calcium phosphate precipitates, and many other chemical incompatibilities may occur
   2) Precipitates can develop because of various factors—e.g., concentration, pH, and phosphate content of amino acid solutions; calcium and phosphorus additives; order of mixing; mixing process; or compounder
h. Caution should be taken when compounding three-in-one solutions because the presence of the lipid emulsion may obscure the presence of any precipitate

M. Parenteral Nutrition Formulas

1. Use a standard formula ordering sheet to specify the protein, calorie, and electrolyte content of each solution
2. PPN
   a. Standard solutions contain
      1) 100 to 150 g dextrose with 1 to 1.5 g amino acids/kg (final concentrations of 1.75 to 3.5% amino acids and 5 to 10% dextrose), along with 500 ml of 10 or 20% lipids and electrolytes, trace elements, and vitamins[20]
   b. Prolonged infusions should be limited to solutions that are lower than 900 mOsm/l
      1) Reports have shown that with the use of three-in-one solutions a higher osmolality may be tolerated
      2) No greater than 10% final concentration of dextrose should be infused peripherally[44]
3. TPN
   a. Standard solutions contain final concentration
      1) 4.25% amino acids
      2) 25% dextrose
      3) Electrolytes, trace elements, vitamins
   b. This provides
      1) 105 calories/100 ml
      2) 85 nonprotein calories
      3) 5 g protein
      4) 106:1 nonprotein-calories-to-nitrogen ratio

    c. Addition of 500 ml 10% lipid emulsion twice weekly provides an average of 157 additional calories per day

  4. Three-in-one

    a. Standard solutions contain

      1) 5% amino acids

      2) 17.5% dextrose

      3) 10% lipid emulsion

    b. This provides

      1) 130 total calories/100 ml

      2) 110 nonprotein calories

      3) 5 g protein

      4) 138:1 nonprotein-calories-to-nitrogen ratio

  5. Nonstandard solutions

    a. Solutions contain varying amounts of amino acids and dextrose

    b. Are indicated when the standard glucose-based or lipid admixture solutions do not provide the adequate amounts or types of calories and protein required or when the patient may not tolerate the load of a standard solution

  6. Formulations for infants and young children

    a. Amino acids such as histidine, tyrosine, cysteine, and taurine, which are nonessential in adults, may be essential for infants and young children

    b. Special amino acid formulations are available to meet these needs[46]

N. Disease-specific Formulations

  1. Renal failure

    a. Indications/considerations for use[1]

      1) Use of specialty amino acid

      2) Commonly believed that nonessential amino acids may be needed to optimize protein synthesis and achieve positive nitrogen balance

      3) During the dialysis process, both essential and nonessential amino acids are removed, and therefore standard amino acid solutions containing both essential and nonessential amino acid are recommended to meet the protein requirements of dialyzed patients

    b. Solution composition

      1) There are four commercially available amino acid products specifically formulated for patients with renal failure

      2) All contain high levels of essential amino acids as well as histidine, considered an essential amino acid in patients with renal dysfunction

      3) One product contains arginine and another contains nonessential amino acids in lower concentrations as compared with general purpose amino acid formulations[20]

  2. Hepatic failure

a. Patients with hepatic failure have abnormal plasma amino acid profiles characterized by high levels of aromatic amino acids and low levels of BCAAs, which have been theorized as contributing to "false neurotransmitter" synthesis and the development of encephalopathy

1) Some patients with hepatic encephalopathy have responded to a specific parenteral nutrient formulation that contains little or no aromatic amino acids and high concentrations of BCAAs

2) The solution is designed to normalize plasma amino acids

3) It has not been clearly demonstrated that these specialized solutions are more helpful than standard solutions[47]

b. Solution composition

1) Increased BCAA and decreased AAA with a high concentration of dextrose, electrolytes, vitamins, and trace elements; dextrose concentration of the nutrient solution is usually 20 to 25%

3. Stress

a. Patients become hypercatabolic secondary to the metabolic state created by trauma, sepsis, and burns; unique nutritional needs and amino acid patterns have been associated with these disease states

1) The plasma amino acid pattern of septic patients shows significant similarities to patients with hepatic failure; high levels of aromatic amino acids and low-normal levels of BCAA are seen

2) It is believed that trauma patients break down BCAA in muscles; the administration of formulas high in BCAA is thought to replenish those depleted stores

3) BCAAs are more easily metabolized than AAAs

b. Solution composition

1) BCAA-enriched formulations have been developed

2) Often a reduced proportion of dextrose calories is used to optimize usable nitrogen intake

3) Lipid emulsion may be added as an additional source of calories[20]

VIII. PREPARATIONS AND STORAGE OF PARENTERAL ADMIXTURES

A. Solution Compounding

1. Nutritional solutions should be compounded in the pharmacy using aseptic technique under a laminar flow hood

2. To prevent three-in-one solutions from separating, stability patterns of the products must be considered

a. The pH of the formulation has to be raised to 5.7 to increase the stability of the lipid emulsion with the protein mixture

b. The usual 4.25% amino acid and 25% dextrose concentrations are compatible with lipid emulsion

c. The amount of electrolytes added must be carefully controlled, as they can significantly affect stability; must avoid the excess of divalent ions[48]

   1) Calcium (up to 2.3 mmol)
   2) Magnesium (up to 10 mmol)
   3) Zinc (up to 20 mg)

B. Storage

1. Nutritional admixtures should be either used immediately after preparation or refrigerated at 4°C until used
2. Acceptable length of time for refrigeration is based on the stability of the admixed components
3. When solutions are stored for more than 24 hours, quality control measures must be initiated to ensure the acceptability of the solutions
4. Lipid emulsions are refrigerated or stored at room temperature

C. Parenteral Nutrition Solutions

1. Must be infused or discarded within 24 hours after hanging

IX. SOLUTION ADMINISTRATION REGIMENS

A. Considerations for Initiation

1. Confirmation of catheter tip location must be done before initiating TPN; before initiating PPN, careful assessment of the peripheral site must be done
2. Solution labels should be carefully checked and compared with physician's orders before administration
3. Solution should be removed from refrigerator 1 hour before hanging
4. Before administration, check solution container for leaks, cracks, clarity, expiration date; with three-in-one solutions, check for pink discoloration or separation of oils

B. Rate of Delivery

1. Rate recommendations
   a. Should be gradually increased to the prescribed rate to avoid hyperglycemia
   b. Gradual rate introduction of approximately 60 to 80 ml/hr for first 24 hours with 20 ml/hr incremental increase every 24 to 48 hours is recommended
   c. PPN does not require tapering and may be initiated at desired rate
2. Consistency and accuracy of infusion rate
   a. TPN must be administered at a constant rate
   b. Changes in rate should be gradual
   c. Maintain consistency and accuracy with an electronic infusion device

C. Discontinuation

1. Occurs when patient is likely to resume full oral intake within 48 hours
2. To avoid potential complications, TPN should not be abruptly discontinued
3. Reduction of TPN infusion rates should be in conjunction with increases in caloric intake by the oral or enteral route
   a. As the TPN is decreased, fluid intake must also be increased
   b. Consumption of half the estimated nutrient requirements should be achieved before discontinuation of TPN
4. Rate reduction considerations
   a. The patient's diagnosis, condition, and length of therapy to evaluate whether tapering is required for discontinuation
   b. Tapering may be accomplished over a few hours by progressive reduction in the rate of infusion (consider glucose intake at the time of weaning)
   c. PPN does not require tapering
5. 10% dextrose in water should be hung at the same rate if the TPN solution is not available or sudden discontinuation occurs

D. Cyclic Regimens

1. Description
   a. Involves the infusion of TPN on a cyclic basis over 8 to 16 hours versus the standard continuous infusion over a 24-hour period
2. Benefits
   a. Improves quality of life through resumption of normal daily activities
   b. Allows the patient freedom from pumps during daytime hours, increased psychological well-being
   c. Allows for increased mobility, which maintains somatic muscle
   d. Allows for more physiological hormonal responses and stimulation of appetite
   e. Prevents or used in treatment of hepatotoxicities induced by continuous TPN; reversal of fatty liver and enzyme elevations and faster albumin level recovery
   f. Prevents or used in treatment of EFAD in patients on fat-free TPN; reduced insulin levels during TPN-free periods allows for lipolysis and release of essential linoleic acid[49]
3. Indications
   a. Patients who have been stable on continuous TPN and require long-term parenteral nutrition
   b. Patients who are on home TPN
   c. Patients who can handle a total infusion volume in a shortened time period
   d. Patients who require TPN for only a portion of their nutritional needs

     e. Patients who have hepatic steatosis or for the prevention of hepatic steatosis

4. Recommendations for initiation/termination

     a. TPN can be transitioned to cyclic administration once tolerance to 24-hour continuous infusion has been obtained; the switch is accomplished by gradual decreases in hours of infusion, usually 1 to 2 hours per day

     b. The hourly rate is determined by dividing the total required volume of TPN by the number of hours the TPN is to be infused; cyclic TPN is usually administered at rates no more than 200 ml/hr

     c. The ability to tolerate the glucose and fluid volume determines how rapidly the solution can be infused; with the average patient receiving 2 to 3 liters, this typically requires a period of 12 to 16 hours to complete; patients receiving 2 liters of fluid may tolerate 8-hour infusions

     d. For patients without complications such as glucose intolerance or a precarious fluid balance, a 12-hour cycling regimen is generally used; when glucose or fluid management is difficult, the infusion time can be lengthened

     e. TPN may need to be initiated gradually unless the goal rate is fairly low; to avoid the complications of abrupt changes in glucose, there must be a period of escalating up to the maintenance rate as well as tapering down from the maintenance rate

          1) Various procedures have been reported with tapering periods ranging from 1 to 2 hours; usually accomplished by reducing the rate by one-half in 15- to 30-minute increments before discontinuing the infusion

     f. Usually infused at night and turned off during the daytime hours; the infusion schedule can be designed around the patient's activity schedule

5. Contraindications/considerations

     a. Cardiovascular status must accommodate the large fluid volume infused during the cyclic phase; patients who are septic and metabolically stressed are not candidates unless it becomes necessary to manage liver injury associated with TPN

     b. Requires twice as many central line manipulations for cyclic TPN versus continuous TPN in each 24-hour period; increased manipulations may increase the risk of infection

6. Monitoring: patients receiving cyclic regimens need careful monitoring for the development of rebound hypoglycemia after cessation of the TPN solution

     a. Test for blood glucose 1 hour after tapering the infusion and anytime a patient develops symptoms associated with hypoglycemia: nausea, tremors, sweating, anxiety, or lethargy

     b. Hyperglycemia can develop during the peak flow rate and is indicated by a blood glucose greater than 250 mg/dL or the presence of glucosuria

1) Always evaluate for an infectious process
2) If hyperglycemia persists, lengthen infusion time
3) Small quantities of insulin can be added to control infusion-related hyperglycemia
4) Percentage of calories derived from fat should be maximized in an attempt to control the blood glucose

c. Inability to control hyperglycemia may require changing to continuous TPN

E. Lipids

1. Administration considerations
   a. Before administration, inspect for frothiness, separation, or oily appearance
   b. The emulsion should be allowed to come to room temperature if it has been refrigerated; administration of cold emulsion can cause pain and blanching of the skin
   c. May be administered in conjunction with TPN through a Y-connection system close to the injection site below any filters or as a separate infusion
   d. May be administered peripherally because of the isotonic nature
   e. Lipids should not be filtered; filtering can result in clogging of the filter and perhaps separation of the emulsion
      1) If a three-in-one solution is being administered, a 1.2-micron filter may be used

2. Rate of delivery
   a. Follow manufacturer's recommendations for rate and dose
   b. Test dose is recommended before the full infusion to allow time to note any adverse reactions
      1) In adults:
         • 10% fat should be infused at a rate of 1 ml/min for the first 15 to 30 minutes
         • 20% fat should be infused at a rate of 0.5 ml/min for the first 15 to 30 minutes
   c. Traditionally, 10% solutions are infused over 4 to 6 hours, and 20% solutions are infused over 6 to 8 hours; slower infusions of 12 hours and up to 24 hours (particularly with three-in-one solutions) have been used more frequently

X. MEDICATION COMPATIBILITY WITH PARENTERAL NUTRITION

A. Parenteral Nutrition Solutions

1. Provide a viable alternative to the intravenous administration of medications, help limit the number of intravenous lines in patients with limited peripheral access, and decrease the volume of fluid administered in patients whose fluid intake is restricted

B. Stability Considerations

1. Parenteral nutrition solutions provide a greater buffering capacity than either dextrose or saline solutions; however, the physical and chemical stability of drugs still pose a major problem
   a. The physical stability of the solution must be considered as well as the physicochemical stability of the additives
   b. Chemical incompatibility may render the medication ineffective
   c. It is not always possible to determine the stability or compatibility of the formulation from available resources due to the complex nature of parenteral nutrition solutions
2. Variables to consider
   a. Base amino acid solution
   b. Concentration of additives
   c. Solution pH, temperature, and length of storage time

C. Compatible Medications

1. Cimetidine, aminophylline, several antibiotics, chemotherapeutic agents, and other medications have been tested for compatibility when mixed with TPN formulas
   a. Several have been shown to be physically compatible based on visual inspection
   b. Insulin, heparin, cimetidine, and rantidine are often added to TPN formulations
2. The routine addition of other drugs to TPN solutions is not advocated because most are not dosed on a continuous basis[50]

XI. VASCULAR ACCESS

A. Peripheral Venous Access

1. Peripheral veins are appropriate for the administration of PPN only
   a. Appropriate vein selection: vein selection should allow for adequate dilution of the hypertonic PPN solution
2. Device selection
   a. The smallest gauge and shortest length cannula should be selected
   b. Over-the-needle catheters are recommended
3. Site preparation
   a. Cleanse the peripheral insertion site aseptically with an antimicrobial solution before cannula placement
   b. Antimicrobial solutions that may be used to prepare the cannula site
      1) Tincture of iodine 1 to 2%
      2) Iodophors
      3) 70% isopropyl alcohol
      4) Chlorhexidine

    c. Cleansing solution is applied in a circular motion starting at the intended site and working outward[51]

    d. To remove excess hair, clipping is recommended; shaving is not recommended because of the potential for causing microabrasions, which increase the risk of infection[51]

4. Dressings

    a. Types of dressings: the following sterile dressings are appropriate to cover the catheter and must be applied aseptically[51]

       1) Gauze: to ensure that the dressing is closed and intact, adhesive material should be applied over the entire gauze surface, securing all edges

       2) Transparent semipermeable membrane (TSM): if placed over gauze, it should be considered a gauze dressing

    b. Dressings should be changed in accordance with the *Intravenous Nursing Standards of Practice*

5. Site observation: frequency of monitoring is determined by the prescribed therapy, patient condition and age, and practice setting; because of the nature of PPN solutions, frequent observation and documentation of the site should include

    a. Signs and symptoms of peripheral catheter complications, including but not limited to erythema/warmth, swelling, pain/tenderness, streak formation, palpable cord, and drainage

6. Nursing interventions include assessment for complications

    a. Discontinuation of catheter

    b. Further treatment and/or medical intervention depends on the degree of phlebitis and severity of the complication

    c. The presence and severity of the complication should be documented in the patient's medical record

    d. Consideration should be given to the completion of an incident report dependent on severity of the complication

    e. Ongoing observation and patient education should be initiated as appropriate

7. Peripheral access site should be rotated in accordance with the *Intravenous Nursing Standards of Practice*

B. Central Venous Catheter (CVC) Access

1. Central venous access is required for administration of TPN solutions

2. Insertion sites include the subclavian vein, internal jugular vein, external jugular vein, femoral vein, basilic or cephalic veins

3. Catheter types/selection considerations

    a. Percutaneously placed central catheters

       1) Commonly used for short-term administration of TPN

       2) Single-lumen catheters are preferred over multilumen because of decreased risk of sepsis

    b. Peripherally inserted central catheters (PICCs): associated with a decreased risk of insertion complications as compared with percutaneously placed central catheters
        1) Appropriate for short- or long-term TPN administration
        2) For long-term use, consideration should be given to placement of a tunneled catheter or implanted vascular access port
    c. Tunneled catheters
        1) Commonly used for long-term TPN administration
    d. Implanted vascular access ports
        1) Appropriate for long-term TPN administration
        2) Consideration must be given to needle change frequency requirements

4. CVC materials/considerations for TPN administration: consider variations in catheter designs and composition that may be beneficial to reduction of infection and/or thrombosis
    a. Polyvinylchloride, polyethylene: material is rigid and easy to insert but highly thrombogenic
    b. Polyurethane: less stiff than polyvinylchloride or polyethylene, so the risk of thrombosis and/or thrombophlebitis is reduced; maintains enough stiffness for easy insertion percutaneously; becomes more flexible with increased body temperature
    c. Silastic
        1) Soft material with a low potential for thrombogenicity; difficult to insert percutaneously
        2) Common material used for long-term catheters
    d. Catheters are available with hydromer, antibiotic, and anticoagulant coatings

5. Patient preparation for catheter insertion
    a. Informed consent for central venous catheterization must be obtained by a physician and should include
        1) Reason for and risks of parenteral nutrition
        2) Explanation of central venous catheterization and associated risks
        3) Alternative treatments, if any
    b. Preinsertion teaching by the nurse may include
        1) Indications for parenteral nutrition
        2) Description of the catheter, explanation of procedure, location of catheter insertion, and where it will be located in the body
        3) Postinsertion considerations

6. Catheter insertion
    a. Site preparation
        1) To remove excess hair, clipping is recommended; shaving is not recommended because of the potential for causing microabrasions
        2) Nurses may be required to perform site preparation when

placement of the central venous catheter occurs outside of the surgical suite; if skin is unusually dirty, cleanse with soap and water before application of an antimicrobial solution

    3) Antimicrobial solutions that may be used to prepare the catheter site
- Tincture of iodine 1 to 2%
- Iodophors
- 70% isopropyl alcohol
- Chlorhexidine

    4) Antimicrobial solution should be applied in a circular motion starting at the intended site and working outward

    5) 70% isopropyl alcohol should not be applied after an iodophor prep, because the alcohol negates the effect of the iodophor

    6) The solution should be allowed to air dry[51]

  b. Central venous catheters may be placed by percutaneous techniques or cutdown techniques

    1) Catheter placement requires the use of mask, sterile gloves, gown, and a surgical scrub

    2) Surgically placed long-term catheters require personnel and site preparation in accordance with operating room policies and procedures

7. Postinsertion considerations

  a. Radiological verification should be done and read promptly after every catheter insertion, before initiation of prescribed therapy[51]

    1) The purpose is to rule out catheter malposition, pneumothorax, hemothorax, or other early complications

  b. Correct tip location is the superior vena cava (SVC)

    1) When placed via a femoral vein, the correct tip location is the inferior vena cava

  c. Physical assessment for any evidence of respiratory compromise such as decreased breath sounds, chest pain, or dyspnea

8. Dressings: sterile dressings and sterile procedures are used for CVC dressing changes

  a. Types of dressings: the following sterile dressings are appropriate to cover the catheter and must be applied aseptically[51]

    1) Gauze: to ensure that the dressing is closed and intact, adhesive material should be applied over the entire gauze surface, securing all edges

    2) TSM: if placed over gauze, it should be considered a gauze dressing

  b. Dressings should be changed in accordance with the *Intravenous Nursing Standards of Practice*

  c. Consideration should be given to the use of sterile gloves and mask when changing the dressings

XII. ADMINISTRATION EQUIPMENT

A. Electronic Infusion Devices

1. Rationale for use with parenteral nutrition: the rate of delivery of parenteral nutritional solutions should be regulated to provide an accurate, consistent rate of delivery
2. Pumps
   a. Description: delivers a specific volume of solution over a specific period of time
      1) Pressure is exerted to expel the fluid
      2) Advances in infusion device technology have provided pumps that allow multiple rate programming and automatic cyclic regimens
      3) Pumps are available in pole mount and ambulatory models
   b. Use with parenteral nutrition: recommended for administration of parenteral nutritional solutions to provide accurate regulation of rate
      1) Pumps are better suited for administration of viscous fluids such as parenteral nutrition
3. Controllers
   a. Description: functions under the principle of gravity and counts drops electronically; flow is dependent on height of solution in comparison with delivery site
   b. Use with parenteral nutrition: acceptable but not preferred for delivery of parenteral nutritional solutions because of potential for inaccurate rate delivery
4. Ambulatory infusion devices: programmable, ambulatory infusion devices are available for use with parenteral nutrition; used most commonly with home TPN to facilitate ease of use and activities of daily living

B. Administration Sets

1. Set change frequency
   a. Should be changed immediately on suspected contamination or when the integrity of the product has been compromised
   b. Should be changed using aseptic techniques
   c. Solution container changes, addition of add-on devices, and other set manipulations should coincide with set change[51]
      1) PPN: administration sets used for PPN are changed in accordance with the *Intravenous Nursing Standards of Practice*
      2) TPN: administration sets used for TPN are changed every 24 hours
         • More frequent set changes are required because of the dextrose and protein content of TPN solutions, which provide a greater potential for bacterial growth and contamination
      3) Lipids: administration sets used for lipid emulsion should be

discarded after each unit, unless additional units are
administered consecutively
  • When lipids are administered consecutively, the
    administration set should be changed every 24 hours
  4) Three-in-one: administration sets should be changed every 24
     hours
2. Luer-Lok devices are recommended to avoid accidental
   disconnection

C. Filters

1. PPN/TPN solutions: parenteral nutrition solutions should be filtered
   with a 0.2-micron filter
2. Three-in-one solutions: should be filtered with no smaller than 1.2-
   micron filter
3. Lipids: are not routinely filtered

XIII. COMPLICATIONS

A. Technical

1. Peripheral catheter-related complications
   a. Phlebitis/thrombophlebitis: related to hyperosmolarity, acidic pH,
      and particulate matter
      1) Addition of heparin 1,000 units, hydrocortisone 5 mg, or
         sodium bicarbonate 1.8 mEq to each liter may decrease the
         incidence of phlebitis/thrombophlebitis[2]
      2) Concurrent infusion of lipid emulsion buffers pH and dilutes
         hypertonic dextrose
      3) Filtration may decrease phlebitis
   b. Infiltration/extravasation: because of the hypertonic nature of PPN
      solutions, sites must be monitored frequently to avoid infiltration
      1) Depending on the solution composition, severe tissue damage
         may occur
2. CVC-related insertion complications
   a. Pneumothorax
      1) When a patient develops dyspnea, chest pain, cyanosis, or shock
         during or following placement of a subclavian or internal
         jugular catheter, tension pneumothorax should be suspected;
         physical examination may reveal decreased breath sounds and
         hyperresonance on the affected side with tracheal deviation to
         the contralateral side and jugular venous distention
         • Occurs in up to 6% of insertions
         • Pain behind the clavicle after insertion is almost always an
           indication of pneumothorax[52]
      2) Management includes insertion of a large-bore needle or chest
         tube

b. Air embolism
1) May occur during insertion when the syringe is removed to thread the catheter or guidewire
2) Symptoms include dyspnea, chest pain, tachypnea, tachycardia, cyanosis, or elevated central venous pressure leading to shock and cardiac arrest
3) Management includes clamping the catheter or extension set as close to the body as possible, lying the patient on his or her left side, and initiating emergency procedures as required
c. Catheter malposition
1) Catheter tip may be misdirected into the jugular, contralateral arm, or azygos vein
   • Hypertonic solutions are not well tolerated in veins more peripheral than the innominate veins or SVC
   • The ideal tip location is in the SVC
2) Management includes repositioning the catheter under sterile conditions with a guidewire or fluoroscopy, or discontinuing the catheter
3) Periodic chest x-rays to verify tip placement are recommended and should be done whenever the function or location of the catheter is questionable
3. CVC-related post-insertion complications
a. Thrombosis/thrombophlebitis
1) Can be related to the hypertonic TPN infusion
2) Can be a result of thrombogenic catheter materials and damage or disruption of the intima of the vein; duration of catheterization and repeated catheterizations are contributing factors
3) Patients receiving TPN are often volume-depleted or subject to low flow states; their blood may be hypercoagulable as a result of sepsis, major surgical trauma, or malignancy
b. Air embolism
1) May occur if the intravenous tubing becomes inadvertently detached from the intravenous catheter, or after the intravenous catheter has been pulled out and before the tract is sealed
2) Preventive measures
   • Luer-Lok or well-secured administration set connections
   • Air-eliminating filters
   • Valsalva maneuver
   • Clamps during tubing changes
   • Ointment and occlusive dressing over insertion site for 24 hours after removal
c. Catheter occlusion
1) May occur as a result of improper flushing protocols; may be treated with urokinase 5,000 U/ml instilled in a quantity equal to the catheter volume

2) May occur as a result of medication precipitates

3) Occlusions specifically related to three-in-one solutions have been successfully treated with the use of ethanol instilled in a quantity equal to the catheter volume[53]

4) Calcium phosphate crystal occlusions have been successfully treated with instillation of 0.1 N-hydrochloric acid (HCl) in a quantity equal to the volume of the catheter; the HCl is proposed to work by lowering the pH, which increases the solubility of the precipitate occlusion[54]

4. Equipment-related complications

  a. Complications may occur as a result of malfunction of electronic infusion devices or administration sets

  b. Adequate knowledge and training related to equipment is necessary

B. Septic Complications

1. Infection associated with parenteral nutrition may be related to microbial contamination of the cannula or the solution

2. Parenteral solution-related complications

  a. TPN solutions are poor growth media; poor bacterial survival has been attributed to the low pH and hypertonicity of amino acid and dextrose solutions; parenteral nutrition may also contain large quantities of acetate, which is bacteriostatic

    1) Addition of albumin has been shown to increase the potential of solutions to support the growth of bacteria and fungi

    2) Fungi, particularly *Candida albicans,* proliferate in standard solutions[55]

  b. Growth of most microorganisms has been found to be significantly higher in three-in-one solutions than in standard solutions

  c. Lipid emulsions provide an excellent media for growth of gram-positive, gram-negative, and fungal species at room temperature

  d. To determine the source of infection, carefully examine

    1) Solutions for particulate matter or turbidity

    2) Tubing

    3) Filter

    4) Connectors for possible leaks or cracks

  e. Change administration set and solution, and culture any fluid remaining in the delivery system

3. Catheter-related complications

  a. Origin of catheter sepsis is most often caused by improper site maintenance; most cases of catheter-related sepsis in the patient receiving TPN are secondary to growth of skin organisms along the outside of the catheter or breaks in a closed system allowing organisms to gain access to the inside of the catheter[46]

  b. Clinically defined as a sepsis episode for which no anatomical septic focus can be identified and that resolves on catheter removal

c. Septicemia is one of the most frequent and potentially serious complications in TPN patients; because of severe and complex medical and surgical conditions being treated, these patients are frequently difficult to assess for catheter-related septicemia

d. Evaluation

    1) Inspect the insertion site for signs of inflammation, edema, or drainage

    2) Laboratory confirmation may be provided by recovery of the same organism from the catheter tip and from a peripheral blood culture

    3) Monitor temperature

    4) Monitor blood and urinary glucose levels; the appearance of hyperglycemia in a previously stable patient who has not spilled glucose generally signals the onset of sepsis

    5) If another source of infection cannot be found, the catheter should be removed

C. Metabolic Complications

1. Refeeding syndrome

  a. Usually represents the initial stage of aggressive and excessive nutritional repletion

    1) Individuals who are in an adaptive starvation phase have somewhat adjusted to their deprived state

    2) Individual's basal energy requirements have decreased and there are fewer energy demands on the metabolic processes

    3) Initiation of nutrition must begin cautiously; an overly aggressive approach can result in catastrophic imbalances

    4) The process is reversed when the body has re-established normal electrolyte and albumin balance[15]

    5) May develop
- Dyspnea
- Hypercapnia
- Tachycardia
- Elevated venous pressure
- Congestive heart failure
- Cardiac arrest

    6) Carefully monitor volume and electrolyte intake and balance; carefully adjust caloric input and source depending on an appropriate mixture of carbohydrate and fat calories

2. Electrolyte imbalances: most common imbalances are related to potassium, phosphorus, and magnesium

  a. During active protein synthesis and anabolism, the level of the aforementioned ions in the plasma may fall

    1) Careful monitoring of laboratory values and general patient condition to detect deficiencies and excesses is required; correct imbalances through a change in the prescription[21]

  b. Phosphorus: hypophosphatemia is commonly found during the initial phases of nutritional support
   1) As TPN is administered, there is a redistribution of phosphate into muscle, protein synthesis begins, and phosphate is driven into the intracellular space as a component of adenosine triphosphate[21]
  c. Potassium: potassium is driven into the intracellular space during TPN administration
   1) Potassium binds to cells in many metabolic processes, and serum potassium can become markedly depleted in aggressive refeeding
   2) Insulin administration further intensifies intracellular potassium and phosphate shifting[21]
  d. Magnesium: driven into the intracellular space during TPN administration
  e. Sodium: to maintain homeostasis, sodium will be driven from the intracellular space into the extracellular space
 3. Trace element deficiencies: patients on TPN are at risk of depletion; avoid by daily supplementation of trace elements
 4. Hyperglycemia/hyperosmolar syndrome
  a. Predisposing factors
   1) Common occurrence as a result of the high dextrose concentration in the TPN solution; occurs when the rate of infusion exceeds the rate at which the body can metabolize glucose
    • Patients with normal insulin response can be expected to tolerate a glucose infusion of 0.5 g/kg/hr
    • Rates up to 1.2 g/kg/hr have been administered without complication[21]
   2) Do not increase the rate of infusion to "catch up" if it is behind schedule
   3) Factors predisposing to glucose intolerance
    • Presence of overt or latent diabetes mellitus
    • Increased age
    • Pancreatitis
    • Hypokalemia
    • Hypophosphatemia
    • Thiamine or B_6 deficiency
    • Some antibiotics
    • Steroids
   4) Conditions of stress, such as sepsis or surgery, result in decreased glucose tolerance and hyperglycemia in as many as 25% of TPN patients[21]
  b. Signs/symptoms
   1) The first sign of hyperglycemia is usually glucosuria; if not treated, it will lead to the development of osmotic diuresis,

followed by hyperosmolar nonketotic acidosis/coma, possibly leading to death

2) Watch for signs and symptoms of glycosuria, dry skin, oliguria, confusion, or lethargy

c. Treat with the addition of insulin; can also be minimized by decreasing the rate of infusion or by supplementing the carbohydrate calories with fat

5. Hypoglycemia
   a. Predisposing factors: may occur if hypertonic glucose infusions flowing at a rapid rate are abruptly terminated or decreased; can be seen after sudden withdrawal of a prolonged highly concentrated glucose solution infusion
      1) Uncommon in adults, but seen frequently in children
      2) Mechanical causes that may lead to hypoglycemia
         • Clogged filters
         • Kinked tubing
         • Piggybacking additional medications
   b. Symptoms
      1) Weakness
      2) Trembling
      3) Diaphoresis
      4) Headache
      5) Chills
      6) Rapid pulse
      7) Decreased consciousness
   c. Prevention
      1) Ensure a constant flow
         • If infused volume falls behind schedule, do not increase the rate to "catch up"
         • The rate should be recalculated to infuse the prescribed amount of solution over the remainder of the 24 hours at a uniform rate; recalculate only if this rate does not exceed 10% of the original rate
      2) Treatment includes instituting an infusion of 10% glucose and frequent measurement of serum glucose levels

6. Vitamin deficiencies: vitamins should be added daily to the solution as most vitamin stores are depleted in malnourished patients; the input of fat-soluble vitamins should be carefully controlled

7. Hyperlipoproteinemia: the overproduction of lipids causing hyperlipidemia may result from infusion of carbohydrates in excess of needs, high infusion rates of lipid emulsions, or reduced utilization of fat

8. EFAD
   a. Signs/symptoms
      1) Dry scaly skin
      2) Hair loss

3) Impaired wound healing
4) Hemolytic anemia
5) Thrombocytopenia
b. Prevent or correct the deficiency with administration of a lipid emulsion

9. Pancreatitis: lipid emulsions may produce symptoms of pancreatitis in inflammatory bowel disease patients; association with TPN is usually the result of either hypercalcemia or hyperlipidemia

10. Liver function abnormalities: hepatic complications are one of the most common metabolic abnormalities associated with parenteral nutrition
   a. Biochemical and morphological findings are related to the duration and composition of the nutritional support as well as the age of the patient
   b. Adults usually have relatively benign biochemical and morphological changes, while hepatic abnormalities in infants and neonates can be progressive and even fatal[21]
   c. Cholestasis and gallbladder disease are potential complications of long-term TPN
   d. Causes
      1) Continuous or excessive dextrose infusion, EFAD, excessive lipid infusion, amino acid imbalance, toxic effects of TPN degradation products, overgrowth of intestinal flora
         • Hepatic damage has been reported in one-third of infants receiving TPN and up to one-half of low birth-weight infants
         • Earliest abnormal finding is an elevated direct or conjugated bilirubin, followed by elevation of other hepatic enzymes[3]
      2) Prevalence increases with duration of TPN; prolonged TPN therapy can lead to irreversible damage
   e. Slight rise in the level of alkaline phosphatase commonly occurs but returns to normal and has no clinical significance

11. Respiratory deterioration
   a. Can occur in patients with pulmonary compromise who are oversupplemented with carbohydrate calories
   b. Dextrose oxidation produces 21% more carbohydrate than fat; manifested as increased carbon dioxide level, respiratory rate, and decreased tidal volume

12. Fluid balance
   a. Dehydration: consequence of failure to meet fluid requirements
   b. Monitor
      1) Pulse
      2) Blood pressures, including orthostatic changes
      3) Condition of mucous membranes
      4) Skin turgor

5) Laboratory tests such as BUN, creatinine, hematocrit, albumin

  c. Excess fluid: results in edema or shortness of breath as a result of excess fluid; make solution more concentrated, and/or extend cyclic period

XIV. PATIENT MONITORING

A. Parameters to Monitor

1. Daily weight
2. Intake and output
3. Vital signs
4. Laboratory tests
   a. Hemoglobin
   b. White cell count
   c. Electrolytes
   d. Serum glucose
   e. Blood urea nitrogen (BUN)
   f. Serum creatinine should be monitored frequently and should be done at least three times per week
   g. Other tests may be required more frequently depending on the patient's condition
5. Periodic tests to monitor nutritional status and abnormalities
   a. Serum albumin
   b. Serum iron
   c. Iron binding capacity (transferrin)
   d. Serum calcium
   e. Magnesium
   f. Phosphorus
   g. Triglycerides
   h. Cholesterol
   i. Transaminase levels, alkaline phosphatase, and bilirubin are important for recognizing the development of liver abnormalities and should be done once a week
6. Glucose tolerance monitoring
   a. Report glycosuria of 2+ or greater; note: verify accuracy of test; after 6 days may be caused by
      1) Infection
      2) Increased flow rate
      3) Drug interference with urinary glucose testing
      4) Copper reduction test false-positive
      5) Vitamin C
      6) Aspirin
      7) Salicylates in large doses
   b. Infusion rates may need to be adjusted, along with addition of insulin

7. Bowel function
8. Appetite
9. Psychological needs

XV. DOCUMENTATION

A. Clinical Monitoring

1. Assessments
2. Weight changes/presence of edema
3. Results of pertinent laboratory tests

B. Observations Regarding Improved Nutritional Status

1. Improved wound healing
2. Skin integrity
3. Stamina

C. Routine Catheter Care

D. Solution Administration

E. Changes in Oral Intake

F. Psychological and Emotional Support Provided

G. Patient and Family Teaching Relative to Nutritional Therapy

H. Evidence of Discharge Planning

XVI. HOME PARENTERAL NUTRITION

A. Rationale for Use

1. Patients requiring extended or permanent intravenous feeding to maintain normal nutrition

B. Discharge Planning

1. Patient must have adequate intelligence to understand and be willing to participate in the program and basic procedures in the home setting; mastery of procedures is facilitated by the patient's or caregiver's literacy
2. Motivation of patient and caregivers
3. Support of family/significant others
4. Physical limitations of patients; need adequate eyesight and manual dexterity to
   a. Manage infusion pumps
   b. Add additives to infusions
   c. Accomplish administration set tubing changes
   d. Care for the catheter

5. Financial and insurance considerations must be carefully evaluated and understood
   a. Insurance coverage for home therapy should be determined before initiation of patient education
   b. Insurance carriers vary in coverage offered for home infusion services
   c. Coverage must be evaluated, and financial planning implemented as needed
6. Venous access requirements
   a. Percutaneously placed catheters may be appropriate for short-term periods (2 to 3 months)
   b. Long-term catheters such as tunneled catheters or implanted vascular access ports are necessary for long-term vascular access; with implanted access ports, factors associated with frequency of needle changes must be considered
   c. The system should be comfortable and must not limit joint mobility or interfere with normal activity or the ability to exercise
   d. Should allow infusion and maintenance procedures to be performed safely and comfortably
   e. Should minimize the risk of infection
7. Patient assessment and consultation with appropriate healthcare and support individuals; communication of all patient information and homecare requirements
8. Coordination of services with home health and home infusion agencies
9. Provision of necessary supplies and storage
10. Appropriateness of home environment

C. Emotional and Psychosocial Issues

1. The influence of TPN on the patient and family will depend on the role and responsibility the patient has played in the family structure and on the family's coping mechanisms
2. Alterations in self-perception and body image related to vascular access devices and attachment to administration equipment for TPN solution administration
3. Alterations in lifestyle, including catheter-related care, TPN infusion and related requirements, social activity changes (most social activities revolve around eating), and potential financial impact
4. Readjustment of priorities and values, secondary to possible alterations in lifestyle, finances, and health-related considerations
5. Dependency on medical equipment and medical personnel
6. With children, home TPN may interfere with normal developmental stages

D. Patient Education

1. Comprehensive curriculum for patient education is tailored to the needs of each individual
   a. Verbal and written instructions of appropriate therapy-related procedures should be provided
   b. The educational process should include demonstration of procedures followed by return demonstrations by the patient or primary caregiver
   c. Evaluation of competency and instruction should be documented
2. Definition of therapy/indication for treatment
3. Solution preparation in the home, including specific drug/nutrient information related to the admixture
4. Infusion administration procedures
   a. Spiking container
   b. Priming administration set/filter
   c. Catheter connection
   d. Use of electronic infusion device
5. Catheter maintenance
   a. Dressing change procedure
   b. Catheter complication monitoring
   c. Catheter protection during bathing/swimming
   d. Techniques for maintaining catheter patency: dose, volume, frequency, method used for drawing up, and injecting solution
6. Daily self-monitoring and significance of alterations
   a. Notify physician if elevated temperature, chills, or sweats are experienced
   b. Urinary glucose and acetone
      1) Generally measured 1 hour after infusion
      2) Notify physician if persistently greater than 2+
   c. Blood sugar monitoring: frequency dependent on stability of patient; attempt to keep glucose less than 200 mg/dL
   d. Weight gain/loss
      1) Measure at same time daily, with the patient wearing similar articles of clothing
      2) Expected weight gain or loss will vary with each patient, depending on rationale for therapy; weight gain therapy has an expected gain of approximately 0.5 to 1.0 pound/week; maintenance therapy is administered to maintain weight at a determined level
      3) Sudden losses or gains are indicators of fluid imbalance
   e. Intake and output/decreased or excessive urine output
      1) Teach to monitor intake and output
      2) Ideally, total intake should be approximately 500 ml greater than total output
      3) If patient develops new or increased peripheral edema or urine

output of less than 600 ml for 2 consecutive days, contact the physician; may indicate dehydration or fluid retention
    4) Urine output greater than 1700 ml/day in the average adult usually means that the patient is getting too much fluid
7. Instruction should be provided on how to manage emergencies until healthcare clinician can be contacted, such as clotted catheters, broken catheters, blood back-up in tubing, and malfunctioning equipment and physical complications such as air embolism
8. Care and storage of supplies
    a. Storage, refrigeration, and preparation of solution
    b. Prescription verification
    c. Expiration verification
    d. Visual inspection of solutions and supplies
    e. Use of syringes, vials, and ampules
    f. Clean work area and place for storage
9. Disposal of supplies: use of puncture-resistant container and procedure for disposal

E. Solution Administration Regimens

1. Continuous
    a. Continuous infusions at a steady rate, 24 hr/day, are not preferred for home infusion because of the limitations it places on the patient and caregiver
    b. Continuous infusion is desirable for patients who cannot tolerate a dextrose load and who have difficulty tolerating large quantities of fluid
    c. If the patient is ambulatory, portable infusion pumps should be considered to allow for activities of daily living
2. Cyclic
    a. Most home TPN patients prefer cyclic infusion and generally choose the evening and/or nighttime for their infusion
    b. Promotes independence and "normal" lifestyle
3. Supplemental infusions
    a. May be appropriate for patients who have limited gut function and/or inadequate oral intake
    b. Some insurance carriers may not reimburse for this type of therapy
4. Lipid emulsion delivery: may be administered concurrently by using a Y-connection below the filter on the parenteral nutrition tubing, or added directly to the TPN solution (three-in-one)

REFERENCES

1. Terry J, Baranowski L, Lonsway R, Hedrick C, eds. *Intravenous Therapy: Clinical Principles and Practice.* Philadelphia, PA: Saunders, 1995:219–248.
2. Holcomb B. Adult parenteral nutrition. In *Applied Therapeutics: The Clinical Use of Drugs,* 6th ed., edited by Young LY. Vancouver, WA: Applied Therapeutics, Inc, 1995.
3. Edwards RC. Pediatric nutrition. In *Applied Therapeutics: The Clinical Use of Drugs,* 6th ed., edited by Young LY. Vancouver, WA: Applied Therapeutics Inc, 1995.
4. Shizgal HM, Knowles JB. Peripheral amino acids. In *Total Parenteral Nutrition,* 2nd ed., edited by Fischer JE. Boston, MA: Little, Brown, 1991.
5. American Society for Parenteral and Enteral Nutrition. Guidelines for the use of parenteral and enteral nutrition. *Journal of Parenteral and Enteral Nutrition* 1993;17(4S):suppl.
6. Miller SJ. Peripheral parental nutrition: Theory and practice. *Hospital Pharmacy* 1991;26:796–801.
7. Grant J. *Handbook of Total Parenteral Nutrition.* Philadelphia, PA: Saunders, 1992.
8. Sax HC, Hasselgren P. Indications. In *Total Parenteral Nutrition,* 2nd ed., edited by Fischer JE. Boston, MA: Little, Brown, 1991.
9. Hill ID, Armando Madrazo-de la Garza J, Lebenthal E. Parenteral nutrition in pediatric patients. In *Clinical Nutrition: Parenteral Nutrition,* 2nd ed., edited by Rombeau JL, Caldwell MD. Philadelphia, PA: Saunders, 1993.
10. Warner BW. Parenteral nutrition in the pediatric patient. In *Total Parenteral Nutrition,* 2nd ed., edited by Fischer JE. Boston, MA: Little, Brown, 1991.
11. Hill GL. Nutritional assessment. In *Total Parenteral Nutrition,* 2nd ed., edited by Fischer JE. Boston, MA: Little, Brown, 1991.
12. Knox LS. Nutritional requirements. In *Nutritional Support Nursing Core Curriculum,* 2nd ed., edited by Kennedy-Caldwell C, Guenter P. Silver Spring, MD: Aspen, 1988.
13. Barbul A. Measurements of relevant nutrition data. In *Total Parenteral Nutrition,* 2nd ed., edited by Fischer JE. Boston, MA: Little, Brown, 1991.
14. Kinney JM. Clinical biochemistry: Implications for nutritional support. *Journal of Parenteral and Enteral Nutrition* 1990;14(5S):148–156.
15. O'Keefe SJD. Parenteral nutrition and liver disease. In *Clinical Nutrition: Parenteral Nutrition,* 2nd ed., edited by Rombeau JL, Caldwell MD. Philadelphia, PA: Saunders, 1993.
16. Dudrick PS, Souba WW. Special fuels in parenteral nutrition. In *Clinical Nutrition: Parenteral Nutrition,* 2nd ed., edited by Rombeau JL, Caldwell MD. Philadelphia, PA: Saunders, 1993.
17. Torosian MH, Daly JM. Solutions available. In *Total Parenteral Nutrition,* 2nd ed., edited by Fischer JE. Boston, MA: Little, Brown, 1991.
18. Dickerson RN, Brown RO, White KG. Parenteral nutrition solutions. In *Clinical Nutrition: Parenteral Nutrition,* 2nd ed., edited by Rombeau JL, Caldwell MD. Philadelphia, PA: Saunders, 1993.
19. Albina JE, Melnik G. Fluid, electrolyte, and body composition. In *Clinical Nutrition: Parenteral Nutrition,* 2nd ed., edited by Rombeau JL, Caldwell MD. Philadelphia, PA: Saunders, 1993.
20. LaFrance RJ, Miyagawa CI. Pharmaceutical considerations in TPN. In *Total Parenteral Nutrition,* 2nd ed., edited by Fischer JE. Boston, MA: Little, Brown, 1991.

21. Von Allmen D, Fischer JE. Metabolic complications. In *Total Parenteral Nutrition,* 2nd ed., edited by Fischer JE. Boston, MA: Little, Brown, 1991.

22. AMA Department of Food and Nutrition. Guidelines for essential trace element preparations for parenteral use: A statement by an expert panel. *Journal of the American Medical Association* 1979;241:2051.

23. AMA Department of Food and Nutrition. Multivitamin preparations for parenteral use: A statement by the Nutrition Advisory Group. *Journal of Parenteral and Enteral Nutrition* 1979;3:258.

24. Demetriou AA, Jones LK. Vitamins. In *Clinical Nutrition: Parenteral Nutrition,* 2nd ed., edited by Rombeau JL, Caldwell MD. Philadelphia, PA: Saunders, 1993.

25. Hiyama DT, Rolandelli R. Short bowel syndrome. In *Clinical Nutrition: Parenteral Nutrition,* 2nd ed., edited by Rombeau JL, Caldwell MD. Philadelphia, PA: Saunders, 1993.

26. Cohen MC, Driscoll DF, Bistrian BR. Parenteral nutrition in patients with cardiac disease. In *Clinical Nutrition: Parenteral Nutrition,* 2nd ed., edited by Rombeau JL, Caldwell MD. Philadelphia, PA: Saunders, 1993.

27. O'Keefe SJD. Parenteral nutrition and liver disease. In *Clinical Nutrition: Parenteral Nutrition,* 2nd ed., edited by Rombeau JL, Caldwell MD. Philadelphia, PA: Saunders, 1993.

28. Georges J. Renal failure. In *Nutritional Support Nursing: Core Curriculum,* 3rd ed., edited by Hennessey KA, Orr ME. Silver Spring, MD: Aspen, 1996.

29. Ziegler TR, Smith RJ. Parenteral nutrition in patients with diabetes mellitus. In *Clinical Nutrition: Parenteral Nutrition,* 2nd ed., edited by Rombeau JL, Caldwell MD. Philadelphia, PA: Saunders, 1993.

30. Gaare JM, Manner T, Wiese S, et al. Nutrition in pulmonary diseases. In *Clinical Nutrition: Parenteral Nutrition,* 2nd ed., edited by Rombeau JL, Caldwell MD. Philadelphia, PA: Saunders, 1993.

31. Norton JA, Thom AK. Parenteral nutrition and the patient with cancer. In *Clinical Nutrition: Parenteral Nutrition,* 2nd ed., edited by Rombeau JL, Caldwell MD. Philadelphia, PA: Saunders, 1993.

32. Kotler DP, Tierney AR, Culpepper-Morgan JA, et al. Effect of home total parenteral nutrition on body composition in patients with acquired immunodeficiency syndrome. *Journal of Parenteral and Enteral Nutrition* 1990;14(5):454–458.

33. Raiten DJ. Nutrition and HIV infection: A review and evaluation of the extant knowledge of the relationship between nutrition and HIV infection. *Nutrition in Clinical Practice* 1991;6(5S):1–94.

34. Frankel WL, Evans NJ, Rombeau JL. Scientific rationale and clinical application of parenteral nutrition in critically ill patients. In *Clinical Nutrition: Parenteral Nutrition,* 2nd ed., edited by Rombeau JL, Caldwell MD. Philadelphia, PA: Saunders, 1993.

35. Bessey PQ. Parenteral nutrition and trauma. In *Clinical Nutrition: Parenteral Nutrition,* 2nd ed., edited by Rombeau JL, Caldwell MD. Philadelphia, PA: Saunders, 1993.

36. Goodwin CW. Parenteral nutrition in thermal injuries. In *Clinical Nutrition: Parenteral Nutrition,* 2nd ed., edited by Rombeau JL, Caldwell MD. Philadelphia, PA: Saunders, 1993.

37. Curtas S. Nutritional assessment. In *Nutritional Support Nursing Core Curriculum,* 2nd ed., edited by Kennedy-Caldwell C, Guenter P. Silver Spring, MD: Aspen, 1988.

38. Fletcher JP, Little JM, Guest PK. A comparison of transferrin and serum prealbu-

min as nutritional parameters. *Journal of Parenteral and Enteral Nutrition* 1987;11:144.

39. Smith LC, Mullen JL. Nutritional assessment and indications for nutritional support. *Surgical Clinics of North America* 1991;71:449M–458.

40. Bower RH. Nutrition and immune function. *Nutrition in Clinical Practice* 1990;5(5):189–195.

41. Jeejeebhoy KN, Detsky AS, Baker JP. Assessment of nutritional status. *Journal of Parenteral and Enteral Nutrition* 1990;14(5S):193–196.

42. Marcuard SP, Dunham B, Hobbs A, et al. Availability of insulin from total parenteral solutions. *Journal of Parenteral and Enteral Nutrition* 1990;14(3):262–254.

43. Rollins CJ, Elsberry VA, Pollack KA. Three-in-one parenteral nutrition: A safe and economical method of nutritional support in infants. *Journal of Parenteral and Enteral Nutrition* 1990;14(3):290–294.

44. Hoheim DF, O'Callaghan TA, Joswiak BJ, et al. Clinical experience with three-in-one admixtures administered peripherally. *Nutrition in Clinical Practice* 1990;5(3):118–122.

45. Thompson B, Robinson LA. Infection control of parenteral nutrition solutions. *Nutrition in Clinical Practice* 1991;6(2):49–53.

46. Alvarado-Highes M, Helms RA. Pediatric parenteral protein formulas. *Hospital Pharmacy* 1989;24:551–555.

47. Hiyama DT, Fischer JE. Nutritional support in hepatic failure: The current role of disease-specific therapy. In *Total Parenteral Nutrition*, 2nd ed., edited by Fischer JE. Boston, MA: Little, Brown, 1991.

48. Jeejeebhoy KN. Lipid emulsions. In *Total Parenteral Nutrition*, 2nd ed., edited by Fischer JE. Boston, MA: Little, Brown, 1991.

49. Bennet KM, Rosen GH. Cyclic total parenteral nutrition. *Nutrition in Clinical Practice* 1990;5(4):163–165.

50. Stranz MH, Sacher Barfood K. Total parenteral nutrition: Compatibility of antibiotic admixtures. *Journal of Intravenous Nursing* 1988;11(1):43–48.

51. Intravenous Nurses Society. Intravenous Nursing Standards of Practice (revised 1998). *Journal of Intravenous Nursing* 1998;21(1):suppl.

52. Flowers JF, Ryan JA, Gough JA. Catheter-related complications of TPN. In *Total Parenteral Nutrition*, 2nd ed., edited by Fischer JE. Boston, MA: Little, Brown, 1991.

53. Pennington CR, Pithie AD. Ethanol lock in the management of catheter occlusion. *Journal of Parenteral and Enteral Nutrition* 1987;8:507–508.

54. Breaux CW, Duke D, Georgeson KE, et al. Calcium phosphate crystal occlusion of central venous catheters used for total parenteral nutrition in infants and children: Prevention and treatment. *Journal of Pediatric Surgery* 1987;22:829–832.

55. Thompson B, Robinson LA. Infection control of parenteral nutrition solutions. *Nutrition in Clinical Practice* 1991;6(2):49–53.

CHAPTER 9

Quality Assurance

Deborah B. Benvenuto, CRNI

I. QUALITY PROGRAMS

A. Overview

1. Quality is a commitment to achieving excellence
   a. Not a singular activity
   b. Variety of behaviors and actions are involved
      1) Occurs on a continuum
      2) Seeks to improve outcomes by improving processes
      3) Cannot be assured but rather managed and improved on
2. Quality is a process that can be measured, monitored, and evaluated
   a. Comparison of actual outcomes against desired outcomes
   b. Challenge of providing high-volume, high-risk therapies safely
      1) Competent expertise, knowledge, and dedicated, detailed monitoring required
      2) Positive patient outcomes ensured
      3) Resultant cost-effective and efficient care
3. Quality programs provide a framework
   a. Identification of areas for improvement
   b. Evaluation of corrective action
   c. Development of accountability by clinicians
   d. Monitoring progress
4. Quality programs should ensure timely, appropriate interventions by identifying accountability
   a. Accountability is defined by knowledge, skills, judgment, and experience expected of practitioners
      1) Assignment to an autonomous group of individuals
      2) Ultimate goal to enhance and ensure positive outcomes
      3) Problem-solving, planning, and process and outcome evaluation
   b. Competency inferred through accountability via application of knowledge and skills
   c. Critical thinking is essential
5. Quality program formats are similar to the nursing process and are ongoing
   a. Assessment

        b. Diagnosis

        c. Planning

        d. Implementation

        e. Evaluation with monitoring of desired outcomes

    6. Participation in a quality program involves several elements

        a. Awareness of factors that identify, evaluate, and measure outcomes

        b. Review of data retrieval, collection, and analysis

        c. Review of methodology for implementing corrective actions based on needed outcomes

        d. Problem identification and reasons for deficiencies

    7. Following are other terms for quality programs

        a. Quality assurance

        b. Total quality management

        c. Performance improvement

            1) Current term for satisfying documentation processes and strategies in organizational efforts to ensure positive patient outcomes

            2) Performance dependent on what is done and how well it is done

            3) Processes involved with organization's approach to improving its performance

              • Process design

              • Performance measurement

              • Performance assessment

              • Performance improvement

            4) Approach based on real work of healthcare professionals and real improvements that can be achieved to benefit patients

        d. Total quality improvement

        e. Continuous quality improvement

B. Criteria

    1. Structure

        a. Resource and framework for care delivery

            1) Organizational

            2) Physical

            3) Human

            4) Financial

        b. Rules of the organization and its domain or governance

    2. Process

        a. Combined tasks and activities directly affecting patient care

        b. Practitioner focused

            1) Specific job description

            2) Role delineation

            3) Defined responsibilities and duties

    3. Outcomes

        a. Positive or negative results of activities or tasks

        b. Patient-focused

  c. Reflective of desired goal of actual care provider
 4. Corrective action
  a. Measures instituted for outcome improvement
  b. Determined by deviation from expected outcomes (deficiencies)
  c. Various methods used
   1) Education
   2) Communication
   3) Criteria change
   4) Performance revision
   5) Desire for change
 5. Re-evaluation
  a. Monitoring outcomes of corrective action
  b. Measurement of corrective action
   1) Reappraisal of problem or deficiency
   2) Comparison of pre-outcome with post-outcome data
   3) Validation of deficiency
  c. Remedial effects
   1) Positive or negative
   2) Validation
   3) Conscientious application
   4) Increased knowledge
   5) Reduced risk for error

II. COMPONENTS OF A QUALITY PROGRAM

A. Knowledgeable Staff

 1. Considered an integral component within a sound quality program
 2. Developed through well-constructed and measurable orientation
  programs, validation of competency, and ongoing education
  a. Orientation to introduce the nurse to organizational and
   departmental structure, policies, and procedures
   1) Familiarizes nurse with specific tasks, duties, and functions
   2) Includes didactic and clinical education
   3) Ranges from several days to several weeks depending on the
    individual
  b. Validation of competency established by organizational and
   departmental policies
   1) Includes accountability, communication, collaboration, and
    autonomy
   2) Emphasizes tasks and functions performed (competencies) with
    high-risk, high-volume ones most essential to validate
    • Proficiency in clinical aspects including clinical judgment and
     practice
    • Guidelines for practitioner
    • Format for design and development of orientation and
     continuing education programs

- Validation at established intervals (usually by the employing organization), such as annually or biannually
3) Involves observation of demonstrated clinical skills, judgment, and expertise; termed "competency" or "certification" of staff
4) Includes certification on national level
   - Method for regulating and protecting specialized practitioners
   - Expert method for ensuring expert quality healthcare delivery to the public
   - Identification of a healthcare professional practicing on a higher, more advanced level than determined by licensure
5) Provides opportunities for recertification
   - Device or documentation tool for re-evaluating and updating skills and competencies of specialists
   - Continued adherence to organizational policies and procedures in compliance with federal and state regulatory laws and the specialty's national guidelines
6) Certain requirements for recertification
   - Documentation of ongoing education
   - Proof of current licensure
   - Validation of clinical experience and current active credentials within specific practice area
   c. Continuing education is vital for maintenance and continued growth of the specialty
   1) Involves active participation in programs and sharing of information with other healthcare professionals
   2) Required for all nurses
      - Proof of continuing education required by many states for relicensure
      - Assurance to the public that practitioner is current with professional practice
   3) Provides new information relative to advances in technology and practice

B. Policies and Procedures

1. Direct practice within a specific organization
   a. Identify acceptable courses of action for various personnel
   b. Reviewed annually
   c. Periodically revised when appropriate
   d. Represent organizational and national standards
2. Policy
   a. Defined as a course or method of action
   b. Must be specific, concise, and clinically sound
   c. Must be achievable within the resources of the organization
   d. Must be written and formally approved by the organization it is designed to serve
   e. Based on state law, federal regulations, standards of practice, and the state of the art in the practice area

f. Must be circulated, revised as necessary

g. Must have documentation present verifying annual review

3. Procedure

    a. Outlines a series of definite steps and responsibilities

    b. Reflects current standards of practice

    c. Complies with federal and state laws

    d. Based on state law, federal regulations, standards of practice, and the state of the art in the practice area

4. Policy and procedure manual

    a. Identifies acceptable courses of action for various personnel

        1) Reviewed annually

        2) Revised periodically when appropriate

    b. Represents organizational standards

    c. Reflects national standards

5. Job description

    a. Describes the functions of a particular role

    b. Further defines tasks and activities necessary to fulfill a role successfully

    c. Clinically sound and performance-based

    d. Provides for self-inventory

    e. Addresses achievable behaviors and actions

        1) Stated in measurable terms using measurable statements

        2) Assists in the identification and resolution of performance problems

    f. Reviewed annually, and revised as necessary

6. Documentation

    a. Describes the care given relative to assessment, intervention, and outcomes

    b. Recorded as part of the patient's medical record

        1) Accurate, succinct description of care rendered to patient

        2) Legible and timely, including facility-approved abbreviations

        3) Initial and ongoing assessments and nursing interventions

        4) Communication of essential findings to physician and others involved in patient's care

        5) Intravenous access device

          • Type of cannula, including brand name

          • Location

          • Gauge and length

          • Date of insertion

          • Site care and condition according to established intervals along with necessary interventions

        6) Patient and caregiver education

        7) Author's signature

    c. Forms approved for use by the healthcare facility

        1) Plans of care

        2) Flow sheets

        3) Monitoring tools

4) Quality control check lists
5) Unusual Occurrence Report (incident report)
- Written description of occurrence
- Risk management tool
- Provides specific facts concerning an event or incident that may result in risk exposure (actual or potential injury)
- Addresses immediate follow-up to determine possible causes
- Internal (e.g., within the healthcare facility) reporting mechanism notifying the organization that such an event has occurred
- Provides opportunity for investigation of the situation in its entirety
- Must be objective, reporting the nature of the occurrence, including assessment of patient's condition before the occurrence with results of the occurrence and/or injury
- Is not referenced in patient's medical record
- May be considered as the only evidence demonstrating that nursing actions met the legal standard of care
6) Adverse drug reaction
- Required by the Food and Drug Administration (FDA)
- Allows monitoring of unusual drug reactions/interactions

III. QUALITY MEASURES: STANDARDS

A. Overview

1. Framework for monitoring care and products used in the delivery of care (i.e., infusion therapy)
   a. Value-driven
   b. Combination of individual, societal, institutional, and professional values
2. Framework from which specific distinctions can be differentiated with litigation
   a. Malpractice
   b. Product failure
   c. Noncompliance
   d. Other occurrences
3. Method for resolving ethical conflicts between the healthcare professional's duty to the patient and position as an employee within the healthcare organization

B. Classification

1. Process standards
   a. Govern actual tasks by describing the functions/tasks to be performed
   b. Observable and measurable

     c. Evaluated through documentation

  2. Structural standards

     a. Mission, philosophy, and goal statements of the organization

     b. Institutional or organizational policies and procedures

       1) Rules that govern action

       2) Non-negotiable

       3) Example: approved drug list

  3. Outcome standards

     a. Focused on the end result and reflective of desired goals

     b. Often expressed in negative terms (i.e., phlebitis rate)

     c. Most frequently linked to process standards

C. Types

  1. Standards of patient care

     a. Focus on the recipient of care

     b. Define expected patient outcome and expectations of the healthcare provider

  2. Standards of professional practice

     a. Focus on the provider of care

     b. Structure and processes used by the healthcare professional

  3. Standards of performance

     a. Evolutionary process originating from organizational job descriptions

     b. Define the levels of performance required for the job

     c. Further assist in the performance evaluation of the nurse

     d. Integrate components of, and conversely correlate with, the healthcare organization's quality or performance programs

     e. Include practice guidelines

       1) Protocols specifying care for a patient in a particular situation

       2) Complementary to procedures and practice guidelines

       3) Basis for clinical decision-making in specific patient care activities

IV. LEGAL ASPECTS

A. Overview

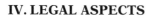

  1. Legal standards are an integral component of a quality program

  2. Two types of legal activities pertinent to intravenous therapy practice are criminal and civil law

     a. Criminal law involves an offense against the general public

       1) Primary emphasis defines behaviors prohibited or controlled by society as a whole

       2) Criminal offenses are prosecuted by a government authority

       3) May result in fines or imprisonment, or both

     b. Civil law applies to the legal rights of private individuals or organizations; includes medical negligence or malpractice

B. Negligence

1. Defined as not performing an activity that a reasonable lay person would comparatively do in a similar situation
2. Carrying out an activity that a reasonable person would not in similar circumstances is considered to be negligent
3. A claim of negligence must meet certain criteria to be considered valid
   a. Must be established that the person had proprietary ownership of the duty/task
   b. Standards of care were not met
   c. Injured party received injury as a result
   d. Proof of breach of duty must be validated without question
4. Malpractice is defined as negligent conduct on the part of a member of a recognized accountable profession
   a. Further defined as a deviation from the professional standard of practice that a qualified healthcare provider in the identical area of practice would follow in a similar situation
   b. May be considered synonymous with professional negligence because failure to act in a reasonable and prudent manner, as defined by the profession, may result in harm to the patient
   c. Denotes stepping beyond one's authority
      1) State Nurse Practice Act defines scope of nursing practice
      2) Performing a procedure outside the boundaries of nursing practice may be ruled illegal and in violation of the State Nurse Practice Act
   d. Common areas of nursing malpractice
      1) Medication administration
      2) Equipment use
      3) Lack of communication
      4) Failure to act; for example, failing to clarify an illegible order for intravenous medication and its administration

C. Torts

1. Civil offense that occurs as a private wrong against another person or property
   a. Usually based on some type of fault
      1) Procedure performed incorrectly
      2) Task that should have been done and was not
   b. Possibly intentional or a result from an act of negligence
2. May be differentiated based on the type of offense
   a. Assault
      1) Coercion of a person or perceived threat by another causing apprehension of being touched in an offensive or potentially injurious way

2) Absence of actual physical contact
  - A competent adult patient refuses to undergo venipuncture but the nurse proceeds to assemble necessary equipment and prepares to perform procedure

b. Battery
  1) Unlawful carrying out of threatened physical harm
  2) Physical contact of a competent adult patient without permission
    - Nurse applies the tourniquet and performs the insertion procedure without patient's permission

c. Coercion
  1) Forcing a person to act in a certain manner
  2) Involves threats or intimidation
    - Competent adult patient does not want a venipuncture
    - Nurse forces patient into accepting an unwanted venipuncture

d. False imprisonment
  1) Act of placing an individual in a confined area against his or her will
  2) Often involves restraints
    - Nurse places a restraint on a patient in an effort to preserve integrity of a venipuncture site, post-insertion
    - The use of the restraint may be contrary to organizational policy

e. Slander
  1) Communication that may damage a person's reputation through the use of false and/or malicious statements
  2) Oral or written

f. Disclosure of confidential information
  1) Act of providing private and confidential information concerning a patient and diagnosis, matters pertaining to his or her care, and prognosis to uninvolved persons
  2) Absence of expressed patient permission

D. Informed Consent

1. The educational process allows the patient to be given sufficient information to fully comprehend the procedure at hand
   a. Intended consequences or expected outcomes of the procedure
   b. Expectations of compliance and behavior of the patient during the procedure
2. Patient freely and willingly consents to the procedure
   a. Capable of granting consent via authorized signature or via a legally recognized, approved, and associated third party
   b. Absence of coercion witnessed by a third party
   c. Usually verbal; written agreement necessary if determined by organizational policy
3. Emergency consent may be obtained when there is an immediate need for consent

a. According to organizational policy, a witnessed telephone or verbal consent may be valid within specified parameters and time constraints

b. Obtain from a person legally authorized to give consent

1) A minor child brought to the emergency department by someone other than the custodial parent; consent must be obtained from the legal guardian unless there is a life-threatening emergency

c. Increased awareness needed in today's era of blended or extended family units versus traditional families; a family member may not be the child's legal guardian

4. Investigational therapies require special informed consent that is obtained by the principal investigator of a research study

E. Rule of Personal Liability

1. Legal responsibility to fulfill an obligation
2. Each person is responsible for his or her own actions

a. The nurse is a knowledgeable professional, capable of independent judgment and actions inherent in professional nursing practice

b. The nurse's role in carrying out or questioning physicians' orders has increased nursing autonomy and legal responsibilities

c. The nurse must be able to evaluate medical orders as they apply to the patient and the intended plan of care

d. The nurse must question any order believed not to be in the patient's best interest before implementation

V. REGULATING AGENCIES

A. Overview

1. Mandates that directly or indirectly impact the role of the healthcare practitioner (intravenous nurse specialist)
2. Federal, state, and professional levels of regulation

B. Food and Drug Administration (FDA)

1. Controls testing, manufacturing, labeling, and distribution of drugs, cosmetics, and medical devices
2. Procedures and forms for reporting occurrences must be contained within the framework of a quality program
3. Reportable occurrences include but are not limited to

a. Malfunctioning infusion equipment
b. Transfusion-related deaths
c. Faulty labeling or packaging
d. Drug-related incidences

C. Occupational Safety and Health Administration (OSHA)

1. Oversees compliance with safety procedures, including occupational exposure to bloodborne pathogens

2. Standard precautions and the use of protective devices fall under the auspices of OSHA

3. Employers bear the responsibility and expense for employee compliance with these mandates

D. Joint Commission on Accreditation of Healthcare Organizations (JCAHO)

1. Has ongoing programs designed to ensure that healthcare organizations provide a high level of quality in patient care and health service delivery

2. Can approve healthcare organizations as Medicare-certified providers

E. State Regulatory Boards

1. State agencies establish policies regarding professional licensure, joint policy statements, and licensing of healthcare facilities

2. State Boards of Nursing are responsible for the development, implementation, and compliance to practice guidelines identified in the State Nurse Practice Act

   a. State Nurse Practice Act varies from state to state

      1) Some delineate and detail nursing functions critically

      2) Others establish broad parameters

   b. Defines the practice of professional and licensed practical/vocational nursing within the specific state

   c. Delineates specific rules as to how the nurse is allowed to legally participate within the profession

   d. Nursing Boards of Registration establish the minimal requirements for licensure (the basic entry mechanism for nursing practice) to be met within the borders of a particular state

   e. The State Board is empowered to suspend or revoke the license of any nurse for violation of specific measures of professional conduct for that specific state

F. Professional Organizations

1. Intravenous Nurses Society (INS)

   a. Developed the *Intravenous Nursing Standards of Practice*

   b. Periodically reviewed and updated when appropriate

      1) Reflective of current clinical principles and practice specific to intravenous nursing

      2) Applicable to all practice settings

   c. Established a credentialing program for the public's protection through the Intravenous Nurses Certification Corporation (INCC)

      1) Certification assures a higher level of knowledge and expertise than licensure

      2) Certified Registered Nurse Intravenous (CRNI) or Certified Licensed Nurse Intravenous (CLNI) as the measure for quality equating to positive patient outcomes

2. Other associations interface with the practice of intravenous/infusion nursing
   a. American Association of Blood Banks (AABB), Association for Professionals in Infection Control and Epidemiology (APIC), and the American Society of Health-System Pharmacists (ASHP)
   b. Participate in developing guidelines beneficial to enhance the practice of intravenous nursing

VI. QUALITY INFUSION PROGRAMS
A. Overview
1. Provision of high-volume, high-risk infusion therapy safely via competent expertise, knowledge, and dedicated, detailed monitoring
2. Ensure positive patient outcomes
3. Opportunities for identifying strategies to implement planned action to positively affect the level of care for patients requiring and receiving infusion therapy
4. Goal development
   a. Ensure the best intravenous care possible
      1) Establish regional, state, and national guidelines as the foundation
      2) Quality controls
      3) Direct compliance by intravenous nurse specialist
      4) Specific plan coordination
      5) Regulation through analysis
   b. Decrease the incidence of intravenous complications
      1) Identify deficiencies
      2) Evaluate corrective actions
      3) Assign accountability
   c. Assure timely, appropriate intervention
      1) Accountability via demonstrable knowledge, skills, judgment, and experience
      2) Documentation
      3) Corrective action and re-evaluation

B. *Intravenous Nursing Standards of Practice*
1. Basis for intravenous practice
   a. Policies and procedures written from the *Intravenous Nursing Standards of Practice*
   b. Outcomes measured by the *Intravenous Nursing Standards of Practice*
   c. Same standards, regardless of practice setting
2. Examples
   a. Cannula selection, site preparation, and site care
      1) Use of gloves
      2) Aseptic technique and standard precautions

3) Use of sterile dressings
4) Minimal patient discomfort
5) Maximum number of attempts

b. Cannula removal, including site rotation, according to the *Intravenous Nursing Standards of Practice*

c. Intravenous set changes

d. Documentation
1) Intravenous device and procedure
  • Prescribed therapy and treatment
  • Observed complications
  • Appropriate nursing assessments
2) Cannula removal for infiltrated site
  • Condition of surrounding tissue
  • Integrity of cannula
  • Name of person removing cannula
3) Signs and symptoms of existing complications
  • Intravenous discontinuation
  • Physician notification
  • Unusual occurrence report

C. Safe Administration of Intravenous Medications

1. Governed by federal and state regulations
2. Dependent on well-established structural components
   a. Approved drug list of the healthcare organization
   1) Additions or deletions approved by pharmacy and other organizational committees
   2) Adheres to healthcare organization policies
   b. IV push drug list
3. Administer for intended therapeutic outcomes
   a. Comply with approved usage guidelines
   b. Adhere to recommended rate and route of administration
   c. Observe drug stability and incompatibility data
   d. Monitor and report side effects, toxicities, and unusual occurrences
   e. Initiate appropriate nursing interventions
   f. Adhere to aseptic technique
   g. Document

D. Safe Administration of Investigational Drugs

1. Determined by specific guidelines, policies, and procedures
2. Controlled usage based on specific criteria
   a. Specific institutional policies and procedures
   b. Medical staff monitoring
   c. Patient consent
   d. Institutional review process
3. Administer under direction of principal investigator
   a. Is a member of the medical staff

b. Is responsible for obtaining informed consent
4. Provide information available regarding investigational drugs
   a. Dosage forms
   b. Strengths available
   c. Actions
   d. Uses; only for approved clinical conditions of the investigation
   e. Side effects
   f. Signs of toxicity
5. Adherence by the professional nurse to the correct validation procedure before administration
   a. Signed informed consent is obtained and on file
   b. Policies and procedures are on file
   c. Drug is approved by the appropriate organizational committee
   d. Drug is on the organization's approved investigational drug list
   e. Review action, dosage, side effects, and symptoms of toxicity

E. Safe Administration of Blood Component Therapy

1. Based on federal and state regulations; law requires transfusion-related deaths be reported to the FDA
2. Determined by organizational policies and procedures
   a. Return blood not initiated within 30 minutes after dispensation from the blood bank
   b. Divide into aliquots, if ordered to be infused over a time period greater than 4 hours
   c. Close patient monitoring for the first 15 minutes after initiation of infusion
   d. Immediate discontinuation at the first sign of a reaction
      1) Tubing disconnected at cannula adapter or hub
      2) 0.9% sodium chloride infusion started using new administration set

F. Safe Administration of Intravenous Antineoplastic Therapies

1. Determined by organizational policies and procedures and recommended guidelines and protocols
2. Includes a published approved list of antineoplastic agents
3. Provides a clear definition of appropriate nursing interventions related to reduction of possible complications
   a. Extravasation protocols
      1) Application of heat or ice to area of extravasation
      2) Cannula removal before or after administration of neutralizing antidotal medication
   b. Spill protocols; e.g., spill of mechlorethamine hydrochloride (Mustargen) neutralized with an equal volume of sodium thiosulfate and 5% sodium bicarbonate
   c. Vesicant drug administration in a multiple drug protocol
   d. Biohazardous cytotoxic waste preparation and disposal

1) No glove material is impervious to all drugs, but considerable protection against inadvertent skin contact is provided
2) Latex is the material of choice for protecting against accidental exposure
3) Disposal of hazardous agents and materials in specially designed containers by qualified and certified waste handlers
4) Waste tracking system

VII. QUALITY INFUSION PROGRAM PROCESS AND OUTCOMES

A. Overview

1. Monitoring by an intravenous nurse specialist is critical to the success of the organization's quality infusion program
2. Important as a method of patient protection
3. The process is most beneficial when operating simultaneously with infusion care delivery
4. A quality infusion program consists of
   a. Establishing standards
   b. Monitoring practice
   c. Evaluating outcomes
   d. Implementing corrective actions
5. Involves risk management
   a. Identifying unfavorable conditions
   b. Investigating unfavorable conditions
   c. Controlling unfavorable conditions
6. Quality model focuses on inspection
   a. Reactive model
   b. Concerned with individual correction and process improvement
   c. All parties are involved in delivery without responsibility and accountability for patient and system outcome
7. Improvement model crosses territorial lines
   a. Active participation by all players
   b. All levels of personnel participating in problem-solving exercises
   c. Concentration on process and customer perceptions

B. Quality Mechanisms

1. Identify the problem and its effect on patient care; e.g., increased phlebitis rate, poor documentation, or excessive use of catheters
2. Review performance criteria and outcomes
   a. Collect data to determine if standards were met
      1) Is retrospective or concurrent
      2) Identifies controllable or uncontrollable variations
         • Controllable variations, such as system deficiencies or lack of knowledge, usually correctable

- Uncontrollable variations such as unpredictable events are usually not correctable
  b. Determine the cause of the problem by comparing actual care with established standards
  c. Develop and implement a plan of action for improvement
    1) Obtain input from individuals responsible for implementing action
    2) Focus on specific issues; be realistic and flexible
    3) Establish a target date for implementation and review
    4) Focus on corrective action
       - Education: providing staff with the knowledge needed to perform appropriately
       - Development of employee skills and abilities
       - Communication of expected outcomes and means to achieve them
       - Development of strategies for change
  d. Re-evaluate to determine if corrective action is effective and improvement in service is obtained

C. Data Retrieval, Collection, and Analysis

1. Documentation of infusion care allows for data retrieval
2. Data may be collected by interview, observation, or visual inspection
3. Solid data analysis depends on equally solid data collection techniques
   a. Various tools may be used for ongoing analysis
      1) Fishbone diagram
         - Groups individual factors under broad categories
         - Includes management, staff mix, materials, and methods
      2) Flow charts: sequence of events within a given time period
      3) Run charts: sequence of events over a pre-established time period
      4) Parieto charting: order of importance in determining priorities
   b. Monitoring tools, such as audits, are used in data collection
4. Tool should establish outcome criteria for the audit and state the expected desired compliance rate
   a. Data are retrievable
   b. Criteria are measurable
   c. Current knowledge is reflected
5. Once completed and analyzed, problems can be identified
   a. Criteria are developed to further evaluate possible causes of the identified problem
   b. Individual and combined factors are examined
      1) Procedural events
      2) Techniques

    3) Equipment
    4) Skills
    5) Patient acuity level
  c. Possible deficiencies are identified
    1) Lack of knowledge
      • Education
      • Review
      • Practice
      • Feedback
    2) Lack of performances
      • Task interference
      • Lack of feedback
      • Indifference
      • Deficiencies
      • Lack of willingness to adapt to change

D. Data Translation

1. Assessing data means translating it into information for use in drawing conclusions about performance
2. Requires the use of indicators quantified by reporting trends
  a. Process indicators are determined by dividing the number of times a process is successfully completed by the number of times the process was performed
  b. Outcome indicators are stated as the number of occurrences divided by the total number of patients at risk
3. Results are classified as either sentinel or rate-based occurrences
  a. Sentinel occurrences are serious, undesirable and unpredictable outcomes that require organizational investigation each time an event occurs; e.g., ruptured central venous access device
  b. Rate-based occurrences refer to events in which a certain proportion of events are representative of care
    1) Intensive review only if rate obtained exceeding pre-set or expected level or if significant trend identified
    2) Examples include medication errors and phlebitis rates
4. Thresholds are established for sentinel and rate-based occurrences
  a. For sentinel events: expected rates for compliance are 100%; for noncompliance, 0%
  b. For rate-based events: expected compliance rates may be set lower than 100% but more than 0%; e.g., a rate-based occurrence threshold of 5% or less is used for phlebitis
5. Conclusions about current performance-based assessments may indicate a need for more intensive measurement and assessment
  a. Interpretive comparison with past performances
  b. Others' performance
  c. Practice guidelines
  d. Scientific literature

e. Best available practice
6. Data assessment must be interdisciplinary when appropriate

E. Corrective Action

1. Necessary when deviation from the expected outcome occurs
2. Two major forms of deficiencies require corrective action
   a. Knowledge
   b. Performance
3. Several methods may be used for corrective action
   a. Education
   b. Communication
   c. Criteria change
   d. Performance review
   e. Desire for change
4. Examples of corrective action
   a. Tamper-proof sharp containers
      1) Installed in patients' rooms
      2) Installed at "shoulder height"
      3) Emptied regularly and when needed
   b. Lack of compliance with standard precautions
      1) Determine availability of necessary equipment
      2) Review organizational policy and procedure with staff
   c. Administration set audit revealing 60% are not properly labeled: provide staff inservice on tubing/label policy
   d. Policy stating continuous nonvesicant antineoplastic medication be infused by an electronic infusion device (EID)
      1) Re-assess control of EIDs
      2) Investigate and develop alternative methods to coordinate and provide instrumentation
      3) Re-assess deployment of EIDs throughout organization
      4) Re-evaluate corrective action

F. Re-Evaluation

1. Evaluation of corrective action is vital to ensure that desired results/outcomes have been achieved and/or maintained
2. Corrective action is measured by reappraising the problem/deficiency
3. Pre-action data are compared with post-action data
4. Deficiency is validated
5. Example: phlebitis rate is greater than that recommended in the *Intravenous Nursing Standards of Practice*
   a. Corrective action is taken
   b. Re-evaluate plan of action after 6 months by re-audit
6. Remedial effects can be positive or negative
   a. Positive effects
      1) Validation
      2) Conscientious application

3) Increased knowledge
4) Reduced risk of error
5) Reduced intravenous hazards
b. Negative effects
1) Development of another plan
2) Need to re-evaluate outcome

G. JCAHO Model for Quality Management

1. Most accepted process for quality management
2. Refer to currently accepted framework for implementation

REFERENCES

Baldwin DR. Quality management. In *Intravenous Therapy: Clinical Principles and Practice,* edited by Terry J, Baranowski L, Lonsway RA, Hedrick C. Philadelphia, PA: Saunders, 1995:47–67.

Dugger B. Intravenous nursing competency: Why is it important? *Journal of Intravenous Nursing* 1997;20(6):287–297.

Intravenous Nurses Society. *Intravenous Nursing Standards of Practice* (revised 1998). *Journal of Intravenous Nursing* 1998;21(1): suppl.

Katz J, Green E. *Managing Quality: A Guide to System-Wide Performance Management in Healthcare,* 2nd ed. St. Louis, MO: Mosby, 1996.

Meisenheimer CG. *Improving Quality: A Guide to Effective Programs,* 2nd ed. Gaithersburg, MD: Aspen Publications, 1997.

Miller RD. *Problems in Hospital Law,* 7th ed. Gaithersburg, MD: Aspen Publications, 1996.

Phillips L. *Manual of IV Therapeutics,* 2nd ed. Philadelphia, PA: FA Davis, 1997.

Schroeder P. *Improving Quality and Performance: Concepts, Programs, and Techniques.* St, Louis, MO: Mosby, 1994.

Terry J, ed. *Intravenous Therapy: Clinical Principles and Practice.* Philadelphia, PA: Saunders, 1995.

1997–1998 Comprehensive Accreditation Manual for Home Care. "Improving Organization Performance." Joint Commission on Accreditation of Health Care Organizations. Oakbrook Terrace, IL: 267–294.

Summary of Centers for Disease Control and Prevention Standard Precautions

Guidelines and Procedures for Establishing Specific Precautions

STANDARD PRECAUTIONS

Guidelines for Use

Use Standard Precautions for the care of all patients.

Procedures for Implementing

- Wash hands after touching blood, body fluids, secretions, excretions, and contaminated items, regardless of whether gloves are worn. Wash hands immediately after gloves are removed, between patient contacts, and whenever indicated to prevent transfer of microorganisms to other patients or environments. Use plain soap for routine hand washing and an antimicrobial or waterless antiseptic agent for specific circumstances.
- Wear clean nonsterile gloves when touching blood, body fluids, excretions or secretions, contaminated items, mucous membranes, and non-intact skin. Change gloves between tasks on the same patient as necessary and remove gloves promptly after use.
- Wear mask, eye protection, or face shield during procedures and care activities that are likely to generate splashes or sprays of blood or body fluids. Use gown to protect skin and prevent soiling of clothing.
- Ensure that used patient care equipment that is soiled with blood or identified body fluids, secretions, and excretions is handled carefully to prevent transfer of microorganisms, or cleaned and appropriately reprocessed if used for another patient.
- Use adequate environmental controls to ensure that routine care, cleaning, and disinfection procedures are followed.

- Handle, transport, and process linen soiled with blood and body fluids, excretions, and secretions in a manner that prevents skin and mucous membrane exposures, contamination of clothing, and transfer of microorganisms.
- Use previously identified techniques and equipment to prevent injuries when using needles, sharps, and scalpels, and place these items in appropriate puncture-resistant containers after use.

(Adapted from Centers for Disease Control and Prevention. Guidelines for isolation precautions in hospitals. Part II: Recommendations for isolation precautions in hospitals. *American Journal of Infection Control* 1996;24(1): 32–52.)

Calculations for Computing Flow Rate

1. Drops per minute:

   To calculate drops per minute (gtt/min), multiply the infusion rate in milliliters per hour (ml/hr) by the drop factor (gtt/ml) and divide by 60 to convert hours (hr) to minutes (min).

   Example: Calculate drops (gtt) of solution per minute (min) if the infusion rate is 120 ml/hr and the drop factor is 10 gtt/ml.

   $$\frac{gtt}{min} = \frac{ml \text{ of solution}}{hr} \times \frac{gtt}{ml} \times \frac{hr}{60 \text{ min}}$$

   $$= \frac{120 \text{ ml}}{hr} \times \frac{10 \text{ gtt}}{ml} \times \frac{hr}{60 \text{ min}}$$

   $$= \frac{(120 \times 10) \text{ gtt}}{60 \text{ min}} = \frac{20 \text{ gtt}}{min}$$

2. Milliliters per hour:

   Example: Calculate the number of milliliters (ml) per hour (hr) to infuse 1000 ml over 8 hours.

   $$\frac{ml}{hr} = \frac{\text{total volume}}{\text{administration time}}$$

   $$= \frac{1000 \text{ ml}}{8 \text{ hours}} = 125 \text{ ml/hour}$$

3. Milligrams per minute:

Example: Calculate the amount of medication to be infused if 2 mg/min are to be infused from 500 ml of solution containing 2 g of medication.

Convert the amount of drug in solution from grams to milligrams:

$$\text{amount of drug} = \text{drug in g} \times \frac{1000 \text{ mg}}{1 \text{ g}}$$

$$= 2 \text{ g} \times \frac{1000 \text{ mg}}{1 \text{ g}} = 2000 \text{ mg}$$

Calculate the infusion rate by multiplying the IV solution volume per total amount of drug by the dose rate, which must be converted from minutes to hours.

$$\frac{\text{ml of solution}}{\text{hr}} = \frac{\text{ml of solution}}{\text{amount of drug}} \times \frac{\text{dose}}{\text{time}}$$

$$= \frac{500 \text{ ml}}{2000 \text{ mg}} \times \frac{\text{dose}}{\text{min}} \times \frac{\text{min}}{\text{hr}} = \frac{0.25 \text{ ml}}{1 \text{ mg}} \times \frac{2 \text{ mg}}{\text{min}} \times \frac{60 \text{ min}}{\text{hr}}$$

$$= \frac{(0.25 \times 2 \times 60) \text{ ml}}{\text{hr}} = \frac{30 \text{ ml}}{\text{hr}}$$

4. Single dose:

Example: Calculate the dose to administer 500 mg of medication from a vial containing 250 mg per 5 ml of medication.

$$\text{dose} = \frac{\text{ml of solution}}{\text{amount of drug}} \times \text{dose ordered}$$

$$= \frac{5 \text{ ml}}{250 \text{ mg}} \times 500 \text{ mg} = \frac{0.02 \text{ ml}}{\text{mg}} \times 500 \text{ mg} = 10 \text{ ml}$$

Adult Laboratory Values

Blood Chemistry/Electrolytes	Normal Values
Arterial Blood Gases	
Base excess	-2 to $+2$
Bicarbonate	22 to 26 mEq/L
$PaCO_2$	38 to 42 mm Hg
PaO_2	80 to 100 mm Hg
pH	7.35 to 7.45
Clotting Times	
Prothrombin	11 to 15 seconds
Partial thromboplastin	
Activated	32 to 46 seconds
Standard	68 to 82 seconds
Complete Blood Count	
Leukocytes (total)	4500 to 11,000/mm^3
Lymphocytes	1500 to 3000/mm^3 (25–33%)
Neutrophils	
Banded (bands)	150 to 400/mm^3 (3–5%)
Segmented (segs)	3000 to 5800/mm^3 (54–62%)
Platelets	150,000 to 300,000/mm^3
Hematocrit	
Males	44 to 52%
Females	39 to 47%
Hemoglobin	
Males	13.5 to 18.0 g/dL
Females	12.0 to 16.0 g/dL
Red Blood Cells	
Males	4600 to 6000/mm^3
Females	4200 to 5400/mm^3
Renal Function	
Blood urea nitrogen (BUN)	10 to 20 mg/dL
Creatinine, serum	0.7 to 1.5 mg/dL

(continued)

Continued

....

Blood Chemistry/Electrolytes	Normal Values
Serum	
Electrolytes	
Calcium	8.9 to 10.3 mg/dL
Chloride	97 to 110 mEq/L
Magnesium	1.3 to 2.1 mEq/L
Phosphate (adults)	2.5 to 4.5 mg/dL
Potassium	3.5 to 5.0 mEq/L
Sodium	135 to 145 mEq/L
Glucose	70 to 110 mg/dL
Osmolality	280 to 295 mOsm/kg
Proteins (total)	6.0 to 8.0 g/dL
Albumin	3.5 to 5.5 g/dL
Globulin	1.5 to 3.0 g/dL

Index

Page numbers in *italics* denote figures; Those followed by a "t" denote tables.